The Washington
Manual® Endocrinology
Subspecialty Consult

The Washington Manual® Endocrinology Subspecialty Consult

Faculty Advisors

William E. Clutter, M.D.
Associate Professor of Medicine
Department of Internal Medicine
Divisions of Endocrinology, Metabolism, and
Lipid Research and Medical Education
Washington University School of Medicine
Barnes-Jewish Hospital
St. Louis, Missouri

Anne C. Goldberg, M.D.
Associate Professor of Medicine
Department of Internal Medicine
Division of Endocrinology, Metabolism, and
Lipid Research
Washington University School of Medicine
Barnes-Jewish Hospital
St. Louis, Missouri

Janet B. McGill, M.D.
Associate Professor of Medicine
Department of Internal Medicine
Division of Endocrinology, Metabolism, and
Lipid Research
Washington University School of Medicine
Barnes-Jewish Hospital
St. Louis, Missouri

The Washington Manual® Endocrinology Subspecialty Consult

Editors:
Katherine E. Henderson, M.D.
Instructor of Medicine
Department of Internal Medicine
Division of Medical Education
Washington University School of Medicine
Barnes-Jewish Hospital
St. Louis, Missouri

Thomas J. Baranski, M.D., Ph.D.
Assistant Professor of Medicine
Departments of Internal Medicine and
Molecular Biology and Pharmacology
Division of Endocrinology, Metabolism, and
Lipid Research
Washington University School of Medicine
Barnes-Jewish Hospital
St. Louis, Missouri

Perry E. Bickel, M.D.
Assistant Professor of Medicine
Departments of Internal Medicine and Cell
Biology and Physiology
Division of Endocrinology, Metabolism, and
Lipid Research
Washington University School of Medicine
Barnes-Jewish Hospital
St. Louis, Missouri

Series Editor
Tammy L. Lin, M.D.
Adjunct Assistant Professor of Medicine
Washington University School of Medicine
St. Louis, Missouri

Series Advisor
Daniel M. Goodenberger, M.D.
Professor of Medicine
Chief, Division of Medical Education
Washington University School of Medicine
St. Louis, Missouri
Director, Internal Medicine Residency Program
Barnes-Jewish Hospital
St. Louis, Missouri

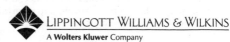
LIPPINCOTT WILLIAMS & WILKINS
A **Wolters Kluwer** Company
Philadelphia · Baltimore · New York · London
Buenos Aires · Hong Kong · Sydney · Tokyo

Executive Editor: Danette Somers
Managing Editor: Tanya Lazar
Project Manager: Nicole Walz
Production Editor: Melissa Jones, Silverchair Science + Communications
Senior Manufacturing Manager: Ben Rivera
Senior Marketing Manager: Kathleen Neely
Cover Designer: QT Design
Compositor: Silverchair Science + Communications
Printer: RR Donnelley & Sons–Crawfordsville

Library of Congress Cataloging-in-Publication Data

The Washington manual endocrinology subspecialty consult / [edited by] Katherine E. Henderson, Thomas J. Baranski, Perry E. Bickel.
    p. ; cm.
Includes bibliographical references and index.
ISBN 0-7817-4378-8
1. Endocrinology--Handbooks, manuals, etc. 2. Endocrine glands--Diseases--Handbooks, manuals, etc. I. Title: Endocrinology subspecialty consult. II. Henderson, Katherine E. III. Baranski, Thomas J. IV. Bickel, Perry E. V. Washington University (St. Louis, Mo.). School of Medicine.
    [DNLM: 1. Endocrine Diseases--Handbooks. 2. Metabolic Diseases--Handbooks. WK 39 W319 2004]
RC649.W28 2004
616.4--dc22

                                                                        2004021747

Contents

Contributing Authors

Amanda F. Cashen, M.D.

Fellow in Oncology
Department of Medicine
Washington University School of
Medicine
Barnes-Jewish Hospital
St. Louis, Missouri

Jeannie Chen, M.D.

Attending
Private Practice
Tucson, Arizona

Michael A. DeRosa, D.O.

Division Chief
Department of Internal Medicine
Division of Endocrinology, Diabetes,
and Metabolism
Western Reserve Care System
Youngstown, Ohio

Lamice R. El-Kholy, M.D.

Physician
University Medical Consultants
Barnes-Jewish Hospital
St. Louis, Missouri

Grace S. Eng, M.D.

Physician
Associated Internal Medicine
Summit Hospital
Oakland, California

Kellie L. Flood, M.D.

Instructor of Medicine
Department of Internal Medicine
Division of Geriatrics and Nutritional
Science
Washington University School of
Medicine
Barnes-Jewish Hospital
St. Louis, Missouri

Jason S. Goldfeder, M.D.

Assistant Professor of Medicine
Department of Internal Medicine
Division of Medical Education
Washington University School of
Medicine
Barnes-Jewish Hospital
St. Louis, Missouri

Katherine E. Henderson, M.D.

Instructor of Medicine
Department of Internal Medicine
Division of Medical Education
Washington University School of
Medicine
Barnes-Jewish Hospital
St. Louis, Missouri

Andrew F. Holt, M.D.

Fellow in Gastroenterology
Department of Internal Medicine
Division of Digestive Diseases
University of Cincinnati College of
Medicine
University Hospital
Cincinnati, Ohio

Michael Jakoby, M.D.

Clinical Assistant Professor of Medicine
Academic Section Head
Department of Internal Medicine
Division of Endocrinology
University of Illinois at Urbana-
Champaign College of Medicine
Carle Foundation Hospital
Urbana, Illinois

Paul A. Kovach, M.D.

Fellow
Department of Internal Medicine
Division of Nephrology
Washington University School of
Medicine
Barnes-Jewish Hospital
St. Louis, Missouri

Janet B. McGill, M.D.

Associate Professor of Medicine
Department of Internal Medicine
Division of Endocrinology, Diabetes,
and Lipid Research
Washington University School of
Medicine
St. Louis, Missouri

Veronica P. McGregor, M.D.

Physician
Private Practice
Clayton, Missouri

Subramaniam Pennathur, M.D.

Assistant Professor
Department of Medicine
Division of Geriatrics and Nutritional
Science
University of Washington School of
Medicine
University of Washington Medical
Center
Seattle, Washington

Bharathi Raju, M.D.

Fellow
Department of Internal Medicine
Division of Endocrinology,
Metabolism, and Lipid Research
Washington University School of
Medicine
Barnes-Jewish Hospital
St. Louis, Missouri

Dominic N. Reeds, M.D.

Clinical Instructor
Department of Internal Medicine
Division of Geriatrics and Nutritional
Science
Washington University School of
Medicine
Barnes-Jewish Hospital
St. Louis, Missouri

Divya Shroff, M.D.

Attending
Department of Internal Medicine
VA Medical Center
Washington, D.C.

Dawn D. Smiley, M.D.

Fellow
Department of Medicine
Division of Endocrinology
Emory University School of Medicine
Emory University Hospital
Grady Memorial Hospital
Atlanta, Georgia

Savitha Subramanian, M.D.

Senior Fellow
Division of Metabolism,
Endocrinology, and Nutrition
University of Washington School of
Medicine
Seattle, Washington

Denise A. Teves, M.D.

Assistant Professor of Endocrinology
Department of Endocrinology and
Metabolism
Medical College of Wisconsin
Zablocki VAMC/Froedtert Hospital
Milwaukee, Wisconsin

Chairman's Note

Medical knowledge is increasing at an exponential rate, and physicians are being bombarded with new facts at a pace that many find overwhelming. The Washington Manual® Subspecialty Consult Series was developed in this context for interns, residents, medical students, and other practitioners in need of readily accessible practical clinical information. They therefore meet an important unmet need in an era of information overload.

I would like to acknowledge the authors who have contributed to these books. In particular, Tammy L. Lin, M.D., Series Editor, provided energetic and inspired leadership, and Daniel M. Goodenberger, M.D., Series Advisor, Chief of the Division of Medical Education in the Department of Medicine at Washington University, is a continual source of sage advice. The efforts and outstanding skill of the lead authors are evident in the quality of the final product. I am confident that this series will meet its desired goal of providing practical knowledge that can be directly applied to improving patient care.

Kenneth S. Polonsky, M.D.
Adolphus Busch Professor
Chairman, Department of Medicine
Washington University School of Medicine
St. Louis, Missouri

Series Preface

The Washington Manual® Subspecialty Consult Series is designed to provide quick access to the essential information needed to evaluate a patient on a subspecialty consult service. Each manual includes the most updated and useful information on commonly encountered symptoms or diseases and highlights the practical information you need to gather before formulating a plan. Special efforts have been made to organize the information so that these guides will be valuable and trusted companions for medical students, residents, and fellows. They cover everything from questions to ask during the initial consult to issues in subsequent management.

One of the strengths of this series is that it is written by residents and fellows who know how busy a consult service can be, who know what information will be most helpful, and can detail a practical approach to patient care. Each volume is written to provide enough information for you to evaluate a patient until more in-depth reading can be done on a particular topic. Throughout the series, key references are noted, difficult management situations are addressed, and appropriate practice guidelines are included. Another strength of this series is that it was written in concert. All of the guides were designed to work together.

The most important strength of this series is the collection of authors, faculty advisors, and especially lead authors assembled to write this series. In addition, we received incredible commitment and support from our chairman, Kenneth S. Polonsky, M.D. As a result, the extraordinary depth of talent and genuine interest in teaching others at Washington University is showcased in this series. Although there has always been house staff involvement in editing The Washington Manual® series, it came to our attention that many of them also wanted to be involved in writing and making decisions about what to convey to fellow colleagues. Remarkably, many of the lead authors became junior subspecialty fellows while writing their guides. Their desire to pass on what they were learning, while trying to balance multiple responsibilities, is a testament to their dedication and skills as clinicians, teachers, and leaders.

We hope this series fulfills the need for essential and practical knowledge for those learning the art of consultation in a particular subspecialty and for those just passing through it.

Tammy L. Lin, M.D., Series Editor
Daniel M. Goodenberger, M.D.,
Series Advisor

Preface

This first edition of *The Washington Manual® Endocrinology Subspecialty Consult* was written largely by Washington University house staff and fellows under the direction of our endocrine faculty. The manual is designed to serve as a guide for students, house staff, and fellows involved in inpatient and outpatient endocrinology consults. It is not meant to serve as a comprehensive review of the field of endocrinology. Rather, it focuses on a practical approach to endocrinopathies commonly seen in consultation, with emphasis on key components of evaluation and treatment.

We would like to thank the following endocrine faculty for their expert editorial advice: Dr. William E. Clutter for the four thyroid disease chapters included in this book (Evaluation of Thyroid Function, Euthyroid Goiter and Thyroid Nodules, Hyperthyroidism, and Hypothyroidism); Dr. Anne C. Goldberg for the Diagnosis, Standards of Care, and Treatment for Hyperlipidemia chapter; and Dr. Janet B. McGill for the Diabetes Mellitus Type 1 and Diabetes Mellitus Type 2 chapters.

K.E.H.
T.J.B.
P.E.B.

Hypothalamic and Pituitary Disorders

Key to Abbreviations

ACE	angiotensin-converting enzyme
ACTH	adrenocorticotropic hormone
ADH	antidiuretic hormone
AIDS	acquired immune deficiency syndrome
ALT	alanine aminotransferase
ARB	angiotensin II receptor blocker
AST	aspartate aminotransferase
AVP	arginine vasopressin
BMD	bone mineral density
BUN	blood urea nitrogen
CMV	cytomegalovirus
CNS	central nervous system
COPD	chronic obstructive pulmonary disease
CT	computed tomography
CVA	cerebrovascular accident
D_5W	5% dextrose solution
DDAVP	desmopressin
DHEA-S	dehydroepiandrosterone sulfate
ECG	electrocardiogram
ENT	ear, nose, and throat
FDA	U.S. Food and Drug Administration
GI	gastrointestinal tract
HIV	human immunodeficiency virus
HLA	human leukocyte antigen
^{131}I	iodine-131
ICP	intracranial pressure
ICU	intensive care unit
IFN	interferon
IGF	insulin-like growth factor
IM	intramuscular, -ly
IV	intravenous, -ly
K^+	potassium
kD	kilodalton
MAOI	monoamine oxidase inhibitor
MRI	magnetic resonance imaging
NAD	nicotinamide adenine dinucleotide
NADH	nicotinamide adenine dinucleotide (reduced form)
NIH	National Institutes of Health
NSAIDs	nonsteroidal antiinflammatory drugs, agents
OH	hydroxy
PCP	*Pneumocystis carinii* pneumonia
PCR	polymerase chain reaction
PET	positron emission tomography
PO	oral
TB	tuberculosis

Pituitary Adenomas

Denise A. Teves

INTRODUCTION

Pituitary tumors constitute 10% of intracranial tumors. They can be benign or malignant, hormone-producing, or functionally inactive. According to their size, they are classified as microadenomas (<10 mm in widest diameter) or macroadenomas (>10 mm in widest diameter). The most frequent primary tumors are pituitary adenomas, which are benign neoplasms arising in the adenohypophysial cells. They can be divided into

- Somatotroph adenomas: Growth hormone (GH)-producing tumors clinically associated with acromegaly or gigantism. They account for approximately 15% of tumors.
- Lactotroph adenomas: Prolactinomas account for approximately 25% of symptomatic pituitary tumors.
- Thyrotroph adenomas (<1% of pituitary tumors): Associated with hyperthyroidism, hypothyroidism, or they can be silent, depending on whether the thyroid-stimulating hormone (TSH) subunits are processed correctly.
- Corticotroph adenomas (approximately 15% of pituitary tumors): Contain ACTH and related peptides. Clinically, they are associated with Cushing's disease or Nelson syndrome (after bilateral adrenalectomy).
- Gonadotroph adenomas, (approximately 10% of pituitary tumors): Result in elevated serum follicle-stimulating hormone (FSH) and, rarely, luteinizing hormone (LH) levels.
- Plurihormonal adenomas (approximately 15% of pituitary tumors): Produce >1 type of hormone. Apart from the frequent occurrence of elevated GH and prolactin (PRL) levels, the most common association of combined endocrine disorders is acromegaly and hyperthyroidism.
- Null cell adenomas (approximately 20% of pituitary tumors): No histologic, immunocytologic, or electron microscopic markers of hormone excess.

Any type of tumor may be clinically nonfunctioning and present with symptoms of sellar and extrasellar mass effect and hypopituitarism. The majority of these tumors are gonadotroph or null cell adenomas.

CAUSES

Pituitary adenomas arise as a result of monoclonal pituitary cell proliferation. Several different mutations have been associated with pituitary adenomas. Activating gsp mutations are present in 40% of GH-secreting adenomas. These are point mutations of the G-protein alpha subunit (Gs alpha) gene, which activate Gs alpha protein and increase cyclic adenosine monophosphate levels, leading to GH hypersecretion and cell proliferation. H-ras gene mutations were identified in metastatic pituitary carcinomas. Pituitary tumor transforming gene is abundant in all pituitary tumor types, especially prolactinomas. In addition to somatic mutations, hypothalamic factors may promote and maintain growth of transformed pituitary adenomatous cells.

PRESENTATION

If the adenoma secretes functional hormones, the patient usually presents with symptoms caused by the hormone excess (see the section Disorders of the Pituitary Hormone Axis). Some patients present with symptoms secondary to mass effects of the adenoma. Most pituitary masses are benign neoplasms, but they may aggressively invade locally into contiguous structures. Large infarcts may lead to partially or totally empty pituitary sella. Most masses arising from within the sella are benign, hormonally functional, or nonfunctional, with a relatively good prognosis, and their invasiveness is relatively limited. In contrast, parasellar masses are often malignant or invasive and have a less favorable prognosis. It is important to differentiate pituitary adenomas from other pituitary lesions.

Differential Diagnosis of Pituitary Tumors

Sellar/Parasellar Cysts

The most common cysts are **craniopharyngiomas**. They are derived from embryonic squamous cell rests of Rathke's cleft. They have a bimodal peak of incidence, occurring predominantly in children between the ages of 5 and 10 years; a second peak occurs in the sixth decade. There is a female preponderance, and most cysts present as calcified sellar/suprasellar masses. Children present with headache, vomiting, visual field deficits, and growth failure. Adults may present with bitemporal hemianopsia, cranial nerve abnormalities (III, IV, VI, and V1), anterior pituitary hormone deficits, and diabetes insipidus (DI).

Chordomas

Chordomas are rare tumors that arise from notochordal remnants within the clivus. They produce bony destruction with local infiltration and tend to recur. They are more common in men ages 30–50 years. They produce cranial neuropathy and diplopia. Endocrine dysfunction is unusual. Calcification is seen in 50% of cases.

Germinomas

Germinomas arise in sellar/suprasellar regions and involve the hypothalamus, chiasm, optic nerves, and pineal region. Patients present with hypopituitarism or pituitary hyperfunction, precocious puberty, DI, visual field defects, and signs of increased intracranial pressure. They metastasize within the CNS in 10% of cases.

Dermoid Tumors

Dermoid tumors are rare developmental tumors in childhood that produce recurrent meningitis from leakage of tumor contents.

Pituitary Metastases

Pituitary metastases occur most commonly in elderly patients and usually arise from breast carcinomas (women) and lung carcinomas. Other sites of primary malignancies that metastasize to the pituitary include GI tract, kidney, prostate, and skin (melanoma). Patients present with anterior pituitary dysfunction, visual field abnormalities, DI, and cranial nerve palsies. A rapidly enlarging mass is highly suggestive of a metastatic lesion.

Aneurysms

Aneurysms can arise from the cavernous sinus, infraclinoid or supraclinoid internal carotid arteries. They may compress the optic nerve or chiasm and produce bitemporal deficits, ocular motor palsies, intense headache, and supraorbital pain. They may extend into the sella and cause direct pituitary compression, producing hypopituitarism and hyperprolactinemia. They are identified by MRI and MR angiography and need to be excluded before transsphenoidal biopsy.

Pituitary Granulomas

- Tuberculous meningitis can involve the sellar and parasellar regions. A tuberculoma may be sellar or suprasellar and is associated with hypopituitarism, visual field changes, and DI.

- Sarcoidosis of the hypothalamic-pituitary region occurs in most patients with CNS involvement and can cause hypopituitarism with or without symptoms of an intrasellar mass. It has a predilection for the hypothalamus, posterior pituitary, and cranial nerves.
- Giant cell granuloma (granulomatous hypophysitis) is a rare noncaseating giant cell granulomata that partially or completely replaces the pituitary gland in the absence of involvement of other organs. It is most common in middle-aged to older women. The cause is unknown. It produces hypopituitarism and hyperprolactinemia.
- Histiocytosis X (HX): It can be a unifocal or multifocal eosinophilic granuloma [Hand-Schüller-Christian disease (HSC) or the more malignant form, Letterer-Siwe disease]. HX has predilection for the hypothalamus, and one-half of patients present with DI. Children can present with growth retardation and anterior pituitary hormone deficits. HSC disease includes the triad of DI, exophthalmos, and lytic bone disease (only 25% of patients present with this triad). Other features of the disease include axillary skin rash and history of recurrent pneumothorax.

Lymphocytic Hypophysitis
Lymphocytic hypophysitis affects mostly women and in 60–70% of cases presents in late pregnancy or during the postpartum period. Other autoimmune diseases (autoimmune thyroiditis) are present in 20–25%. It can present as an enlarging intrasellar/suprasellar mass, hypopituitarism, DI, and/or visual impairment (56–70%). Partial recovery of pituitary function and resolution of the sellar mass can occur spontaneously or with use of corticosteroids and hormone replacement. The diagnosis is confirmed by resolution of the mass over time. Surgery is needed if visual or compressive symptoms develop.

Pituitary Abscess
Pituitary abscesses are rare and occur from direct extension of adjacent infection in the sphenoid sinuses and other CNS infections. Most abscesses arise in previously healthy pituitary glands, but one-third are associated with pituitary adenomas or craniopharyngiomas. Gram-positive streptococci or staphylococci may be isolated, or, rarely, Aspergillus, *Candida albicans*, or *Entamoeba histolytica*. Patients present with visual compromise, hypopituitarism, and DI (50%). MRI shows ring enhancement and a central isointense cavity with contrast.

Intrapituitary Hemorrhage and Infarction
Intrapituitary hemorrhage and infarction is caused by ischemic damage to the hypophyseal-portal system, and pituitary insufficiency is clinically apparent when 75% of the gland is damaged. The damage is limited to the anterior lobe, and the posterior pituitary function remains intact. In pregnancy, the pituitary gland enlarges in response to estrogen stimulation and makes it vulnerable to arterial pressure changes. Sheehan's syndrome, described after severe postpartum hemorrhage, is less commonly seen.

Pituitary Carcinoma
Pituitary carcinomas are rare tumors and may produce GH, ACTH, or PRL or may be clinically nonfunctioning. The diagnosis can only be established when the lesion metastasizes.

Disorders of the Pituitary Hormone Axis

Prolactinomas
Hyperprolactinemia produces amenorrhea and galactorrhea in women and decreased libido and impotence in men. Macroadenomas also produce visual symptoms secondary to compression of the optic chiasm, cranial neuropathies and hypopituitarism (see Chap. 2, Prolactinoma).

GH-Secreting Tumors

- Acromegaly: The insidious progression over years often results in a delay in diagnosis (6–10 years). Symptomatic cardiac disease is present in 20% (hypertension occurs in 50%, left ventricular hypertrophy, arrhythmias, cardiac failure) and it accounts for 60% of deaths. Diabetes mellitus can develop in 10–25% of patients. There is a 2- to 3-fold increased rate of developing colon cancer and premalignant polyps (see Chap. 3, Acromegaly).

- Gigantism: It should be considered in children >3 SD above the normal mean height for age or >2 SD above normal mean parental height. It is due to excess of GH secretion before the epiphyses close.

ACTH-Secreting Tumors (Cushing's Disease)

See also Chap. 14, Cushing's Syndrome. The classic features of centripetal obesity, hirsutism, and plethora are not always present. Children can present with generalized obesity and poor linear growth. Patients develop fat depots over the thoracocervical spine (buffalo hump), supraclavicular region, cheeks, and temporal regions (moon facies). Gonadal dysfunction is common, with menstrual irregularities in women and loss of libido. Hirsutism (vellus hypertrichosis of face) and acne are common. Psychiatric abnormalities occur in 50% of patients (depression, lethargy, paranoia, psychosis). Long-standing Cushing's disease can produce osteoporotic vertebral collapse, rib fractures, and aseptic necrosis of femoral and humeral head. Hypercortisolism produces skin thinning, bruising with minimal trauma, red-purple striae >1 cm in diameter (usually found on the abdomen, upper thighs, and arms), and proximal muscle weakness of the lower limb and shoulder girdle (inability to climb stairs or rise from a deep chair). Hypertension occurs in 75% of patients. Infections are more common (poor wound healing, reactivation of tuberculosis, onychomycosis). Glucose intolerance occurs, and overt diabetes mellitus is present in more than one-third of patients.

TSH-Secreting Tumors

TSH-secreting tumors are usually large macroadenomas, and >60% are locally invasive. Patients present with visual field abnormalities, cranial nerve palsies, headache, hyperthyroidism (palpitations, arrhythmias, weight loss, tremors), and goiter.

Gonadotropin-Producing Pituitary Tumors (Clinically Nonfunctioning Tumors)

Gonadotropin-producing pituitary tumors are usually macroadenomas, and patients present with visual disturbance, symptoms of hypopituitarism, or headache. Some tumors produce elevated FSH, LH, or alpha subunit concentration, and patients present with hypogonadism related to gonadal down-regulation.

Pituitary Apoplexy

An endocrine emergency, pituitary apoplexy results from spontaneous hemorrhage into a pituitary adenoma or after head trauma. It evolves over 1–2 days, with severe headache, neck stiffness, and progressive cranial nerve damage, cardiovascular collapse, change in consciousness, bilateral visual disturbances, hyperglycemia, fever, CNS hemorrhage, and coma. Acute adrenal insufficiency may also be superimposed. Pituitary imaging reveals intra-adenomal hemorrhage and stalk deviation. Most patients recover spontaneously but experience long-term pituitary insufficiency. Ophthalmoplegia may resolve spontaneously, but signs of reduced visual acuity and altered mental status are indications for transsphenoidal surgical decompression.

Hypopituitarism

In congenital forms of hypopituitarism, an earlier age of onset will result in greater severity of thyroid, gonadal, adrenal, growth, or water disturbances. The corticotrophs and thyrotrophs are most resistant to mass effects and the last to lose function. ACTH deficiency produces hypotension, shock, hypoglycemia, nausea, vomiting, fatigue, and dilutional hyponatremia. Serum cortisol and ACTH can be determined before glucocorticoid administration. A cosyntropin stimulation test can be done several weeks after the onset of ACTH deficiency (see Chap. 11, Adrenal Insufficiency, for further details about this test). Hypothyroidism becomes apparent weeks after pituitary insufficiency. TSH is not elevated in secondary hypothyroidism, and free T_4 is used for follow-up. Patients develop coarse and cold skin and delayed ankle reflex relaxation. Even in the absence of symptoms, T_4 should be administered (glucocorticoids should be replaced first). Sexual dysfunction related to gonadotropin deficiency is common: Women present with abnormal menses or amenorrhea with no elevation of LH or FSH levels, and men present with sexual dysfunction and low testosterone. Sex hormone replacement is important to prevent osteoporosis even though sexual function may not be normalized. GH deficiency is present when ≥2 hormones are deficient. PRL deficiency is rare and occurs when the anterior pituitary is completely destroyed, as in apoplexy.

Local Effects of Sellar Masses

Headaches are common and they do not correlate with the size of the adenoma. Upward compression and pressure on the optic chiasm may result in bitemporal hemianopsia, loss of red perception, scotomas, and blindness. Lateral invasion may impinge on the cavernous sinus, leading to lesions of the III, IV, VI, and V1 cranial nerves, producing diplopia, ptosis, ophthalmoplegia, and facial numbness. Uncinate seizures, personality disorders, and anosmia occur if temporal and frontal brain lobes are invaded by the expanding parasellar mass. Direct hypothalamic involvement produces recurrent vomiting with or without extrapyramidal or pyramidal tract involvement, precocious puberty, hypogonadism, DI, sleep disturbances, dysthermia, and appetite disorders (obesity, hyperphagia, anorexia, adipsia, compulsive drinking).

MANAGEMENT

Diagnostic Evaluation

The screening tests for functional pituitary adenomas include the following.

Prolactinomas
Elevated serum PRL levels (although a mild elevation should be confirmed on serial samples).

Acromegaly
Elevated IGF-1 levels, GH nadir >1 mcg/L during an oral glucose tolerance test are consistent with acromegaly (see Chap. 3, Acromegaly).

Cushing's Disease
High 24-hour urine free cortisol or failed dexamethasone suppression tests (cortisol levels are not suppressed with low dose but are suppressed with the high dose), high normal ACTH levels (but they are inappropriately elevated for the plasma cortisol), elevated late-night plasma and salivary cortisol levels are diagnostic of Cushing's disease. CRH testing produces a rise in plasma ACTH and cortisol levels in contrast to ectopic ACTH secretion. The most reliable way to differentiate pituitary from ectopic ACTH secretion is by inferior petrosal sinus sampling (measuring ACTH levels in the venous blood draining the pituitary).

TSH-Secreting Tumors
High T_4, T_3, and alpha subunit with high or inappropriately normal TSH and a pituitary tumor seen in MRI confirm the diagnosis. Thyrotropin-releasing hormone (TRH) stimulation distinguishes between TSH overproduction by a TSH-secreting tumor (TSH response to TRH is blunted) and thyroid hormone insensitivity (TSH rises in response to TRH). The molar ratio of alpha subunit to TRH is high (>1) in 85% of patients.

Hypopituitarism

* To evaluate adrenal insufficiency, check 8 A.M. cortisol, ACTH levels, and cosyntropin stimulation test (if it is inconclusive, the insulin tolerance test can be done).
* To evaluate hypothyroidism, check serum free T_4.
* For GH deficiency, perform insulin-induced hypoglycemia and arginine–GH-releasing (GHRH) tests.
* For gonadotropin deficiency, obtain LH, FSH, testosterone in men, PRL (hyperprolactinemia is associated with hypogonadism). Gonadotropin-releasing hormone

stimulation test rarely differentiates causes of gonadotropin deficiency and is usually not indicated.

Imaging Studies

Tumors of the pituitary gland are best diagnosed with MRI focused on the pituitary (contiguous sections detect lesions of 1–3 mm). MRI detects tumor effect on soft tissue structures, cavernous sinus or optic chiasm, sphenoid sinus, and hypothalamus. T1-weighted sections with gadolinium distinguish most pituitary masses. T2-weighted images are important for diagnosing high-signal hemorrhage. During pregnancy, the gland should not exceed 10–12 mm. A thickened stalk may indicate the presence of hypophysitis, granuloma, or atypical chordomas. Microadenomas enlarge the sella turcica and can grow upward toward the optic chiasm. MRI can distinguish pituitary adenomas from other masses. Pituitary CT allows visualization of bony structures, including the sellar floor and clinoid bones. CT recognizes calcifications of craniopharyngiomas that are not evident on MRI.

Treatment and Follow-Up

Nonfunctioning Pituitary Adenomas

The risk of significant tumor enlargement is low for microadenomas. MRI may be repeated at yearly intervals for 2 years, and, if there is no evidence of growth of the lesion, the interval between scans may subsequently be lengthened. Surgery is not indicated unless growth is demonstrated. Macroadenomas have already indicated a propensity for growth, and if the lesion is asymptomatic, MRI can be repeated at 6 and 12 months and then yearly, and surgery may be deferred unless there is evidence of growth. If the macroadenoma is accompanied by compression of the optic chiasm, cavernous sinus invasion, or pituitary hormone deficiencies, surgery should be performed and irradiation of the mass considered (especially gamma-knife, external beam radiation therapy). Ten percent of these tumors respond to bromocriptine with tumor size reduction.

Prolactinoma

Treat with dopamine receptor agonists such as bromocriptine (see Chap. 2, Prolactinoma).

Acromegaly

Transsphenoidal surgery is the treatment of choice, and 70% of patients achieve GH levels <5 ng/mL and have normal IGF-1 levels, but recurrence rate is 5–10%. After use of conventional radiation, GH levels <5 ng/mL are achieved in 40% of patients by 5 years and 60–70% by 10 years (see Chap. 3, Acromegaly).

Cushing's Disease

Transsphenoidal surgery is the mainstay of treatment, and cure is expected in 80–90% of patients, with a 5–10% recurrence rate. The hypothalamus-pituitary-adrenal axis (HPA) may be suppressed for up to 1 year. Radiotherapy is used for patients not cured by surgery and those with bilateral adrenalectomy or with Nelson's syndrome. 61% of patients are in remission by 12 months and 70% by 24 months. At the time of surgery, patients should be treated with corticosteroids for any potential or confirmed HPA axis deficit. On postoperative day 5, plasma cortisol should be measured at 9 A.M., with the patient having omitted hydrocortisone for 24 hours: A nonsuppressed plasma cortisol postoperatively suggests residual tumor activity or an ectopic source of ACTH. Medical therapy can provide some benefit and includes

- Ketoconazole (Nizoral) (doses 200–1200 mg/day). It blocks cortisol synthesis, and 90% of patients normalize cortisol levels without a rise in ACTH levels.
- Other medications (less effective) are metyrapone (Metopirone), aminoglutethimide (Cytadren), and mitotane (Lysodren) (see Chap. 14, Cushing's Syndrome).

TSH-Secreting Adenomas

Transsphenoidal surgery is the treatment of choice but rarely results in cure. Most cases respond well to octreotide acetate (Sandostatin, Sandostatin LAR) with tumor shrinkage, but in one-third of patients tachyphylaxis may develop. Radiation therapy is adjunctive when surgery is not curative. For treatment of hyperthyroidism, propranolol, radioactive iodine thyroid ablation, thyroidectomy, methimazole, or propylthiouracil are used.

KEY POINTS TO REMEMBER

- Most pituitary masses are benign neoplasms but may aggressively invade contiguous structures.
- Pituitary adenomas can produce symptoms due to local effects (headache, visual disturbances, cranial neuropathies of III, IV, VI, V1 if they impinge the cavernous sinus) or to hormone secretion (acromegaly, Cushing's disease, hyperthyroidism).
- Pituitary apoplexy is an endocrine emergency that results from hemorrhage into a pituitary adenoma.
- Pituitary masses most commonly are pituitary adenomas, but other etiologies need to be excluded.

REFERENCES AND SUGGESTED READINGS

Freda P, Post KD. Differential diagnosis of sellar masses. *Endocrinol Metab Clin North Am* 1999;28:81–117.

Freda P, Wardlaw S. Diagnosis and treatment of pituitary tumors. *J Clin Endocrinol Metab* 1999;84:3859–3866.

Katsnelson L, Alexander JM, Klibanski A. Clinically nonfunctioning pituitary adenomas. *J Clin Endocrinol Metab* 1993;76:1089–1094.

Maccagnen P, et al. Conservative management of pituitary apoplexy: a perspective study. *J Clin Endocrinol Metab* 1995;80:2190–2197.

Melmed S. Evaluation of pituitary masses. In: DeGroot LJ, Jameson JL, eds. *Endocrinology*, 4th ed. Philadelphia: WB Saunders, 2001:282–288.

Melmed S. Functional pituitary anatomy and histology. In: DeGroot LJ, Jameson JL, eds. *Endocrinology*, 4th ed. Philadelphia: WB Saunders, 2001:167–182.

Melmed S, Kleinberg D. Anterior pituitary. In: Larsen PR, et al., eds. *Williams textbook of endocrinology*, 10th ed. Philadelphia: WB Saunders, 2003:177–179.

Molitch M. Evaluation and treatment of the patient with a pituitary incidentaloma. *J Clin Endocrinol Metab* 1995;80:3–6.

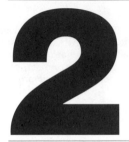

Prolactinoma

Denise A. Teves and
Veronica P. McGregor

INTRODUCTION

Prolactinomas are the most frequent secretory pituitary tumors, occurring with an annual incidence of 6/100,000. They account for 40–50% of pituitary adenomas. The female:male ratio for microprolactinomas (tumors <10 mm in widest diameter) is 20:1 and for macroadenomas (>10 mm in widest diameter) is 1:1. Macroprolactinomas have a greater propensity to grow and are larger in men. Tumor size correlates with serum prolactin (PRL) levels. PRL levels >200 ng/mL are indicative of a macroprolactinoma. The risk of progression from PRL-secreting microadenoma to macroadenoma is 7%. Prolactinoma is the most frequent pituitary tumor occurring in the multiple endocrine syndrome.

The **hypothalamus** exerts a predominantly inhibitory influence on PRL secretion through PRL inhibitory factors (e.g., dopamine). Alterations of D2 dopamine receptors seem to occur in prolactinomas. 10% of prolactinomas also secrete other hormones. The most frequent mixed tumors are growth hormone (GH)/PRL-secreting adenomas. Pituitary PRL-secreting carcinomas are extremely rare, but aggressive, neoplasms that invade the sphenoidal and cavernous sinuses and give rise to distant metastases.

CAUSES

An alteration in the neuroendocrine mechanisms regulating PRL secretion results in modestly elevated PRL levels [25–150 ng/mL (normal values, 5–20 ng/mL)].

Differential Diagnosis for Hyperprolactinemia

Medications

Drugs that are D2 dopamine receptor antagonists: antipsychotics [risperidone (Risperdal), phenothiazines, haloperidol (Haldol)], metoclopramide (Octamide), antihypertensives [methyldopa (Aldomet), reserpine (Serpasil)]. Verapamil (Calan) may raise serum PRL concentrations by an unknown mechanism. Other drugs include tricyclic antidepressants, serotonin reuptake inhibitors, estrogens, opiates, and cocaine.

Physiologic Causes

Physiologic causes include pregnancy and nipple stimulation.

Lactotroph Adenomas (Prolactinomas)

Lactotroph adenomas arise from monoclonal expansion of a cell that has undergone somatic mutation.

Lactotroph Hyperplasia

Lactotroph hyperplasia is due to stalk compression, leading to decreased inhibition of the lactotroph cells. This may occur due to tumors of the hypothalamus (craniopharyngiomas, metastatic breast carcinoma), infiltrative diseases (sarcoidosis), section of the hypothalamic-pituitary stalk in head trauma, or pituitary adenomas.

Hypothyroidism

Basal serum PRL is normal in most hypothyroid patients. In the few hypothyroid patients who have elevated basal serum PRL concentrations, the values return to normal when the hypothyroidism is corrected.

Chest Wall Injury and Spinal Cord Lesions

Chest wall injuries or irritative lesions (e.g., herpes zoster) activate neural reflexes similar to nipple stimulation, thereby increasing PRL levels.

Chronic Renal Failure

Patients with chronic renal failure may have a 3-fold increase in PRL secretion due to decreased clearance of PRL. In the setting of renal failure, medications (e.g., metoclopramide) can cause markedly elevated PRL levels (>500 ng/mL). PRL levels return to normal after renal transplantation.

Cirrhosis

Basal PRL levels are increased in 5–20% of patients with cirrhosis, possibly due to alterations in hypothalamic dopamine generation.

Adrenal Insufficiency

Glucocorticoids have a suppressive effect on PRL gene transcription and release.

Idiopathic Hyperprolactinemia

In some patients with PRL concentrations between 20–100 ng/mL, no cause can be found. Many of these patients have undetectable lactotroph microadenomas. Long-term follow-up of these patients revealed that in one-third, PRL levels returned to normal; in 10–15%, PRL levels rose to 50% over baseline; and in the remaining patients, PRL levels remained stable.

Macroprolactinemia ("Big Prolactin")

A small amount of a 25-kD glycosylated form of PRL (instead of the normal 23-kD nonglycosylated PRL) can circulate in aggregates. This PRL can be distinguished from hyperprolactinemia by gel filtration or polyethylene glycol precipitation. In a series of such patients, none had a history of amenorrhea, few had oligomenorrhea or galactorrhea, and none had adenomas seen on MRI.

Hook Effect (Prozone Effect)

Measurement of serum PRL levels is important in the differentiation of prolactinomas from nonfunctioning adenomas. Immunoradiometric assay is frequently used for measurement of serum PRL levels. It has good sensitivity and precision with a short incubation time. Falsely low values have been reported with this technique when a large amount of antigen (PRL) is present that saturates the antibodies. In the setting of a pituitary macroadenoma, PRL concentrations between 20 and 200 ng/mL might lead the clinician to conclude that the adenoma is nonfunctioning because macroadenomas can increase PRL levels to this range due to stalk compression. Hook effect (prozone effect) artifact should be considered and excluded by performing an additional determination of a 1:10 dilution of serum. If the diluted specimen gives the same value (or even a higher value) then the diagnosis of macroprolactinoma can be made, which will change the management of the patient.

PRESENTATION

Clinical Manifestations

Signs and symptoms of an expanding pituitary lesion include: headache (common in patients with macroadenoma and ameliorates after tumor shrinkage) and diminished visual acuity and visual field defects. Ophthalmoplegia may occur when tumors expand laterally and invade the cavernous sinus. Rhinorrhea may occur if the tumor invades the sphenoidal or ethmoidal sinuses or after rapid drug-induced tumor shrinkage.

The history should focus on a search for medications, symptoms of hypothyroidism, renal disease or cirrhosis, headache, and visual symptoms. The physical exam should look for bitemporal field loss and signs of hypothyroidism or hypogonadism. PRL is secreted periodically. The finding of a mildly elevated PRL level requires confirmation in several samples. A careful history of drug ingestion is recommended. Routine blood tests such as a thyroid-stimulating hormone (TSH) and blood chemistry panel can exclude hypothyroidism, chronic renal failure, and liver cirrhosis. Serum PRL levels <100 ng/mL that progressively drop to within normal limits during multiple samplings exclude the diagnosis of hyperprolactinemia. Serum PRL levels >200 ng/mL are indicative of macroprolactinoma. When there is no obvious cause of hyperprolactinemia, MRI with gadolinium enhancement provides the best anatomic detail of the hypothalamic-pituitary area. Large nonsecreting tumors can cause modest elevations in PRL due to stalk compression (PRL elevation <150 ng/mL), whereas PRL-secreting macroadenomas have much higher levels of PRL (>250 ng/mL). Visual field testing (Goldmann perimetry) should be obtained in patients with tumors that are adjacent to or pressing on the optic chiasm.

Premenopausal Women
Premenopausal women present with secondary hypogonadism (infertility, oligomenorrhea, or amenorrhea). Hyperprolactinemia accounts for 10–20% of cases of amenorrhea (excluding pregnancy) in this group of women. A serum PRL >100 ng/mL is associated with overt hypogonadism and causes hot flashes and vaginal dryness. Mild hyperprolactinemia (20–50 ng/mL) can cause infertility even if there is no abnormality of the menstrual cycle. Women with amenorrhea may have lower spine and forearm bone mineral density scores. They may present with galactorrhea, but most premenopausal women do not.

Postmenopausal Women
Postmenopausal women are already hypogonadal. Because they are markedly hypoestrogenemic, galactorrhea is rare. Hyperprolactinemia in this group is recognized after a prolactinoma is large enough to produce headaches or impair vision. Seborrhea and moderate hirsutism may be present. These symptoms may be accompanied by elevation of androstenedione and dehydroepiandrosterone sulfate, suggesting a stimulatory effect of PRL on adrenocortical androgen secretion.

Men
Men present with hypogonadotropic hypogonadism and symptoms of decreased libido, impotence, infertility, gynecomastia, and, rarely, galactorrhea. Hyperprolactinemia results in decreased testosterone secretion, which in turn produces decreased energy, libido, muscle mass, and body hair and promotes osteoporosis.

MANAGEMENT

Indications for therapy depend on the effects of the tumor size and effects of hyperprolactinemia. Invasion or compression of the stalk or optic chiasm or symptoms due to hyperprolactinemia are indications to initiate therapy. In 95% of patients, microprolactinomas do not enlarge over a 6-year period of observation. Because it is unlikely that a prolactinoma will grow significantly without a concomitant increase in serum PRL levels, most patients with microadenomas can be observed safely with serial PRL levels. If PRL levels rise significantly, repeat scanning is indicated.

Medical Therapy

Bromocriptine
Bromocriptine (Parlodel) is an ergot derivative D2 receptor agonist. It can be administered orally once or twice a day at doses of 2.5–20 mg/day and produces reduction in PRL levels to the normal range in 60–100% of cases. Women resume regular ovulatory menses, and galactorrhea disappears after 2–3 months of therapy. For macroprolactinomas, the reduction in tumor size is usually associated with improved visual fields, reduction of hyperprolactinemia, and improvement in other pituitary functions (due to reduced mass effects). Most series suggest that bromocriptine therapy has little or

no effect on later surgical results for microadenomas; however, in patients with macroadenomas, bromocriptine treatment lasting >6–12 weeks has been associated with perivascular fibrosis in the tumor, thus complicating complete tumor resection. The most common side effects of bromocriptine are nausea and vomiting. Orthostatic hypotension may occur when initiating therapy. Between 5% and 10% of patients either do not respond to bromocriptine or have only minimal responses. To overcome resistance to treatment, other dopamine agonists have been developed.

Cabergoline

Cabergoline (Dostinex) is a nonergot D2 receptor agonist with a long half-life and can be given orally at a dose of 0.25–1 mg twice a week. Several studies have shown that cabergoline is at least as effective as bromocriptine in lowering PRL levels and reducing tumor size, and some studies showed superior success rate to that of bromocriptine. Side effects are much less frequent and less severe than with bromocriptine.

Other Dopamine Agonists

Pergolide (Permax Tablets) (approved for treatment of Parkinson's disease but not for hyperprolactinemia) can be given once a day, but there are limited data showing tumor size reduction. Quinagolide (Norprolac) (can be given once daily) is another potential therapy. 50% of patients with resistance to bromocriptine respond to quinagolide, but it is not yet approved for use in the United States.

Surgery

Pituitary surgery is recommended for patients with microprolactinomas or macroprolactinomas who are refractory to or intolerant of dopamine agonists, for those in whom medical treatment is unable to shrink the adenoma, or for patients with cystic or rapidly expanding tumors. Pituitary surgery aimed at debulking the tumor mass and preventing tumor expansion is indicated for women with macroprolactinoma who wish to become pregnant. Transsphenoidal surgery is the preferred technique for treating microadenomas in patients who do not wish to receive lifelong medical therapy.

Radiotherapy

Radiotherapy is limited to patients with macroprolactinomas refractory to medical treatment and surgery. It is occasionally used in conjunction with medical treatment. Approximately 30% of patients achieve normal serum PRL levels gradually over a period of years.

PROLACTINOMAS AND PREGNANCY

Patients with prolactinomas wishing to become pregnant should be referred to specialists in high-risk obstetrics and endocrinology, because these patients may need to be pretreated with bromocriptine to achieve fertility. Pregnancy rates of 37–81% have been reported in patients with prolactinoma. The drug should be discontinued once pregnancy is achieved. No teratogenic effects of bromocriptine have been reported when it is discontinued within a few weeks of conception. In women with **microprolactinomas**, pregnancy and delivery is usually uneventful. Women with **macroprolactinomas** who desire pregnancy should be pretreated with bromocriptine for a sufficient period of time to cause substantial tumor shrinkage. Once this has occured and pregnancy is achieved, the drug should be discontinued.

During pregnancy, the normal pituitary increases in size due to marked lactotroph hyperplasia due to the effect of estrogen on PRL synthesis. The risk of tumor expansion is <5.5% for microprolactinomas and 15.5–35.7% for macroprolactinomas. Prepregnancy transsphenoidal surgical debulking of a large macroadenoma reduces the risk of serious tumor enlargement. Monitoring periodic PRL levels in pregnant patients is of no benefit as PRL levels do not always rise during pregnancy and may not rise with tumor enlargement. Visual field testing is limited to patients who become symptomatic. Repeat scanning is reserved for patients with symptoms of tumor enlargement and reinstitution of bromocriptine at the lowest effective dose during pregnancy is the treatment of choice for patients with symptomatic tumor enlargement, because any type of surgery during pregnancy results in 1.5-fold increase in fetal loss in the first trimester and 5-fold increase in the second trimester. Transsphenoidal surgery or delivery (if pregnancy is far enough advanced) should be performed if there is no response to bromocriptine and vision is progressively worsening.

KEY POINTS TO REMEMBER

- PRL levels >200 ng/mL are indicative of a macroprolactinoma.
- The most common clinical manifestations of prolactinomas are infertility, oligomenorrhea, amenorrhea, and galactorrhea. Macroadenomas can also produce headaches and visual field defects.
- A careful history of medications that elevate PRL levels; physical exam to test for signs of hypothyroidism, hypogonadism, and bitemporal field loss; and routine blood tests to exclude chronic renal failure and liver cirrhosis are important in the differential diagnosis of hyperprolactinemia.
- The initial treatment for patients with microprolactinomas and macroprolactinomas is medical with either bromocriptine or cabergoline. Cabergoline produces less frequent side effects but is more expensive.
- In a woman with a large macroadenoma who desires pregnancy, prepregnancy transsphenoidal surgery to debulk the tumor reduces the risk for serious tumor enlargement. Bromocriptine given for a sufficient period to shrink the tumor can also reduce the chance of clinically important enlargement.

REFERENCES AND SUGGESTED READINGS

Abrahamson MJ, Snyder PJ. Causes of hyperprolactinemia. In: Rose BD, ed. *UpTo-Date*. Wellesley, MA: UpToDate, 2004.

Bevan J, et al. Dopamine agonists and pituitary tumor shrinkage. *Endocrin Rev* 1992;13(2):220–240.

Faglia G. Prolactinomas and hyperprolactinemic syndrome. In: De Groot L, Jameson JL, eds. *Endocrinology*, 4th ed. Philadelphia: WB Saunders, 2001:329–342.

Melmed S, Kleinberg D. Anterior pituitary. In: Larsen PR, et al., eds. *Williams textbook of endocrinology*, 10th ed. Philadelphia: WB Saunders, 2003:177–279.

Molitch M. Medical treatment of prolactinomas. *Endocrinol Metab Clin North Am* 1999;28:143–169.

Molitch M, et al. Therapeutic controversy: management of prolactinomas. *J Clin Endocrinol Metab* 1997;82(4):99–1000.

Petakov MS, et al. Pituitary adenomas secreting large amounts of prolactin may give false low values in immunoradiometric assays: the hook effect. *J Endocrinol Invest* 1998;21:184.

Snyder PJ. Clinical manifestations and diagnosis of hyperprolactinemia. In: Rose BD, ed. *UpToDate*. Wellesley, MA: UpToDate, 2004.

3

Acromegaly

Dominic N. Reeds

INTRODUCTION

Acromegaly is a disorder characterized by overproduction of growth hormone (GH), most commonly as a result of a pituitary adenoma. When these tumors occur before puberty, they may cause hypogonadism with failure of growth-plate closure, resulting in gigantism. Acromegaly, when occurring post-pubertally, is insidious, with an average lag time of almost 10 years from disease onset to diagnosis. The incidence of acromegaly is low—3 cases/million people/year. Recently, abuse of GH by athletes and patients seeking "the fountain of youth" has led to an increase in the incidence of drug-induced acromegaly.

CAUSES

Acromegaly is usually a result of an adenoma derived from somatotroph cells in the anterior pituitary gland. These cells normally secrete GH, stimulated by GH-releasing hormone (GHRH) from the hypothalamus and inhibited by both somatostatin from the hypothalamus and IGF-1 from peripheral tissue. Most of the effects of GH are mediated through IGF-1, a growth and differentiation factor made in the liver. GH and IGF-1 cause growth of bone and cartilage and lead to impaired glucose tolerance and changes in protein and fat metabolism. Overproduction of GH, and the consequent increased synthesis of IGF-1, results in the clinical findings outlined below.

Differential Diagnosis

The differential diagnosis of acromegaly includes other causes of elevated GH levels. Exogenous use of GH should be considered in adolescent patients and body builders. Nonpituitary GH-secreting tumors are extremely rare. Familial forms of acromegaly include multiple endocrine neoplasia, McCune-Albright syndrome, and Carney's syndrome.

PRESENTATION

Patients present with skeletal overgrowth and soft tissue enlargement. The most frequent signs and symptoms are

- Dermatologic: Excessive sweating, oily skin, more or enlarging skin tags
- Musculoskeletal: Arthralgias; osteoarthritis of large weightbearing joints; larger hat, ring, or shoe size; enlarged gaps between the teeth; kyphoscoliosis
- Endocrine: Hypothyroidism, including cold intolerance, weight gain, and fatigue; hypogonadism, including menstrual irregularities, reduced libido, and infertility; diabetes mellitus
- Neurologic: Headache, carpal tunnel syndrome, peripheral paresthesias, visual disturbances
- Pulmonary: Obstructive sleep apnea
- Cardiac: Increased left ventricular mass, hypertension
- GI: Organomegaly, polyps
- Renal: Hypercalciuria

MANAGEMENT

Diagnostic Evaluation

The initial lab tests to be ordered in a patient suspected of having acromegaly should be IGF-1 and GH levels. A GH level <0.4 mcg/L and IGF-1 level within the normal range (adjusted for age and gender) exclude the diagnosis of acromegaly. If either of these tests is abnormal, a 2-hour oral glucose tolerance test should be performed as follows:

1. Draw baseline glucose and GH levels
2. Patient consumes 75 g of oral glucose
3. Draw GH and glucose levels every 30 minutes for 2 hours

If the GH level falls to <1 mcg/L during the oral glucose tolerance test, acromegaly is excluded. False positives may occur in patients with diabetes, chronic hepatitis, renal failure, and anorexia.

The initial imaging study should be a head MRI with and without gadolinium contrast to evaluate for pituitary adenoma.

Treatment

Patients with acromegaly have premature mortality, with an increased incidence of insulin resistance, left ventricular hypertrophy, hypertension, and death due to cardiovascular disease. Studies have shown that reducing GH levels improves survival in patients with acromegaly. Acromegaly appears to be associated with an increased risk for development of colonic carcinoma, and it is recommended that colonoscopy be performed in all patients. The goal of therapy is a GH level <2 mcg/L or an IGF-1 level in the age- and sex-adjusted normal range. A reduction in GH can be achieved with surgery, medical therapy, and/or radiotherapy.

Surgery

Surgery results in the most rapid reduction in GH levels; however, its efficacy depends on (a) the size of the adenoma and (b) the experience of the surgeon. Surgery is the treatment of choice for microadenomas, which are cured surgically in 90% of cases. Results for macroadenomas are more disappointing, with <50% cured by surgery alone.

Medical Therapy

Somatostatin analogues, including octreotide (Sandostatin) and lanreotide (Somatuline), are more effective agents for treatment of acromegaly. They act as agonists on somatostatin receptors on the tumor and achieve adequate IGF-1 suppression in up to 50% of patients. Dosing is titrated based on the patient's GH and IGF-1 levels. These drugs may be administered as monthly depot injections. Dopamine agonists, bromocriptine (Parlodel) and cabergoline (Dostinex), inhibit secretion of GH by stimulating dopaminergic receptors on the adenoma. Bromocriptine is effective in <20% of patients with acromegaly; however, cabergoline appears to be more efficacious. The GH receptor antagonist pegvisomant (Somavert) was recently approved for clinical use. This drug results in normalization of IGF-1 levels in 89% of patients; however, a significant rise in GH levels is seen. This rise in GH levels has not been shown to increase tumor size; however, two patients have required surgery for rapidly enlarging pituitary tumors while receiving pegvisomant.

Radiotherapy

Both conventional fractionated radiotherapy and stereotactic radiotherapy (gammaknife) have been used to treat pituitary adenomas, including GH-secreting adenomas. Treatment with gamma-knife therapy appears to provide faster normalization of GH levels with less damage to surrounding brain tissue. Up to 60% of patients develop hypopituitarism after therapy. Radiation therapy should not be used as primary therapy for acromegaly unless the patient is unwilling or unable to undergo surgery.

KEY POINTS TO REMEMBER

* Acromegaly is a rare condition with a long lag time between disease onset and diagnosis.
* Abuse of GH may result in similar clinical features.
* Ask about an increase in shoe size and ring size.
* Surgery is the initial treatment of choice when the tumor appears resectable.
* Radiotherapy and medical therapy provide adjunctive support and are able to achieve normalization of IGF-1 levels in up to 90% of patients.

REFERENCES AND SUGGESTED READINGS

Abosch A, et al. Transsphenoidal microsurgery for growth hormone secreting pituitary adenomas: initial outcome and long-term results. *J Clin Endocrinol Metab* 1998;83(3):3411–3418.

Abs R, et al. Cabergoline in the treatment of acromegaly: a study in 64 patients. *J Clin Endocrinol Metab* 1998;83:374–378.

Bates AS. An audit of outcome of treatment in acromegaly. *QJM* 1993;86:293–299.

Jaffe CA, Barkan AL. Treatment of acromegaly with dopamine agonists. *Endocrinol Metab Clin North Am* 1992;21:713–735.

Landolt AM, Haller D, Lomax N, et al. Stereotactic radiosurgery for recurrent surgically treated acromegaly: comparison with fractionated radiotherapy. *J Neurosurg* 1998;88:1002–1008.

Melmed S, Casanueva FF, Cavagnini F, et al., for the Acromegaly Treatment Consensus Workshop Participants Guidelines for Acromegaly Management. Guidelines for acromegaly management. *J Clin Endocrinol Metab* 2002;87(9):4054–4058.

Melmed S, Vance ML, Barkan AL, et al. Current status and future opportunities for controlling acromegaly. *Pituitary* 2002;5(3):185–196.

Molitch ME. Clinical manifestations of acromegaly. *Endocrinol Metab Clin North Am* 1992;21:597–615.

Newman CB, et al. Safety and efficacy of long-term octreotide therapy of acromegaly: results of a multicenter trial in 103 patients—a clinical research center study. *J Clin Endocrinol Metab* 1995;80:2768–2775.

Orme SM, McNally RJ, Cartwright RA, et al., for the United Kingdom Acromegaly Study Group. Mortality and cancer incidence in acromegaly: a retrospective cohort study. *J Clin Endocrinol Metab* 1998;83(3):2730–2734.

Sheppard MC. Primary medical therapy for acromegaly. *Clin Endocrinol* 2003;58:387–399.

Trainer PJ, et al. Treatment of acromegaly with the growth-hormone receptor antagonist pegvisomant. *N Engl J Med* 2000;342:1171–1177.

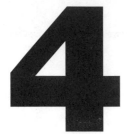

Diabetes Insipidus

Amanda F. Cashen and
Divya Shroff

INTRODUCTION

Diabetes insipidus (DI) is a disorder of water balance caused by nonosmotic renal losses of water. DI results from deficient arginine vasopressin (AVP) secretion (central) or end organ unresponsiveness to AVP (nephrogenic). Patients present with polyuria and, if water intake is inadequate, dehydration and hypernatremia.

AVP, also called antidiuretic hormone (ADH), is released from cells in the posterior pituitary gland and acts to increase water permeability at the distal tubule and collecting duct of the nephron, enhancing water reabsorption at these sites. Decreased production or activity of AVP prevents water reabsorption in the nephron, leading to dilute urine and free water loss.

CAUSES

Differential Diagnosis

The differential diagnosis of polyuria (24-hour urine volume >3 L) includes hypotonic polyuria (primary polydipsia and DI) and solute diuresis. Solute diuresis is commonly caused by diuretic medications or hyperglycemia and can be distinguished from hypotonic polyuria by history and presence of high urine osmolality. If a polyuric patient's plasma osmolality or serum sodium concentration is greater than normal during ad libitum fluid intake, primary polydipsia is virtually excluded.

The differential diagnosis of **hypernatremia** includes other causes of free water loss—for example, insensible losses from the skin or respiratory tract, vomiting or diarrhea, or diuretic use. As with DI, hypernatremia develops when the patient does not drink enough water to compensate for the water loss.

There are 2 basic abnormalities that lead to DI (Table 4–1):

1. **Central DI**—Destruction of the AVP-producing cells of the posterior pituitary gland results in decreased circulating levels of AVP. Complete deficiency of AVP is rare, and circulating AVP levels will usually increase in response to a strong osmotic stimulus such as fluid deprivation.
2. **Nephrogenic DI**—Nephrogenic DI is caused by impaired renal response to AVP, usually due to an abnormality in the renal collecting ducts. Nephrogenic DI may be *partial*, so that increased circulating levels of AVP can overcome the impaired renal response, or *severe*, in which case the renal tubule does not respond to any concentration of AVP.

In both central and nephrogenic DI, serum osmolality increases as a result of the inability of the kidney to concentrate urine. Increased serum osmolality triggers the thirst mechanism, and water intake increases to compensate for water loss in urine. However, if the patient's thirst is impaired, or if access to water is restricted, severe hyperosmolality can develop.

PRESENTATION

Symptoms

Primary symptoms are thirst and polyuria, with a daily urine volume >3 L; symptoms of hypernatremia (weakness, altered mental status, coma, seizures) may develop with significant volume contraction.

TABLE 4-1. CAUSES OF DIABETES INSIPIDUS (DI)

Central DI	Head trauma (may remit after 6 mos)
	Postsurgical (develops 1–6 days after surgery and often disappears, recurs, or becomes chronic)
	Tumors—Craniopharyngioma, pinealoma, meningioma, germinoma, glioma, benign cysts, leukemia, lymphoma, metastatic breast or lung
	Infections—TB, syphilis, mycoses, toxoplasmosis, encephalitis, meningitis
	Granulomatous disease—Sarcoidosis, histiocytosis X, Wegener's granulomatosis
	Cerebrovascular disease—Aneurysms, thrombosis, Sheehan's syndrome, cerebrovascular accident
	Idiopathic—Sporadic or familial (rare autosomal dominant trait)
Nephrogenic DI	Congenital—Rare inherited disorder due to inherited mutations in the AVP receptor (X-linked recessive) or in the water channel of the renal tubule (autosomal recessive)
	Acquired—Much more common and less severe
	Medications [lithium, amphotericin B (Abelcet), demeclocycline (Declomycin), cisplatin, aminoglycosides, rifampin (Rifadin), foscarnet (Foscavir), methoxyflurane (Penthrane), vincristine (Oncovin)]
	Electrolyte disorders (hypercalcemia, hypercalciuria, hypokalemia)
	Chronic tubulointerstitial diseases (polycystic kidney disease, medullary sponge kidney, obstructive uropathy, papillary necrosis)
	Sickle cell disease and trait
	Multiple myeloma, amyloidosis
	Sarcoidosis

AVP, arginine vasopressin.
From Fried LF, Palevsky PM. Hyponatremia and hypernatremia. *Med Clin N Am* 1997;81(3):585–609, with permission.

Signs

The physical exam is usually normal unless dehydration has developed.

Laboratory Evaluation

Labs reveal dilute urine with a specific gravity <1.010 and urine osmolality <300 mOsm/kg in the setting of hypertonicity and polyuria. Hypernatremia is usually mild unless there is an associated thirst abnormality or barrier to obtaining water.

MANAGEMENT

Establishing a Diagnosis of Diabetes Insipidus

1. Measure urine and plasma osmolality. In cases of DI, the urine should be inappropriately dilute for the degree of serum osmolality, usually urine osmolality <300 mOsm/kg and specific gravity <1.010 with plasma osmolality >295 mOsm/kg.
2. Measure serum calcium and potassium. A finding of hypokalemia or hypercalcemia points toward a diagnosis of nephrogenic DI.
3. In the setting of polyuria, a fluid deprivation test may be performed to distinguish between DI and primary polydipsia. (NOTE: If significant hypertonicity is already present, this test is unnecessary and potentially dangerous as it can precipitate symptomatic hypernatremia.) The test should begin in the morning, and body weight, plasma osmolality, serum sodium concentration, urine osmolality, and

urine volume should be followed hourly. Fluids are withheld until body weight decreases by 5%, plasma osmolality and sodium concentration reach the upper limits of normal, or a stable hourly urinary osmolality (variation of <5% over 3 hours) is established. If urine osmolality does not reach 300 mOsm/kg before these parameters are achieved, primary polydipsia is excluded. In patients with partial DI, urine osmolality will be greater than plasma osmolality although the urine will remain submaximally concentrated. In patients with severe DI, the urine osmolality will remain less than the plasma osmolality.

4. Once a diagnosis of DI has been established, administration of desmopressin can be used to distinguish between central and nephrogenic DI. In patients with central DI, the urine osmolality will increase by >50% in response to desmopressin. Patients with nephrogenic DI exhibit little or no change in urine osmolality in response to desmopressin.

TREATMENT

The treatment of DI has 2 goals: (a) replace the water deficit and (b) treat the underlying abnormality in water balance.

Managing the Water Deficit

The patient's water deficit can be calculated with the following formula:

$$\text{Water deficit (L)} = [\,0.6 \text{ (men) or } 0.5 \text{ (women)}\,] \times \text{lean body weight (kg)} \times \left[\frac{\text{plasma } [Na^+] - 140}{140}\right]$$

The water deficit, in addition to ongoing water loss, should be replaced with D_5W or oral water at a rate that will bring the serum sodium concentration to the normal range in approximately 48 hours. A gradual correction of the sodium concentration (0.5 mEq/L/hour) is recommended to avoid cerebral edema. Water can be given more quickly if the hypernatremia has developed acutely or if the patient is symptomatic. If the patient is hypotensive due to volume contraction, normal saline should be used initially until the blood pressure is restored. As the hypernatremia is being corrected, serum sodium concentration and urine output should be followed closely.

Correcting the Chronic Water Loss

Central DI: The agent most commonly used to treat central DI is the AVP analogue DDAVP (desmopressin). AVP can be used for diagnosis or acute therapy, but its hypertensive effects and short half-life limit its long-term usefulness. DDAVP has a longer half-life, almost no pressor activity, and few side effects. It may be administered intranasally at a dose of 5–20 mcg once or twice daily. Oral DDAVP is available in 0.1- and 0.2-mg tablets (patients generally require 0.1–0.8 mg/day in divided doses) and is less expensive than the intranasal preparation. DDAVP given IV, IM, or subcutaneously (SC) is 5–10 times more potent than intranasal DDAVP. Chlorpropamide (Diabinese) (an oral hypoglycemic agent) may also be useful in the treatment of partial central DI as it can potentiate AVP-mediated water reabsorption and stimulate hypothalamic AVP release.

Nephrogenic DI: Because the kidney is unresponsive to ADH, DDAVP is not an effective treatment for nephrogenic DI. If nephrogenic DI is acquired, the concentration defect usually improves quickly with discontinuation of the offending drug or correction of the electrolyte disorder. Otherwise, nephrogenic DI is usually controlled with a sodium-restricted diet and a thiazide diuretic. Thiazides cause an overall reduction in electrolyte-free water excretion by stimulating proximal tubular sodium reabsorption and diminishing sodium delivery to more distal sites. Patients on this therapy should be monitored for hypovolemia and hypokalemia. Amiloride (Midamor) is the treatment of choice for lithium-induced DI and works by blocking the action of lithium on the renal distal tubules and collecting ducts. NSAIDs can be a useful adjunct to treatment because they increase water reabsorption and urine osmolality, thereby reducing electrolyte-free water clearance and urine volume.

FOLLOW-UP

Patients with central DI who are treated with DDAVP should be followed for the development of hyponatremia. Occasional withdrawal of the DDAVP should be performed to confirm recurrence of polyuria, and serum sodium concentration should be checked periodically. When a patient with DI loses access to water, as may occur during a medical emergency or surgery, he or she is at high risk of dehydration. Under these circumstances, urine output and serum sodium concentration should be followed closely.

KEY POINTS TO REMEMBER

- DI results from deficient AVP secretion and/or release or end-organ unresponsiveness to AVP.
- To establish a diagnosis of DI, the urine should be inappropriately dilute for the degree of serum osmolality.
- Treatment of DI should be aimed at replacing the patient's water deficit and treating the underlying cause.
- Central DI is most commonly treated with DDAVP.
- DDAVP is not an effective treatment for nephrogenic DI, which is typically controlled with a sodium-restricted diet and a thiazide diuretic.

REFERENCES AND SUGGESTED READINGS

Fried LF, Palevsky PM. Hyponatremia and hypernatremia. *Med Clin North Am* 1997;81(3):585–609.

Hockaday TDR. Diabetes insipidus. *BMJ* 1972;2(807):210–213.

Palevsky PM. Hypernatremia. In: Greenberg A, ed. *Primer on kidney diseases*. San Diego: Academic Press, 1998:64–71.

Robertson GL. Antidiuretic hormone. Normal and disordered function. *Endocrin Metab Clin North Am* 2001;30(3):671–694.

Robertson GL. Diabetes insipidus. *Endocrin Metab Clin North Am* 1995;24:549–572.

Robertson GL. Disorders of the neurohypophysis. In: Braunwald E, et al., eds. *Harrison's principles of internal medicine*, 15th ed. New York: McGraw-Hill, 2001:2054–2056.

Singer I, Oster JR, Fishman LM. The management of diabetes insipidus in adults. *Arch Intern Med* 1997;157:1293–1301.

Syndrome of Inappropriate Antidiuretic Hormone Secretion

Amanda F. Cashen and
Divya Shroff

INTRODUCTION

The syndrome of inappropriate antidiuretic hormone secretion (SIADH) is the most common cause of normovolemic hyponatremia, yet it remains a diagnosis of exclusion. SIADH results from the inappropriate release of antidiuretic hormone (ADH) from the pituitary gland or from an ectopic source. **Hallmarks of SIADH** are hypo-osmolar hyponatremia and relatively concentrated urine in the setting of normovolemia and normal renal, thyroid, and adrenal function. The incidence of hyponatremia overall is 1–4% and is associated with a 7- to 60-fold increase in mortality, although the underlying etiology may play a role in mortality.

ADH, also known as arginine vasopressin (AVP), is a key component of the homeostatic mechanisms that regulate water balance. ADH is released from cells in the neurohypophysis in response to increased serum osmolality or decreased intravascular volume. Nausea is also a potent stimulus for ADH release. In the kidneys, ADH increases water permeability at the distal tubule and collecting duct of the nephron, enhancing water reabsorption at these sites. With excess ADH, dilutional hyponatremia develops because water cannot be excreted normally. Inappropriate release of ADH from the pituitary is defined as occurring despite serum hypotonicity and in the absence of volume depletion. SIADH can also occur with ectopic production of ADH from a malignancy or inflamed tissue.

CAUSES

The causes of SIADH are summarized in Table 5-1.

Differential Diagnosis

The differential diagnosis of SIADH includes other etiologies of hypo-osmolar hyponatremia.

- **Subclinical hypovolemia**, which is defined by a urine sodium level <20 mEq/L, an increase in serum creatinine and uric acid, and an increase in plasma renin and aldosterone levels.
- **Reset osmostat syndrome** in which, unlike classic SIADH, the patient has the ability to dilute urine normally in response to the water load and concentrate urine in response to dehydration. The primary etiology for this is malnutrition. These patients are primarily asymptomatic; therefore, the only therapy indicated is correction of the underlying condition.

PRESENTATION

As with other causes of hyponatremia, symptoms are dependent on the degree of hyponatremia and the rapidity at which it developed. It is rare to have symptoms with serum sodium levels of ≥125 mEq/L, but at levels of 125–130 mEq/L patients may complain of GI upset with nausea, vomiting, or diarrhea. At levels of ≤125 mEq/L, patients may present with neuropsychiatric signs and symptoms, ranging from muscular weakness,

TABLE 5-1. CAUSES OF THE SYNDROME OF INAPPROPRIATE ANTIDIURETIC HORMONE SECRETION

CNS (excess ADH release)
  Acute intermittent porphyria
  Bleeding (hematoma/hemorrhage)
  CVA
  Delirium tremens
  Guillain-Barré syndrome
  Head trauma
  Hydrocephalus
  Infections (meningitis/encephalitis/abscess)
  Tumors
Medications
  Bromocriptine mesylate (Bromocriptine)
  Carbamazepine (Carbatrol, Tegretol)
  Chlorpropamide (Diabinese)
  Clofibrate (Abitrate, Atromid-S)
  Cyclophosphamide (Cytoxan, Neosar)
  Desmopressin (DDAVP)
  Ecstasy
  Haloperidol (Haldol)
  Nicotine
  Opiates
  Oxytocin (Pitocin, Syntocinon)
  Phenothiazines
  Selective serotonin reuptake inhibitors (SSRIs)
  Tricyclic antidepressants (TCAs)
  Vinblastine (Velban)
  Vincristine (Oncovin)
Miscellaneous
  HIV
  Nausea
  Neuropsychiatric disorders (increased thirst, ADH release at lower osmolality, increased renal sensitivity to ADH)
  Pain
  Postoperative state (excessive amounts of electrolyte free water)
Neoplasms (ectopic ADH secretion)
  Duodenal carcinoma
  Lymphoma
  Mesothelioma
  Olfactory neuroblastoma
  Pancreatic carcinoma

(continued)

TABLE 5-1. *(Continued)*

Prostate carcinoma
Small cell of lung
Thymoma
Pulmonary diseases
   Bronchiectasis
   COPD
   Cystic fibrosis
   Pneumonia (PCP, TB, aspergillosis)
   Positive pressure ventilation

ADH, antidiuretic hormone.

headache, lethargy, ataxia, and psychosis to cerebral edema, increased ICP, seizures, and coma. Signs of either volume overload or depletion are not consistent with SIADH and should prompt evaluation of other causes of hyponatremia.

MANAGEMENT

Diagnostic Evaluation

As SIADH is a diagnosis of exclusion, other causes of hyponatremia must be ruled out, including normotonic (pseudohyponatremia with increased lipids or protein) and hypertonic hyponatremia (hyperglycemia and other solutes). Once a hypotonic state has been diagnosed, the algorithm below can be followed.

1. Measure serum osmolality: A low (<280 mOsm/kg) serum osmolality is consistent with SIADH.
2. Measure urine osmolality and urine sodium concentration: An inappropriately elevated urine osmolality (>200 mOsm/kg) and urine sodium concentration (>20 mEq/L) are consistent with SIADH.
3. Assess the patient's volume status: The patient should appear clinically euvolemic. Volume overload or depletion should prompt evaluation for an alternative diagnosis.
4. Assess renal, adrenal, and thyroid function with serum creatinine, serum cortisol, and thyroid-stimulating hormone measurements. These measurements must be normal to establish the diagnosis of SIADH.

Supplemental diagnostic criteria include

- Abnormal water load test, which is defined as the inability to excrete at least 80% of a water load (20 mL/kg water ingested in 10–20 minutes) after 4 hours and/or the failure to dilute urinary osmolality to <100 mOsm/kg. This test should be administered after the serum sodium level is >125 mEq/L through water restriction and/or saline administration.
- Plasma ADH level inappropriately raised relative to plasma osmolality.
- No significant correction of serum sodium with volume expansion, but improvement after fluid restriction.
- Low-normal or subnormal serum BUN, creatinine, uric acid, and albumin levels.

Treatment

Most cases of SIADH are self-limited, and the key is to correct the underlying etiology. The cornerstone of treatment for SIADH is **fluid restriction**, usually to 500–1000 mL/ day, so that free water excretion in the urine exceeds dietary intake. Treatment for acute symptomatic hyponatremia is managed similarly to other causes by administering **normotonic or hypertonic fluids** as indicated by symptoms and sodium level. A loop diuretic can be added to increase free water excretion. The goal is to raise the serum sodium level by 0.5 mEq/hour to a maximum increase of 12 mEq/L in the first 24 hours. In patients with severe confusion, convulsions, or coma, 200–300 mL of 3–5% NaCl solution may be given IV over 3–4 hours. Serum sodium levels should be monitored at least every 4 hours during IV fluid replacement to monitor for over-correction. Raising the serum sodium concentration too rapidly may precipitate central pontine myelinolysis, a neurologic disorder characterized by dysarthria, dysphagia, and flaccid paralysis. For cases of SIADH that are not self-limited or are refractory to fluid restriction, demeclocycline (Declomycin) may be administered. Demeclocycline (Declomycin) inhibits the renal effect of ADH and can correct serum sodium concentration without fluid restriction. Initial dosing is 600 mg daily in 2–3 divided doses, with an onset of action 3–6 days after treatment initiation. It should be given 1–2 hours after meals. The major side effect is renal toxicity.

Prognosis

Prognosis is dependent on the underlying etiology. Drug-induced causes are rapidly and completely corrected as are pulmonary and CNS infections. The extent of underlying malignancy determines the outcome, though any form of treatment can cause improvement.

KEY POINTS TO REMEMBER

- SIADH is a diagnosis of exclusion.
- A low serum osmolality in conjunction with an inappropriately elevated urine osmolality and urine sodium are consistent with SIADH.
- The cornerstone of treatment is fluid restriction.
- Normotonic or hypertonic fluids can be administered in cases of acute symptomatic hyponatremia, but care should be taken not to correct the serum sodium level too rapidly.

REFERENCES AND SUGGESTED READINGS

Abboud CF. Endocrinology. In: Prakash UB, ed. *Mayo Clinic internal medicine board review*. Philadelphia: Lippincott Williams & Wilkins, 2002:212–214.

Adrogue HJ, Madia NE. Hyponatremia. *N Engl J Med* 2000;342:1581–1589.

Fried LF, Palevsky PM. Hyponatremia and hypernatremia. *Med Clin North Am* 1997;81:585–609.

Kovacs L, Robertson GL. Syndrome of inappropriate antidiuresis. *Endocrinol Metab Clin North Am* 1992;21(4):859–875.

Kumar S, Berl T. Sodium. *Lancet* 1998;352:220–228.

Robertson GL. Antidiuretic hormone. *Endocrinol Metab Clin North Am* 2001;30(3):671–694.

Sorensen JB, Andersen MK, Hansen HH. Syndrome of inappropriate secretion of antidiuretic hormone (SIADH) in malignancy disease. *J Int Med* 1995;238(2):97–110.

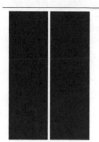

Thyroid Disorders

Evaluation of Thyroid Function

Savitha Subramanian

INTRODUCTION

The thyroid gland participates in a negative feedback loop with the hypothalamus and the anterior pituitary gland. Thyrotropin-releasing hormone (TRH) is secreted by hypothalamic neurons and stimulates thyrotropin or thyroid-stimulating hormone (TSH) secretion from the anterior pituitary. TSH enables secretion of thyroxine (T_4) from the thyroid, which is converted in the peripheral tissues to triiodothyronine (T_3). Circulating T_4 and T_3 negatively inhibit TRH and TSH secretion. The hypothalamic-pituitary axis detects subtle variations in free thyroid hormone levels and acts to correct them.

EVALUATION

Clinical evaluation should include **palpation** of the thyroid gland. The thyroid gland is best palpated from behind the patient. The size, shape, and consistency of the gland are noted, and the presence of tenderness or nodules is identified. Auscultation for a bruit is performed when the thyroid gland is enlarged.

LABORATORY TESTS FOR THYROID FUNCTION

Thyroid-Stimulating Hormone

The TSH is a sensitive measurement for hypo- and hyperthyroidism. Ultrasensitive immunometric TSH assays are able to detect plasma TSH levels to 0.02 mIU/L. This enables the clinician to distinguish between the profound suppression seen in hyperthyroidism as opposed to mildly suppressed levels seen in subclinical hyperthyroidism or nonthyroidal illnesses. Although measurement of TSH is a good initial screening tool, abnormal levels are not specific for a particular thyroid disease. This is because TSH secretion is affected by minimal changes in thyroid hormone levels, and changes in plasma TSH levels may lag behind changes in plasma T_4. Hence, the **TSH should not be used alone for diagnosis**, but in combination with free thyroid hormone levels. It should also not be used when plasma T_4 levels are rapidly changing such as after recent treatment of hyperthyroidism.

Low or Suppressed Thyroid-Stimulating Hormone Levels
Low or suppressed TSH levels (<0.1 mIU/L) occur in hyperthyroidism due to various causes, pituitary disease, severe nonthyroidal illness, and with high doses of steroids or dopamine infusion.

Mildly Elevated Thyroid-Stimulating Hormone Levels
Mildly elevated TSH levels ($\leq$ 20 mIU/L) are seen occasionally in mild (subclinical) hypothyroidism and in the recovery phase of nonthyroidal illness.

Recommended Settings for Measurement of Thyroid-Stimulating Hormone
Measurement of TSH is useful for

- Diagnosis of hyperthyroidism or primary hypothyroidism
- During maintenance therapy for primary hypothyroidism

- Monitoring TSH-suppressive therapy in thyroid cancer
- General evaluation of thyroid function as part of screening, evaluation of hypercholesterolemia, and for exclusion of thyroid disease

Settings for which Measurement of Thyroid-Stimulating Hormone Is Not Recommended

- Pituitary or hypothalamic disease
- After a recent change in thyroid status, such as a recent levothyroxine dose adjustment, because TSH levels take approximately 6 weeks to equilibrate
- First trimester of pregnancy when there is a drop in TSH [with normal free T_4 (FT_4) levels]

Free T_4

T_4 is the principal hormone secreted by the thyroid gland, and 99.98% of the hormone is tightly bound to plasma proteins [primarily thyroxine-binding globulin (TBG)]. Bioavailable or FT_4 fractions are miniscule. Plasma FT_4 may be measured by immunoassay, directly in serum by equilibrium dialysis, or by calculating the FT_4 index (FTI). FT_4 immunoassays are estimates of the actual free hormone concentrations. Equilibrium dialysis is most reliable, but results are not readily available. The FTI is less expensive and is measured as a product of the total T_4 and T_3 resin uptake, but is less reliable and hence seldom used today.

Measurement of free T_4 is usually used for

- Diagnosis of hyperthyroidism or primary hypothyroidism, in conjunction with the TSH
- To diagnose central (secondary) hypothyroidism
- Monitoring T_4 replacement therapy for central hypothyroidism

Total T_4

The total T_4 measures free and bound T_4. T_4 is bound to TBG and other plasma proteins such as albumin and pre-albumin. Hence, changes in T_4-binding proteins will cause a change in T_4 levels. Levels of total T_4 may be increased in hyperthyroidism and decreased in hypothyroidism, but not always. Disadvantages of this test are that elevated total T_4 levels may occur in otherwise euthyroid people. At present, free hormone levels are preferred over total measurements.

Causes of increased total T_4 in euthyroid patients include TBG excess (as in pregnancy), nonthyroidal illness, and drugs such as amiodarone (Cordarone, Pacerone) or propranolol (Inderal, Proprandol). Total T_4 levels are decreased in euthyroid patients on phenytoin (Dilantin) therapy and in iodine deficiency.

Free and Total T_3

T_4 is converted to T_3, the biologically active form of thyroid hormone. Although the amount of free T_3 (FT_3) in plasma is miniscule, it is the biologically active form of thyroid hormone along with FT_4. Levels are high in hyperthyroidism. Plasma FT_3 measurements have low sensitivity and specificity for diagnosing hypothyroidism and should never be used alone. FT_3 assays are technically difficult, and therefore expensive, due to low circulating amounts of the hormone. Total T_3 levels, on the other hand, may be helpful when a patient has hyperthyroidism secondary to elevated T_3 alone (T_3 toxicosis). Measurement of total T_3 poses problems similar to measuring total T_4 due to alterations in protein binding. Hence, total T_3 levels are seldom used alone.

Thyroglobulin

Thyroglobulin (Tg) is the secretory protein of thyroid follicular cells. The Tg concentration in serum is dependent on thyroid cell mass, and levels are decreased after surgery or destruction of the thyroid with radioiodine therapy. **The main use of measuring thyro-**

globulin is to help detect recurrence of cancer in patients with differentiated thyroid cancer who have undergone total thyroidectomy. The presence of Tg antibodies in a patient's serum limits the usefulness of this test (see the section Thyroid Autoantibodies).

Thyroid Autoantibodies

Autoimmune thyroid disease (AITD) includes Graves' disease and Hashimoto's thyroiditis. AITD is characterized by cellular and humoral immune responses to thyroid antigens. These autoantibodies involve thyroid peroxidase (TPO), Tg, and the TSH receptor (stimulating or inhibitory). TPO and Tg antibodies (TgAb) are often present in sera of patients with autoimmune thyroid disease, but occasionally patients may have negative test results.

Thyroid antibody testing is useful in the following situations:

- Detection of anti-TPO antibodies is thought to be the most sensitive test for AITD, because the antibodies occur in >90% of these patients. It may also be useful in predicting the progression of subclinical hypothyroidism.
- In the absence of thyroid neoplasia, measurement of **TgAb** is rarely needed in iodine-replete areas because patients with undetectable anti-TPO antibodies and detectable TgAb rarely develop thyroid disease. **In patients with differentiated thyroid cancer, TgAbs are measured whenever a serum Tg is ordered.** This is because the presence of even low concentrations of TgAbs interferes with the Tg assay, making Tg measurements unreliable in this setting.
- TSH receptor antibodies (also known as thyroid-stimulating immunoglobulins or TSI): Measurement of TSI in diagnosing autoimmune thyroid disease is not needed in a typical patient with Graves' hyperthyroidism. The diagnosis of hyperthyroidism is usually made without these tests. On occasion, these tests may be used to evaluate the cause of hyperthyroidism when the diagnosis is unclear, such as in patients with unilateral exophthalmos, apathetic or masked hyperthyroidism seen commonly in elderly patients, or to predict neonatal Graves' disease in mothers with high TSI levels in the third trimester.

IMAGING STUDIES OF THE THYROID

Radioactive Iodine Uptake

Radioactive iodine uptake detects the fractional uptake of tracer doses of radioiodine (I^{131} or I^{123}) by the thyroid gland. It involves oral administration of radioiodine followed by measurement of radioactivity over the thyroid gland 24 hours later. This test is used to assist dosing of I^{131} for treatment of Graves' disease or toxic multinodular goiter. It may also be used to distinguish between causes of high and low radioactive iodine uptake thyrotoxicosis (see Chap. 8, Hyperthyroidism).

Radioisotope Thyroid Scan

Radioisotope thyroid scan uses technetium-99m pertechnate, which is taken up by thyroid cells and may be helpful in delineating thyroid anatomy and determining its functional activity. Scanning detects hypofunctioning ("cold"), isofunctioning ("warm"), or hyperfunctioning ("hot") nodules. However, this test has low sensitivity and specificity and is seldom indicated in diagnosis of thyroid disease.

Ultrasonography

High-resolution ultrasound of the thyroid is a noninvasive test gaining popularity among endocrinologists to delineate thyroid anatomy. It differentiates solid from cystic nodules and may be used to guide fine-needle biopsy of nonpalpable nodules. Ultrasound detects incidental thyroid nodules, which occur in 20–35% of the general population. Currently, ultrasound is a sensitive test, but has low specificity to detect thyroid cancer, which precludes widespread use of this test.

TABLE 6-1. DRUGS AND THYROID FUNCTION

Drug effect	Drug
↓ TSH secretion	Dopamine, dobutamine, glucocorticoids, octreotide
↑ FT$_4$ and total T$_4$ secretion	Iodine (amiodarone, radiographic contrast)
↓ FT$_4$ secretion	Lithium, iodine, amiodarone, radiographic contrast
Altered T$_4$ transport	↑ TBG—estrogens, tamoxifen, raloxifene, heroin, methadone
	↓ TBG—androgens, anabolic steroids, glucocorticoids, nicotinic acid
	Displacement from protein-binding sites—Furosemide (IV in high doses), salicylates, mefenamic acid, salsalate, heparin and low-molecular-weight heparin (*in vitro* only)
Altered T$_4$ metabolism	↑ Hepatic metabolism—phenytoin, rifampin, estrogen
	↓ T$_4$ →T$_3$ conversion—PTU (high doses), amiodarone, glucocorticoids
Cytokines (hypo- or hyperthyroidism)	Interleukin-2, interferon-alpha
↓ T$_4$ absorption from the gut	Cholestyramine, ferrous sulfate, calcium containing products, sucralfate, soy products, aluminum hydroxide

FT$_4$, free thyroxine; PTU, propylthiouracil; T$_3$, triiodothyronine; TBG, thyroxine-binding hormone; TSH, thyroid-stimulating hormone; ↑, increased; ↓, decreased.
Adapted from Surks MI, Sievert R. Drugs and thyroid function. *N Engl J Med* 1995;333(25):1688–1694.

Fine-Needle Aspiration Cytology

Fine-needle aspiration cytology provides the most direct information about a thyroid nodule. It is safe, fast, inexpensive, and virtually free of complications when performed by an experienced clinician. Diagnostically useful specimens are obtained in 80% of cases. The procedure should be repeated if the specimen is unsatisfactory, preferably under ultrasound guidance.

DRUGS AFFECTING THYROID FUNCTION

Many drugs affect thyroid function in different ways (Table 6-1). Drugs can directly inhibit TSH secretion, affect transport of thyroid hormones, or alter metabolism of thyroid hormones.

KEY POINTS TO REMEMBER

- TSH is the best screening test to evaluate patients with suspected thyroid disease.
- TSH should be used in conjunction with free thyroid hormone testing to establish a diagnosis and to assess severity of thyroid disease.
- Clinicians should be aware of the effects of drugs on thyroid function tests.
- Although imaging studies are seldom used for diagnosis of thyroid disease, fine-needle aspiration cytology is an effective method for quick diagnosis of thyroid nodules.

REFERENCES AND SUGGESTED READINGS

Baloch Z, et al. Guidelines Committee, National Academy of Clinical Biochemistry. Laboratory medicine practice guidelines. Laboratory support for the diagnosis and monitoring of thyroid disease. *Thyroid* 2003;13(1):19–67.

Clutter WE. Endocrine disorders. In: Ahya S, Flood K, Paranjothi S, eds. *Washington manual of medical therapeutics*, 30th ed. Philadelphia: Lippincott Williams & Wilkins, 2001:473–490.

Dayan CM. Interpretation of thyroid function tests. *Lancet* 2001;357(9256):619–624.

Kane LA, Gharib H. Thyroid testing. A clinical approach. In: Braverman LE, ed. *Diseases of the thyroid*, 2nd ed. Totowa, NJ: Humana Press Inc., 2003:39–52.

Ladenson P, Singer P, et al. American Thyroid Association guidelines for detection of thyroid dysfunction. *Arch Intern Med* 2000;160:1573–1575.

Larsen PR, et al. Thyroid physiology and diagnostic evaluation of patients with thyroid disorders. In: Larsen PR, et al., eds. *Williams textbook of endocrinology*, 10th ed. Philadelphia: WB Saunders, 2003:331–373.

Stockigt JR. Free thyroid hormone measurement. A critical appraisal. *Endocrinol Metab Clin North Am* 2001;30:265–289.

Surks MI, Sievert R. Drugs and thyroid function. *N Engl J Med* 1995;333(25):1688–1694.

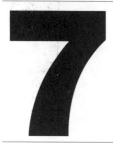

Euthyroid Goiter and Thyroid Nodules

Savitha Subramanian

INTRODUCTION

Euthyroid goiter refers to an enlarged thyroid gland with normal biochemical parameters. There are three common forms of euthyroid goiter: **diffuse goiter**, a **solitary nodule**, and **multinodular goiter (MNG)**.

EUTHYROID DIFFUSE GOITER

Diffuse goiters are thought to be the initial phase of development into a MNG. They are more prevalent in iodine-deficient areas. Although the underlying pathogenesis is unclear, Hashimoto's thyroiditis is a common cause of diffuse enlargement of the thyroid.

Clinical Presentation

Patients with a diffuse goiter are usually asymptomatic. Pressure symptoms are absent. Palpation to assess for the presence of nodules is the key aspect of evaluation. Laboratory evaluation should include a thyroid-stimulating hormone (TSH) measurement. Measurement of thyroid peroxidase antibodies is helpful to diagnose Hashimoto's thyroiditis. Management involves careful clinical follow-up. Although some groups use levothyroxine suppression therapy to decrease size of the gland, we do not advocate this treatment method. Surgery may be indicated for cosmetic reasons.

SOLITARY THYROID NODULES

Palpable thyroid nodules occur in approximately 5–7% of the population. With increasing availability of imaging modalities, the prevalence of nonpalpable thyroid nodules is approximately 20–50% in the general population by ultrasound. The critical question when a thyroid nodule is detected is whether it is malignant or not. Thyroid cancer accounts for only 0.4% of all cancer deaths and for approximately 5 deaths per million people in the United States each year. Its clinical importance, by contrast, is out of proportion to its incidence, and cancers of the thyroid must be differentiated from the much more frequent benign adenomas and MNGs.

Clinical Presentation

The usual presentation of solitary thyroid nodules is a lump noted in the neck either by the patient or the clinician. Symptoms of rapidly increasing size, male sex, co-existent dysphagia, dysphonia, pain, or family history of multiple endocrine neoplasia (MEN) syndromes increase the risk of malignancy. On palpation, the size and consistency of the nodule are noted. Nodules >4 cm in size, fixation to surrounding structures, and presence of associated lymphadenopathy are worrisome for cancer.

Diagnostic Evaluation

Fine-Needle Aspiration Cytology

Fine-needle aspiration cytology (FNAC) is the most important diagnostic modality in evaluation of a thyroid nodule. Cytologically, nodules can be classified as benign, malig-

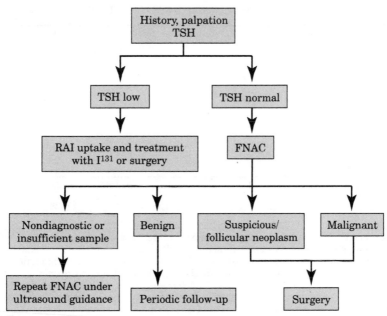

FIG. 7-1. Evaluation of a solitary thyroid nodule. FNAC, fine-needle aspiration cytology; RAI, radioactive iodine; TSH, thyroid-stimulating hormone.

nant, indeterminate, or suspicious follicular neoplasms, and as an insufficient sample (Fig. 7-1). The pitfall of FNAC is the possibility of a false-negative result, which occurs in approximately 5% of samples. The procedure should be repeated when the sample is insufficient, and success is dependent on the skill of the clinician.

Other Studies

Thyroid ultrasound is a relatively new modality being used by endocrinologists for imaging thyroid nodules. It may be used for guided FNAC. However, the ultrasound may pick up incidental nodules. A radionuclide thyroid scan may be indicated on rare occasions to determine whether a nodule in a hyperthyroid patient is causing the hyperthyroidism and is therefore benign, or whether it is a hypofunctioning nodule in a patient with coexisting Graves' disease and should be biopsied to exclude carcinoma. CT scan and MRI have no role in the evaluation of a solitary thyroid nodule.

Laboratory Evaluation

The TSH is a good initial screening test because nodules associated with hyperthyroidism are rarely malignant. In the setting of a family history of MEN syndromes, calcitonin levels are obtained. Obtaining routine calcitonin levels in all patients with a thyroid nodule is controversial. There is no role for routine assessment of thyroglobulin or thyroglobulin antibodies.

Differential Diagnosis

See Table 7-1.

Management

Fig. 7-1 outlines an algorithmic approach for management of a solitary thyroid nodule based on FNAC.

TABLE 7-1. DIFFERENTIAL DIAGNOSIS OF A SOLITARY THYROID NODULE

Adenoma

Dominant nodule in a multinodular goiter

Carcinoma

Hashimoto's thyroiditis

Colloid cyst

Parathyroid cyst or adenoma

Thyroglossal cyst

Nonthyroidal lesions: laryngocele, aneurysm, inflammatory or neoplastic lymph nodes, cystic hygroma

Adapted from Pacini F, DeGroot LJ. Thyroid nodules. Thyroid disease manager, http://www.thyroidmanager.org.

Surgery is indicated for malignant lesions; however, treatment of a nodule with indeterminate cytology is a controversial issue. Most clinicians refer patients for surgery, because nodules labeled as suspicious follicular neoplasms harbor malignancy in up to 20%, especially in high-risk individuals. The extent of surgery is another debatable issue. In young, low-risk patients, lobectomy is preferred because most of these nodules are benign; however, complete thyroidectomy should be performed when malignancy is noted on histologic exam of the nodule. Lobectomy is associated with fewer surgical complications than complete thyroidectomy and avoids the need for levothyroxine replacement.

Thyroid Malignancy

Thyroid cancer is an uncommon malignancy arising from follicular epithelium or parafollicular thyroid cells. Thyroid epithelial cancers may be well differentiated or anaplastic. Differentiated thyroid cancers—follicular and papillary—account for approximately 94% of all thyroid cancers. Medullary thyroid cancer arising from the parafollicular C cells account for approximately 5%, and the remaining 1% include anaplastic and primary lymphoid malignancies. The risk of differentiated thyroid cancer is higher in patients who have received external beam radiation, especially in early childhood. It may also occur as part of several inherited syndromes (e.g., familial adenomatous polyposis).

Treatment

Care of patients with thyroid malignancies is best performed in consultation with an endocrinologist. Primary management is surgical. Total thyroidectomy is the preferred method in tumors >1 cm, tumors extending beyond the thyroid, or when there are metastases. Unilateral lobectomy may be sufficient in patients with well-encapsulated papillary carcinomas <1 cm in size. For follicular cancers, most guidelines recommend total thyroidectomy.

After surgery, patients should receive I^{131} adjuvant therapy to destroy any residual thyroid tissue and microscopic or metastatic disease.

Follow-Up

After I^{131} ablation, patients need lifelong therapy with thyroid hormone. The TSH is maintained between 0.1 and 0.4 mIU/L in patients with low risk for recurrence. High-risk patients, such as those with metastatic disease, need further suppression to levels <0.1 mIU/L. Long-term follow-up also includes whole body I^{131} scans to detect residual thyroid tissue that takes up the iodine. This can be discontinued after two negative scans. Thyroglobulin (with antibodies) is measured at each visit; after near-total thyroidectomy and successful I^{131} ablation, there should be no detectable thyroglobulin in the patient's plasma, making it a useful tumor marker.

Medullary thyroid cancer is treated surgically; patients need lifelong therapy with thyroid hormone at regular replacement doses with maintenance of normal plasma TSH levels. Testing for MEN syndromes is warranted (see Chap. 31, Multiple Endocrine Neoplasia Syndromes). Treatment of anaplastic thyroid cancer is usually palliative due to its high fatality rates.

Incidentally Detected Thyroid Nodules

With increasing use of imaging, thyroid nodules are incidentally noted in approximately 25–30% of asymptomatic individuals. Nonpalpable nodules of the thyroid are extremely common, and autopsy studies report a 50% prevalence of thyroid nodules.

Management

Low-risk individuals (e.g., no history of irradiation, young age) can be clinically followed with palpation or imaging every 6 months to 1 year if the nodule is <1 cm. An increase in size of the nodule over time warrants FNAC to rule out malignancy. Nodules >1 cm on presentation should be biopsied. FNAC is also warranted in patients with a family history of thyroid cancer or with history of head/neck irradiation. Further management is based on cytology.

MULTINODULAR GOITER

Evaluation

Evaluation of an MNG is similar to a solitary nodule if there is a dominant nodule or suspicious area. Only dominant nodules are biopsied. Euthyroid MNGs are followed clinically.

Management

Surgery is indicated for

- Presence of cancer
- Increasing size with pressure symptoms
- Cosmetic reasons

Because most patients with MNG are elderly with coexisting medical problems, the benefits of surgery should be carefully weighed against the risks. If surgery is performed, a subtotal thyroidectomy with removal of most thyroid tissue is preferred because recurrence is common. Radioactive iodine may be used in some patients with large goiters who are a poor risk for surgery. There is no evidence of a beneficial role for T_4 suppression therapy in MNG in iodine-sufficient areas such as the United States.

KEY POINTS TO REMEMBER

- Euthyroid diffuse goiters are most commonly due to Hashimoto's thyroiditis.
- Multinodular goiters are usually asymptomatic, but require treatment when pressure symptoms occur.
- Single thyroid nodules are usually benign, but a small percentage harbor malignancy.
- FNAC is the mainstay of evaluation of a solitary thyroid nodule.
- Incidental thyroid nodules occur in 20–30% of general population.

REFERENCES AND SUGGESTED READINGS

Burguera B, Gharib H. Thyroid incidentalomas. Prevalence, diagnosis, significance, and management. *Endocrinol Metab Clin North Am* 2000;29(1):187–203.
Hegedus L, et al. Management of simple nodular goiter: current status and future perspectives. *Endocr Rev* 2003;24(1):102–132.

Pacini F, DeGroot LJ. Thyroid nodules. Thyroid Disease Manager, http://www.thyroid-manager.org.

Richter B, Neises G, Clar C. Pharmacotherapy for thyroid nodules. A systematic review and meta-analysis. *Endocrinol Metab Clin North Am* 2002;31(3):699–722.

Ross DS. Nonpalpable thyroid nodules—managing an epidemic. *J Clin Endocrinol Metab* 2002;87(5):1938–1940.

Sherman SI. Thyroid carcinoma. *Lancet* 2003;361(9356):501–511.

Singer PA. Evaluation and management of the euthyroid nodular and diffuse goiter. In: *Disease of the thyroid*, 2nd ed. Totowa, NJ: Humana Press, 2003.

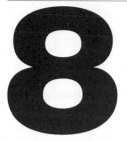

Hyperthyroidism

Savitha Subramanian and
Andrew F. Holt

INTRODUCTION

Hyperthyroidism refers to hyperfunctioning of the thyroid gland. Symptoms are caused by secretion of excess thyroid hormone. Hyperthyroidism affects 2% of women and 0.2% of men during their lifetimes.

CAUSES

Graves' disease is the most common cause of hyperthyroidism. Approximately 60–80% of patients with hyperthyroidism have Graves' disease. In women, the annual incidence is approximately 0.5/1000, making it one of the most common autoimmune disorders in the United States. The peak age of onset is between 40 and 60 years. The ratio of males to females is approximately 1:10. Among the different races, whites and Asians have similar prevalence, whereas it is lower for blacks.

The second leading cause of hyperthyroidism is **toxic multinodular goiter (MNG)**. It arises from a long-standing simple goiter, and thus usually affects patients > age 50 years. It occurs as a result of transition of a nontoxic multinodular thyroid gland into an autonomous functional state.

A third, less common form of hyperthyroidism is caused by a single, autonomous, hyperfunctioning nodule. The nodule is a benign tumor (adenoma) in the thyroid that is intrinsically normal. Other causes of hyperthyroidism include drugs (e.g., iodine), subacute thyroiditis, painless thyroiditis, and surreptitious ingestion of thyroid hormone preparations. On rare occasions, thyrotoxicosis may be caused by ectopic thyroid tissue or by thyroid-stimulating hormone (TSH)–secreting pituitary adenomas (Table 8-1).

Pathophysiology

Graves' disease is an autoimmune disorder caused by antibodies against the TSH receptor, which stimulate the thyroid gland and thereby cause hyperfunction. These antibodies cause thyroid hypersecretion as well as hypertrophy and hyperplasia of thyroid follicles. Lymphocytic infiltration is seen and results in a diffuse goiter. Antibodies to the TSH receptor can be found in approximately 80% of patients. Ocular manifestations seen in Graves' disease (Graves' ophthalmopathy) are caused by edema and inflammation of the extraocular muscles and by an increase in orbital connective tissue and fat. Edema occurs due to the hydrophilic action of glycosaminoglycans secreted by fibroblasts, and inflammation occurs secondary to infiltration by lymphocytes and macrophages.

Toxic MNG develops in the setting of a nontoxic MNG over time. Functional autonomy of one or more of the nodules results in hyperthyroidism, but the exact mechanism of this change is not known. Solitary functioning nodules occur due to somatic mutations in the TSH receptor gene, resulting in progressive growth and, occasionally, increasing function of the adenoma.

Differential Diagnosis

Distinction between the various forms of hyperthyroidism is important for choice of therapy (Table 8-2). Graves' disease can be differentiated by the presence of unique

TABLE 8-1. CAUSES OF HYPERTHYROIDISM

Graves' disease
Toxic multinodular goiter
Toxic adenoma
Iodine and drugs containing iodine (e.g., amiodarone, iodinated contrast agents)
Subacute thyroiditis
Painless thyroiditis
Surreptitious thyroid hormone ingestion
Ectopic thyroid tissue (struma ovarii)
TSH-secreting pituitary adenoma

TSH, thyroid-stimulating hormone.

signs from other forms (although these signs are not present in all patients); recent pregnancy, anterior neck pain or recent iodine excess, such as amiodarone (Cordarone, Pacerone) or imaging studies with contrast, suggest causes other than Graves' disease. Rarely, radioactive iodine (RAI) uptake is needed to distinguish between conditions causing increased radioiodine uptake and low uptake.

PRESENTATION

Clinical Presentation

Patients with hyperthyroidism typically present with a characteristic array of signs and symptoms. Manifestations depend on severity of the disease, age of the patient, and the underlying cause (Table 8-3). Mild hyperthyroidism may be detected only on laboratory

TABLE 8-2. DIFFERENTIAL DIAGNOSIS OF THYROTOXICOSIS

Condition	Clinical features	TSH	FT$_4$	RAIU
Graves' disease (clinical)	Diffuse nontender goiter; may be N	↓↓	↑↑	↑
Toxic multinodular goiter	Nodular goiter	↓	N or ↑	Focally ↑ in areas of nodules
Toxic adenoma	Single nodule	↓	N or ↑	Focally ↑ in area of nodule, ↓ in other areas
Subacute thyroiditis	Tender, firm goiter	↓	N or ↑	↓
Postpartum (painless) thyroiditis	N size gland or diffuse goiter, painless	↓ (transient) then ↑	N or ↑	↓
Iodine-induced hyperthyroidism	N size gland or goiter	↓	N or ↑	↓
Ectopic thyrotoxicosis (factitious, struma ovarii)	N thyroid, painless	↓↓	N or ↑	↓

FT$_4$, free thyroxine; N, normal; RAIU, radioactive iodine uptake; TSH, thyroid-stimulating hormone; ↓, decreased; ↑, increased.

TABLE 8-3. MANIFESTATIONS OF HYPERTHYROIDISM

Symptoms

    Hyperactivity, nervousness

    Heat intolerance, increased sweating

    Fatigue, weakness

    Weight loss with increased appetite

    Palpitations

    Eye complaints[a] (dryness, bulging eyes)

    Dyspnea

    Increased stool frequency, diarrhea

    Oligomenorrhea or amenorrhea, loss of libido

Signs

    Sinus tachycardia, atrial fibrillation (10%)

    Goiter—multinodular or diffuse

    Fine tremor, hyperreflexia

    Warm, moist skin

    Bruit over thyroid[a]

    Graves' ophthalmopathy[a] (see Table 8-4)

    Hair loss

    Muscle weakness and wasting

    Congestive (high-output) heart failure, exacerbation of coronary artery disease

    Palmar erythema, onycholysis

    Periodic paralysis (primarily in Asian men), psychosis

[a]Exclusive to Graves' disease.
Adapted from Weetman AP. Graves' disease. *N Engl J Med* 2000;343:1236–1248.

evaluation. In the elderly, hyperthyroidism may present as weight loss, fatigue, or exacerbation of congestive heart failure or coronary artery disease. A high index of suspicion is required to make the diagnosis (apathetic or masked hyperthyroidism).

    Graves' disease presents similarly to any form of thyrotoxicosis but has some unique features (Table 8-4). Most patients have a **diffuse goiter**, sometimes accompanied by a bruit. Clinically evident Graves' **ophthalmopathy** is seen in 50% of patients with Graves' disease. The most frequent signs are eyelid retraction or lag, periorbital edema, and proptosis. **Localized dermopathy** occurs commonly in the pretibial area (pretibial myxedema), but can occur in other sites after trauma.

Laboratory and Imaging Studies

The most sensitive and best initial screening test for hyperthyroidism is measurement of the serum TSH by an immunometric assay (see Chap. 6, Evaluation of Thyroid Function). **A TSH >0.1 mIU/L excludes clinical hyperthyroidism.** A second- or third-generation immunoassay with detection limits of at least 0.1 mIU/L is used. Estimation of plasma free thyroxine (FT_4) levels helps to ascertain the degree of hyperthyroidism. An elevated plasma FT_4 level with a suppressed TSH establishes the diagnosis of clinical hyperthyroidism. Thyroid-stimulating immunoglobulins (TSI) may be detected in plasma of patients with Graves' disease but may be undetectable or absent, and these are not useful for diagnosis in most cases.

TABLE 8-4. MANIFESTATIONS OF GRAVES' DISEASE

Diffuse goiter

Ophthalmopathy

    Retrobulbar pressure or pain

    Periorbital edema, scleral injection

    Exophthalmos (proptosis)

    Extraocular muscle dysfunction

    Exposure keratitis

    Optic neuropathy (rare)

Localized dermopathy (pretibial myxedema)

Adapted from Weetman AP. Graves' disease. *N Engl J Med* 2000;343:1236–1248.

Normal plasma FT_4 with a TSH suppressed to 0.1 mIU/L in the setting of symptoms suggestive of hyperthyroidism may be seen with **triiodothyronine (T_3) toxicosis**, or hyperthyroidism due to elevated plasma T_3 levels. Measurement of plasma T_3 levels is indicated in such cases.

Occasionally, a thyroid scan may be used to distinguish among Graves' disease, toxic or "hot nodules," and thyroiditis as causes of thyrotoxicosis (see Table 8-2). Imaging studies of the thyroid gland, such as thyroid ultrasound, CT scanning, or MRI of the neck, are not used for the diagnosis of hyperthyroidism.

MANAGEMENT

Treatment

Hyperthyroidism is easily treatable. Some forms of hyperthyroidism require only symptomatic therapy. Current modalities available for definitive treatment of hyperthyroidism include **RAI ablation, antithyroid medications**, or **subtotal thyroidectomy**. The choice of treatment depends on the clinical situation, including the cause of thyrotoxicosis, preference of clinician and patient, cost, and the demographics of the patient.

Symptom Relief

Symptoms of hyperthyroidism can be managed with beta-adrenergic blocking drugs. These drugs effectively relieve tachycardia, anxiety, and tremors. They can be used while patients wait for definitive treatment or until transient forms of hyperthyroidism resolve. All beta-blockers are equally effective, and longer acting preparations, such as propranolol (Inderal) (long-acting 60–320 mg PO qd), atenolol (Tenormin) (50–100 mg PO qd), or metoprolol (Metoprolol) (50–100 mg PO bid), are preferred. The dose is titrated to relieve symptoms. Verapamil (Calan) (40–80 mg PO tid) may be used in patients when beta-blockers are contraindicated.

Definitive Therapy

Radioactive Iodine

RAI is the preferred treatment in adults for hyperthyroidism caused by Graves' disease in the United States. It is also used for treatment of toxic adenomas and toxic multinodular goiters. **It is safe and cost effective; the only major side effect of treatment is hypothyroidism.** There is no evidence of increased risk of birth defects or infertility with RAI treatment, and radiation exposure to the gonads is low. RAI is absolutely contraindicated in pregnant and lactating women, and pregnancy testing should be performed immediately before treatment in appropriate women. Antithyroid medications should be stopped for approximately 1 week before treatment because these drugs inhibit accumulation of iodine by the thyroid. It is generally recommended that women should avoid pregnancy for 6 months after therapy. The dose of I^{131}, the isotope used for treatment, is usually approximately 8–10 mCi.

FOLLOW-UP. Generally, hypothyroidism occurs in 3–12 months; hence, treated patients should initially be followed every 4–6 weeks. Transient increase in FT_4 levels may occur after 1–2 weeks post-RAI treatment due to release of stored hormone from the thyroid. This may cause worsening of symptoms, especially in patients with underlying heart disease. Plasma FT_4 should be followed (not TSH), and prompt levothyroxine replacement should be instituted when hypothyroidism develops. When thyroid function normalizes, follow-up is performed annually. Up to 20% of patients will need a second dose of RAI after initial treatment, as evidenced by persistent symptoms or persistently suppressed TSH measurements. Higher doses are needed in MNG and toxic adenomas, and post-ablative hypothyroidism is uncommon. RAI treatment may exacerbate Graves' eye disease, especially in smokers, though existing evidence is unclear.

Antithyroid Drugs

Antithyroid drug therapy with thionamides is the preferred treatment choice in Europe, Japan, and other parts of the world. Methimazole (Tapazole) and propylthiouracil (PTU) are the two thionamide drugs commonly used in the United States to treat hyperthyroidism. Both drugs inhibit thyroid peroxidase and thus block production of thyroid hormone. However, they do not prevent release of pre-formed thyroid hormone, and, hence, it may take several weeks to render a patient euthyroid. In larger doses, PTU also blocks the peripheral deiodination of T_4 to T_3. The dose of methimazole varies from 10–40 mg/day, and PTU from 200–600 mg/day. Methimazole is long-acting and is given once daily; PTU is given in 3 or 4 divided doses.

FOLLOW-UP. Thyroid function is assessed every 4–6 weeks for the first few months. The dose of the thionamide can be reduced when euthyroid status is achieved for maintenance therapy. The drugs are continued until the disease undergoes spontaneous remission. This occurs in 20–40% patients treated for 6 months to 10 years. Drug tapering or withdrawal may be tried after 1 year of therapy to see if remission has occurred. Common side effects of these medications are rash (5%), fever, GI upset, and arthralgias; serious side effects include agranulocytosis (0.5%), vasculitis, and hepatic necrosis and require discontinuation of the drugs. Patients should be warned of symptoms of agranulocytosis (e.g., fever, sore throat) and be advised to stop the drug immediately and seek prompt medical attention should these symptoms develop.

Subtotal Thyroidectomy

Surgery offers definitive cure of hyperthyroidism. Currently, surgery is reserved for special situations: **patient preference, pregnant women who have not responded to drug therapy, large or symptomatic goiters, and when there is a question of malignancy.** Patients are prepared for surgery with a thionamide to make them euthyroid and beta-blockers for symptomatic relief. Patients should be as close as possible to clinical and biochemical euthyroidism before surgery, as evidenced by normal FT_4 levels (TSH levels are not used because levels remain suppressed for longer periods). Complications of surgery include hypothyroidism, hypoparathyroidism, and recurrent laryngeal nerve damage, which occur in 1–2% patients. The thionamide is stopped postoperatively, whereas beta-blockers are continued for 5–7 days. Thyroid function tests should be obtained a few weeks after surgery to monitor for hypothyroidism.

Complications of Thyrotoxicosis

Hypothyroidism occurs due to treatment of the underlying cause and is easily managed (see Chap. 9, Hypothyroidism). Occasionally, **congestive heart failure** or **exacerbation of coronary artery disease** may occur in uncontrolled hyperthyroidism, which requires urgent therapy.

Thyroid storm (or thyrotoxic crisis) is a rare but life-threatening situation characterized by an acute exacerbation of hyperthyroidism. Manifestations are those of marked hypermetabolism and a hyperadrenergic response. Symptoms include fever, confusion, delirium, GI symptoms (nausea, vomiting, diarrhea, or rarely jaundice), arrhythmias, congestive heart failure, or coma. Precipitating factors include surgery (especially on the thyroid), parturition, radioiodine therapy of partially treated or untreated hyperthyroidism, iodinated contrast agents, and acute illness (stroke, diabetic ketoacidosis, infection). Mortality is high, and urgent therapy in an intensive care setting with treatment of precipitating factors and measures to decrease thyroid hormone synthesis are the mainstays of treatment.

- **PTU,** 300 mg PO q6h, should be started immediately (oral or nasogastric tube) after drawing confirmatory tests (TSH, FT_4). This is the drug of choice because it inhibits peripheral conversion of T_4 to T_3.
- 1–2 hours later, **saturated solution of potassium iodide**, 1–2 drops q12h, or iopanoic acid, 0.5 mg q12h, is given to block thyroid hormone synthesis.
- Adrenergic effects are controlled with **propranolol**, 40–60 mg orally q6h (or 2 mg slow IV q4h), with dose adjusted to prevent tachycardia while avoiding bradycardia and hypotension. IV **verapamil** may be used in the setting of severe heart failure or asthma.
- Additional measures—**Glucocorticoids** (hydrocortisone) may have additive effects; antibiotics are used if there is suspicion of infection; hydration, cooling, and analgesics provide symptomatic relief; treatment of precipitating cause.

Special Situations

Treatment of Ophthalmopathy Secondary to Graves' Disease

Mild to moderate eye disease often resolves spontaneously with treatment. Some general measures, such as use of artificial tears and a simple eye ointment at night to prevent exposure keratitis, are helpful. Severe ophthalmopathy (worsening diplopia, exposure keratitis, optic neuropathy) requires treatment with glucocorticoids and, occasionally, surgical decompression of the orbits.

Toxic Multinodular Goiter

Toxic MNG usually occurs in older people with a long-standing nodular goiter. Hyperthyroidism may be precipitated by a large iodine load, such as after iodinated contrast agents or drugs such as amiodarone. Radioiodine is the treatment of choice because many of these patients are older with complicating medical problems. Doses of RAI used are likely to be much larger than those used in Graves' disease due to variations in sensitivity of the gland to iodine uptake. In large glands, particularly those with retrosternal extension, or in patients with obstructive symptoms, surgery is the preferred method of treatment.

Solitary Toxic Nodule

Toxic adenomas are almost always follicular adenomas and rarely malignant. Hyperthyroidism may be managed with RAI or surgery (especially for large adenomas). Antithyroid drugs may be used in preparation before either of these modalities.

Hyperthyroidism due to Amiodarone (Iodine-Induced Hyperthyroidism)

Amiodarone, a commonly used anti-arrhythmic drug, contains 37% iodine. Amiodarone can cause hypo- or hyperthyroidism. Hyperthyroidism occurs due to the iodine load from the drug or due to the drug's destructive effects on the thyroid gland. These effects may develop either rapidly or after a few years of treatment. Antithyroid drugs are the treatment of choice and are used in higher than usual doses (methimazole, 40–60 mg/day). Occasionally, steroids are used. In refractory cases, surgery is the final option.

Subacute Thyroiditis

See Chap. 9, Hypothyroidism.

Mild (or Subclinical) Hyperthyroidism

Mild (or subclinical) hyperthyroidism refers to the combination of normal FT_4 levels with a suppressed TSH of <0.1 mIU/L. Subtle symptoms or signs of hyperthyroidism may be present. This situation may occur due to an endogenous excess of thyroid hormone (due to Graves' disease or a toxic MNG) or may be exogenous, due to treatment with levothyroxine (for primary hypothyroidism or in thyroid cancer). An estimated 5% of people with endogenous subclinical hyperthyroidism progress to clinical hyperthyroidism. Patients > age 60 years with a serum TSH <0.1 mIU/L are at a 3-fold greater risk for developing atrial fibrillation. These patients may also be at higher risk for bone loss and osteoporosis, though the data are less well defined.

Management of patients with mild hyperthyroidism depends on the clinical setting. In patients with low TSH due to T_4 therapy, dose reduction is appropriate, except in patients with a history of thyroid cancer. In older patients or those with known heart disease, appropriate treatment is justified. In younger patients with no goiter and with no symptoms or signs, semiannual thyroid function testing is performed.

Pregnancy and Hyperthyroidism

Pregnancy is complicated by Graves' disease in approximately 1/500 women and presents a special problem. Untreated hyperthyroidism in pregnancy can result in miscarriages, preterm labor, pre-eclampsia, and low birth weight. Human chorionic gonadotropin (hCG) is a weak stimulator of the thyroid gland, and this results in a fall in TSH levels and normal FT_4 levels during the first trimester of pregnancy. These changes are transient, resolve with progression of pregnancy, and do not require treatment. An exacerbation of this setting is seen with hyperemesis gravidarum. The high maternal hCG levels are thought to be the cause of the hyperthyroidism. Severe cases may be treated with beta-blockers and PTU.

In pregnant women with Graves' disease, RAI is absolutely contraindicated; PTU and methimazole used in low doses are equally effective (100 mg tid or 2.5–5 mg qd, respectively). Methimazole has been associated with the development of a rare fetal scalp defect, and hence is not commonly used during pregnancy in the United States. Severity of the disease declines with progression of pregnancy, and the dosage requirement may fall. **Treatment is aimed at maintaining the FT_4 levels at the upper end of normal range because this results in the lowest risk of fetal hypothyroidism.** Surgery in the midtrimester may be performed in case of allergic reaction to antithyroid drugs. Breast-feeding is not contraindicated during treatment with PTU because the drug is not concentrated in breast milk.

KEY POINTS TO REMEMBER

- Graves' disease is the most common cause of hyperthyroidism.
- Ocular manifestations and dermopathy are seen only in Graves' disease.
- RAI, the preferred treatment for hyperthyroidism in the United States, is safe, and close monitoring for hypothyroidism is required.
- RAI therapy results in definitive treatment of hyperthyroidism in 80% of cases, some require repeat treatment.
- Thioamides may also be used for treatment of hyperthyroidism, with careful monitoring for side effects.
- Propylthiouracil is the drug of choice in pregnancy complicated by Graves' disease and is dosed to maintain FT_4 levels close to upper limit of normal.
- Mild or subclinical hyperthyroidism in the elderly increases the risk of atrial fibrillation and, possibly, osteoporosis.

REFERENCES AND SUGGESTED READINGS

Bahn RS, Heufelder AE. Pathogenesis of Graves' ophthalmopathy. *N Engl J Med* 1993;329:1468–1475.

Clutter WE. Endocrine disorders. In: Ahya S, Flood K, Paranjothi S, eds. *Washington manual of medical therapeutics*, 30th ed. Philadelphia: Lippincott Williams & Wilkins, 2001:473–481.

Cooper D. Hyperthyroidism. *Lancet* 2003;362:459–468.

Davies TF, Larsen PR. Thyrotoxicosis. In: Larsen PR, et al., eds. *Williams textbook of endocrinology*, 10th ed. Philadelphia: WB Saunders, 2003:374–421.

Ginsberg J. Diagnosis and management of Graves' disease. *CMAJ* 2003;168(5):575–585.

Mestman JH. Hyperthyroidism in pregnancy. *Endocrinol Metab Clin North Am* 1998; 27(1):127–149.

Toft AD. Clinical practice: subclinical hyperthyroidism. *N Engl J Med* 2001;345(7): 512–516.

Weetman AP. Graves' disease. *N Engl J Med* 2000;343:1236–1248.

Woeber KA. Update in the management of hyperthyroidism and hypothyroidism. *Arch Intern Med* 2000;160:1067.

Hypothyroidism

Savitha Subramanian and
Andrew F. Holt

INTRODUCTION

Hypothyroidism is defined as deficient production of thyroid hormone by the thyroid gland. Primary hypothyroidism, the most common cause, occurs due to factors affecting the thyroid gland itself, and, therefore, its production of hormone, resulting in elevation of thyroid-stimulating hormone (TSH) and a fall in free thyroxine (FT_4) levels.

EPIDEMIOLOGY

Resistance to thyroid hormone is rare. Central hypothyroidism (due to pituitary TSH deficiency or hypothalamic disorders) also is uncommon. Primary hypothyroidism (thyroid failure), in contrast, is a prevalent disease worldwide. It can be endemic in iodine-deficient regions, but is also a common disease in iodine-replete areas. Primary hypothyroidism accounts for approximately 99% of cases, with <1% due to TSH deficiency. Clinically apparent acquired hypothyroidism affects approximately 2% of adult women and approximately 0.2% of adult men. Mild hypothyroidism may exist in 7–15% of the elderly population.

CAUSES

The most common etiology of hypothyroidism is autoimmune or Hashimoto's thyroiditis, followed by radioiodine treatment and surgery. Certain drugs, such as amiodarone (Cordarone, Pacerone), lithium, and iodine-containing medications can precipitate hypothyroidism in some patients, especially those with an underlying autoimmune thyroiditis. Secondary hypothyroidism occurs due to TSH deficiency from pituitary or sellar lesions, trauma, or irradiation and, rarely, TSH receptor defects. Deficiency of thyrotropin-releasing hormone (TRH) causes tertiary hypothyroidism. Causes of hypothyroidism are listed in Table 9-1.

PATHOPHYSIOLOGY

Autoimmune (Hashimoto's) thyroiditis, the most common cause of hypothyroidism, occurs due to destruction of the thyroid gland by cell- and antibody-mediated immunologic factors. More than 90% of patients have autoantibodies directed against thyroid peroxidase or thyroglobulin (Tg). It is histologically characterized by marked diffuse lymphocytic infiltration of the thyroid gland. Normal thyroid architecture is destroyed, and variable degrees of fibrosis and absence of colloid are seen. The size of the thyroid gland may be enlarged, normal, or diminished.

PRESENTATION

Clinical Presentation

Hypothyroidism can affect all organ systems, and the manifestations depend on the degree of hormone deficiency. Symptoms and signs occur due to a generalized slowing of metabolic processes or due to accumulation of glycosaminoglycans in tissue interstitial spaces.

TABLE 9-1. CAUSES OF HYPOTHYROIDISM

Primary hypothyroidism
   Loss of functional thyroid tissue
      Chronic lymphocytic thyroiditis (Hashimoto's thyroiditis)
      Radiation (I^{131} for Graves' disease or external irradiation)
      Subtotal thyroidectomy
      Subacute thyroiditis (silent and postpartum thyroiditis)
      Thyroid dysgenesis
   Functional defects in thyroid hormone biosynthesis and release
      Congenital defects in thyroid hormone biosynthesis
      Iodine deficiency and iodine excess
      Drugs: antithyroid medications, lithium, interferon-alpha, interleukin-2
Central (hypothalamic/pituitary) hypothyroidism
   Loss of functional tissue
      Tumors (pituitary adenoma, craniopharyngioma, metastases)
      Trauma (surgery, irradiation)
      Vascular (ischemic necrosis, hemorrhage, stalk interruption)
      Infections (abscess, TB)
      Infiltrative diseases (e.g., sarcoidosis, hemochromatosis)
      Chronic lymphocytic hypophysitis
      Congenital
   Functional defects in TSH biosynthesis and release
      Mutations in genes encoding for TRH receptor
      Drugs: dopamine, glucocorticoids
Other
   Thyroid hormone resistance

TRH, thyrotropin-releasing hormone; TSH, thyroid-stimulating hormone.
Adapted from Weirsinga WM. Adult hypothyroidism. Thyroid disease manager, http://www.thyroidmanager.org.

Symptoms
The most frequent symptoms (Table 9-2) of overt hypothyroidism include unexplained weight gain, increased fatigue, constipation, cold intolerance, and menstrual irregularities. The weight gain experienced is usually modest and seldom causes obesity; appetite is reduced. Decreased peristalsis results in the frequent complaint of constipation. Slowing of intellectual functions, difficulty in concentration, and memory defects are common, and in elderly patients may be mistaken for senile dementia. Lethargy and somnolence are prominent. Stiffness and aching of muscles are common and are worsened by cold temperatures. In adult women, severe hypothyroidism may be associated with diminished libido, failure of ovulation, and severe menorrhagia.

Signs
Physical features include puffy face, dull affect, hoarse voice, and delayed reflexes. Skin is very rough, dry, pale, and cool. The cardiac silhouette may be enlarged; bradycardia, diastolic hypertension, and decreased cardiac output may occur. Whether atherosclerosis is worsened by hypothyroidism is controversial. **However, worsening angina during therapy for hypothyroidism may occur.** The ECG may reveal low volt-

TABLE 9-2. SYMPTOMS AND SIGNS OF HYPOTHYROIDISM

Symptoms	Signs
Fatigue, tiredness, lethargy, muscle aches	Dry, pale, coarse skin with a yellowish tinge
Dry skin	Puffy face and extremities
Hair loss	Bradycardia
Cold intolerance	Diastolic hypertension
Weight gain	Delayed tendon reflexes
Constipation	Carpal tunnel syndrome
Difficulty concentrating	Pleural and pericardial effusions
Hoarse voice	Nonpitting edema (myxedema)
Menstrual irregularities	Alopecia areata
Paresthesias	Vitiligo

age QRS complexes and T-wave abnormalities, which show improvement with therapy. Delayed muscle contraction and relaxation cause slowness of movement and delayed tendon jerks.

Laboratory Abnormalities

Occasionally, a megaloblastic anemia may occur as part of an autoimmune picture (pernicious anemia, autoimmune thyroiditis, gluten enteropathy). Elevated serum cholesterol and triglycerides (due to decreased lipid clearance) and elevated creatine kinase are seen. Hyponatremia may occur due to reduced free water clearance. Patients with severe hypothyroidism may have increased serum prolactin levels. Treatment with thyroid hormone corrects serum prolactin and TSH levels.

MANAGEMENT

Diagnosis

Hypothyroidism should be suspected in anyone with a suggestive history, and evaluation should be directed toward confirming the presence and identifying the cause.

Laboratory Testing

As with most thyroid conditions, TSH is the best initial screening test because primary hypothyroidism is the cause in >90% of patients. When an elevated TSH is discovered, the test should be repeated with a FT_4 level. The TSH is not helpful in patients with central hypothyroidism, in acutely ill patients (nonthyroidal illness), or in patients taking drugs that decrease TSH secretion (see Chap. 6, Evaluation of Thyroid Function).

In primary hypothyroidism, the combination of a low FT_4 level with elevated TSH levels is diagnostic. **A normal TSH level excludes primary hypothyroidism.** When the TSH is elevated with a normal FT_4, **subclinical hypothyroidism** is diagnosed. This picture may also occur in nonthyroidal illness. Thyroid autoantibodies may be positive in Hashimoto's thyroiditis.

Central hypothyroidism should be suspected: (a) in patients with a history of known pituitary or hypothalamic disease, such as surgery, trauma, or irradiation; (b) when other pituitary hormonal deficiencies are noted; and (c) when a pituitary or sellar mass is detected. In central hypothyroidism, the TSH may be low or normal, and hence cannot be used for diagnosis. A low FT_4 is diagnostic in these patients. Distinction between hypothalamic and pituitary causes is performed by MRI of the sellar and suprasellar regions.

Treatment

Hypothyroidism is treated with the synthetic thyroid hormone levothyroxine (Synthroid, Levoxyl). The drug is inexpensive and available as the sodium salt. Levothyroxine has a half-life of 7 days and, therefore, can be given once daily. Levels in blood remain nearly constant once steady state is reached. Approximately 80% of an orally administered dose is absorbed, and absorption occurs from all parts of the small intestine. Treatment of primary hypothyroidism is monitored by measuring TSH, and secondary hypothyroidism by measurement of plasma FT_4 levels.

Initial Treatment

Adult replacement doses are usually in the range of 1–2 mcg/kg/day. The initial dose is individualized based on the patient's age, weight, and cardiac status. An average starting dose is in the range of 50–100 mcg/day. Dosage adjustments are made every 6–8 weeks (because TSH is slow to reequilibrate to a new T_4 status) in increments of 25–50 mcg. Levothyroxine requirements decrease with age. In patients with ischemic heart disease, levothyroxine is started at a lower dose of 25 mcg/day, with gradual increments of 25 mcg every 4–6 weeks.

Administration, Drug Interactions, and Formulations

Levothyroxine is given before meals at least 2 hours from other medications. If bedtime dosing is used, it is taken 2 hours after the last meal. Oral levothyroxine is incompletely absorbed. Absorption of levothyroxine is affected by concurrent administration of iron, calcium, aluminum preparations, soy products, sucralfate, or cholestyramine and by malabsorptive states. Patients taking these medications may need higher doses of T_4. Patients taking rifampin (Rifadin) and anticonvulsants such as phenytoin (Dilantin), phenobarbital, and carbamazepine (Tegretol) need higher doses of levothyroxine to maintain a normal TSH due to increased levothyroxine metabolism. Frequent dose changes may indicate poor compliance with therapy.

Several different branded and generic formulations of levothyroxine are marketed in the United States. Though there is little evidence for variable bioavailability among different levothyroxine preparations, it would be prudent for a patient to remain on the same preparation. If substitution occurs, a TSH measurement 6–8 weeks after starting therapy with the new formulation is recommended.

Follow-Up

In patients receiving a stable dose of levothyroxine, annual TSH testing is appropriate. Levothyroxine requirements decrease with age. Pregnancy causes an increase in levothyroxine requirement, with return to pre-pregnancy doses after delivery. In patients with central hypothyroidism, a levothyroxine dose that maintains FT_4 levels in the mid-range of normal is appropriate.

Side Effects of Levothyroxine Therapy

The most common side effect is **iatrogenic thyrotoxicosis** due to excess replacement. Most cases are managed by reducing the daily dose without interrupting therapy. Serious problems that occur with treatment are **exacerbation of ischemic heart disease**, which may cause worsening angina, myocardial infarction, and, sometimes, death. These problems may be avoided by initiating treatment at low doses with close monitoring and by changing the levothyroxine dose in small increments.

Occasionally, adrenal insufficiency may co-exist with hypothyroidism, and when this is unrecognized and levothyroxine is started, **exacerbation of adrenal failure** may occur. Adrenal insufficiency must be suspected in patients who have symptoms and laboratory findings that are suggestive (see Chap. 11, Adrenal Insufficiency) or in patients with central hypothyroidism.

Complications of Hypothyroidism

Myxedema Coma

Myxedema coma occurs in the setting of long-standing profound, untreated hypothyroidism. It is usually seen in older patients and is precipitated by concurrent illness, especially in cold weather, and characterized by hypothermia, bradycardia, severe hypotension, seizures, and coma. Diagnosis is difficult, and, due to increased mortality rates, prompt treatment should be instituted on clinical grounds after laboratory tests for thyroid function have been drawn, even if the results are not yet available.

TREATMENT. Thyroid hormone (T_4) is administered as an IV bolus at a dose of 50–100 mcg q6–8h to replete thyroid hormone reserve, followed by a daily dose of IV T_4 75–100 mcg. Oral preparation should be given as soon as the patient is able to eat. We do not recommend use of triiodothyronine (T_3) for treatment of myxedema coma. Hydrocortisone, 50 mg IV q6–8h, is administered concomitantly to avoid precipitating adrenal failure. Careful monitoring for exacerbation of heart disease is important. **This mode of therapy is instituted in seriously ill patients only and is not warranted in any other situation.**

Adequate supportive measures, such as correction of hypothermia, ventilatory support, and hydration with normal saline or hypertonic saline should be instituted, as well as treatment of coexisting conditions if present.

Special Situations

Mild (Subclinical) Hypothyroidism
Mild (subclinical) hypothyroidism refers to the condition in which patients have no clinical manifestations of hypothyroidism, a normal FT_4, but a mildly increased plasma TSH concentration. The incidence is thought to be 5–15%, and the causes are similar to overt primary hypothyroidism. Patients who are likely to progress to overt hypothyroidism are patients older than age 60 years, patients with a goiter, those with TSH >10 mIU/L, pregnant women, and those with circulating autoantibodies.

Treatment of mild hypothyroidism is indicated

- in the presence of hypercholesterolemia warranting therapy,
- to prevent progression to overt hypothyroidism,
- in pregnant women, and
- in patients with underlying heart disease to improve myocardial function.

Levothyroxine is the drug of choice, and dose requirements are typically one-half that of overtly hypothyroid patients.

Hypothyroidism and Surgery
Urgent surgery can be performed on untreated hypothyroid patients without major adverse events. However, elective surgery should be deferred until euthyroid status is achieved.

Hypothyroid patients undergoing surgery can have their levothyroxine dose held until they are able to eat (due to the 7-day half-life of the drug). However, IV replacement should be considered if oral intake is delayed by >1 week after surgery. IV replacement is approximately 50% of the oral dose.

Hypothyroidism in Pregnancy
Pregnancy results in an increase in serum T_4-binding globulin concentrations during the first trimester due to reduced clearance by the liver and an estrogen-stimulated increase in its synthesis. Serum total T_4 and T_3 concentrations also correspondingly rise, along with a minimal increase in FT_4 levels. Levels decrease after the first 14–16 weeks of gestation.

Pregnant women with pre-existing primary hypothyroidism have minimal thyroid reserve and are unable to raise their total T_4 and T_3 concentrations. This results in a rise in TSH and, therefore, an increase in levothyroxine requirements during the first trimester. The dose increase needed to maintain a normal TSH is approximately 40–50% of the pre-pregnancy dosage of levothyroxine. Patients with hypothyroidism who become pregnant should have their TSH checked immediately after conception. When dose adjustments are being made, the TSH should be checked every 4 weeks, and several dosage increments may be required. After appropriate dosing is achieved, TSH should be measured every trimester. The levothyroxine dose should be decreased to the pre-pregnancy dose immediately after delivery.

Nonthyroidal Illness (Sick Euthyroid Syndrome)

Thyroid function tests are altered in acute nonthyroidal illness without true thyroid dysfunction. **Thyroid function tests are often unreliable in the acutely ill patient**, and evaluation of these patients poses a unique challenge. Thus, thyroid function testing should not be performed in critically ill patients unless there is a high index of suspicion for thyroid disease, and TSH should only be interpreted with FT_4 measurements.

Changes that occur in thyroid function with illness are as follows:

LOW T_3 SYNDROME. The most common change in thyroid tests is a fall in plasma T_3 levels. This occurs due to decreased 5' deiodinase activity, the enzyme that converts T_4 to T_3. This change is reversible and does not require treatment.

LOW T_4 SYNDROME. Critically ill patients frequently have a low plasma total T_4 concentration. This is caused by decreased binding of T_4 to TBG and, in severe illness, due to the presence of circulating binding inhibitors. These patients have a normal FT_4 concentration in plasma when measured by equilibrium dialysis. However, immunoassay methods normally used to measure FT_4 levels in most clinical labs show decreased FT_4 levels.

THYROID-STIMULATING HORMONE. Plasma TSH levels may be normal in nonthyroidal illness. On occasion, levels may be suppressed, but seldom to levels seen in clinical hyperthyroidism. TSH secretion is also decreased by many drugs such as glucocorticoids and dopamine (see Chap. 6, Evaluation of Thyroid Function). Plasma TSH can also be elevated, especially during the recovery phase of nonthyroidal illness, up to 20 mIU/L.

All patients noted to have thyroid function abnormalities during illness should be re-evaluated after recovery from illness.

Effects of Specific Illnesses

PSYCHIATRIC ILLNESS. Patients hospitalized with acute psychosis have elevated T_4 levels, usually with a normal TSH level. This resolves in 7–10 days. Patients with depression have mildly elevated FT_4 levels and a low basal TSH.

CUSHING'S SYNDROME. Cushing's syndrome results in low T_3 and decreased TSH secretion.

Thyroiditis

Thyroiditis refers to a group of disorders resulting from inflammation of the thyroid gland. The following sections discuss the causes and treatment of the various forms of thyroiditis.

AUTOIMMUNE OR HASHIMOTO'S THYROIDITIS. See the section Pathophysiology.

POSTPARTUM (SILENT) THYROIDITIS. Painless postpartum thyroiditis results from lymphocytic infiltration of the thyroid gland in the postpartum period. It typically occurs in the first 6 months of the postpartum period. The incidence is believed to be approximately 10% in the United States.

Painless postpartum thyroiditis is characterized by transient hyperthyroidism, hypothyroidism, or both. Diagnosis is made from history, by thyroid function testing, and by the presence of anti–thyroid peroxidase antibodies (present in only 50% of patients). Most patients have a nontender, firm goiter. Distinction from Graves' disease may be difficult and can be made by waiting 3–4 weeks because postpartum thyroiditis results in spontaneous improvement. RAI uptake is low with thyroiditis (see Chap. 8, Hyperthyroidism) and may be performed in women who are not nursing. Treatment of hyperthyroidism is with beta-blockers due to the transient nature. Symptomatic hypothyroidism is treated with replacement therapy with levothyroxine for 2–3 months followed by discontinuation for 4–6 weeks and re-evaluation. Hypothyroidism may be permanent in 25% of women. Women with a history of postpartum thyroiditis have a higher risk of developing hypothyroidism in later life.

SUBACUTE THYROIDITIS. Painful subacute thyroiditis is a self-limiting condition resulting in inflammation of the thyroid gland, with transient hyperthyroidism due to release of preformed thyroid hormone, followed by transient hypothyroidism. It is, in fact, the most common cause of thyroid pain. This frequently occurs after an upper respiratory tract infection and is thought to have a viral etiology (de Quervain's or granulomatous thyroiditis).

Subacute thyroiditis usually starts with a sore throat, fatigue, and malaise followed by anterior neck pain and swelling. The thyroid gland is firm, moderately enlarged, and usually exquisitely tender. Symptoms of hyperthyroidism occur in approximately 50% of patients. NSAIDs or salicylates are the mainstay of treatment. Corticosteroids are used in severe, refractory cases with a slow taper. There is no role for thionamides or RAI in this setting. Transient hypothyroidism may be treated with levothyroxine for 3–6 months.

ACUTE INFECTIOUS THYROIDITIS. Acute infectious thyroiditis refers to bacterial, fungal, mycobacterial, or parasitic infections of the thyroid gland. The thyroid gland is resistant to infection due to its thick capsule, and infection of the thyroid is therefore rare. It may occur in the immunosuppressed, elderly, or debilitated patients, or in patients with underlying thyroid disease. Patients are acutely ill, with fever, chills, dysphagia, anterior neck pain, and swelling. The thyroid is tender. Patients are usually biochemically euthyroid. Diagnosis is made by fine-needle aspiration, with Gram's stain and culture of the aspirate. Antibiotics and drainage of abscess are the mainstays of treatment.

REIDEL'S THYROIDITIS. Reidel's thyroiditis results from fibrosis of the thyroid gland. The etiology is unknown. Patients present with a painless, hard, fixed goiter. Patients are initially euthyroid, but hypothyroidism develops when the entire thyroid gland becomes fibrosed. Treatment is primarily surgical, although therapy with glucocorticoids and methotrexate may be tried early in the course of the disease.

KEY POINTS TO REMEMBER

- Hashimoto's thyroiditis is the most common cause of hypothyroidism.
- A normal TSH concentration rules out primary hypothyroidism.
- Worsening of symptoms of coronary disease may occur during levothyroxine therapy for hypothyroidism.
- Subclinical hypothyroidism should be treated on a case by case basis.
- Thyroid hormone requirements increase during pregnancy.
- Subacute thyroiditis is the most common cause of thyroid pain.
- Thyroid function tests should be checked in acutely ill patients only when the index of suspicion for thyroid disease is high.

REFERENCES AND SUGGESTED READINGS

Burrow GN, Fisher DN, Larsen PR. Maternal and fetal thyroid function. *N Engl J Med* 1994;331:1072.

Clutter WE. Endocrine disorders. In: Ahya S, Flood K, Paranjothi S, eds. *Washington manual of medical therapeutics*, 30th ed. Philadelphia: Lippincott Williams & Wilkins, 2001:473–481.

Cooper DS. Clinical practice. Subclinical hypothyroidism. *N Engl J Med* 2001;345(4):260–265.

Ladenson PW. Problems in the management of hypothyroidism. In: Braverman LE, ed. *Diseases of the thyroid*, 2nd ed. Totowa, NJ: Humana Press, 2003:161–176.

Langton JE, Brent GA. Nonthyroidal illness syndrome: evaluation of thyroid function in sick patients. *Endocrinol Metab Clin North Am* 2002;31(1):159–172.

Pearce EN, Farwell AP, Braverman LE. Thyroiditis. *N Engl J Med* 2003;348(26):2646–2655.

Roberts CG, Ladenson PW. Hypothyroidism. *Lancet* 2004;363(9411):793–803.

Toft AD. Drug therapy: thyroxine therapy. *N Engl J Med* 1994;331(3):174–180.

Weirsinga WM. Adult hypothyroidism. Thyroid disease manager, www.thyroidmanager.org.

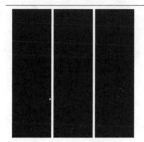

Adrenal Disorders

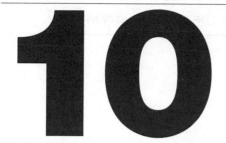

Adrenal Incidentalomas

Grace S. Eng

INTRODUCTION

Adrenal incidentalomas are masses found incidentally during radiographic imaging of the abdomen. By definition, patients do not present for evaluation of signs or symptoms of adrenal disease. Ready access to and use of high-resolution radiographic imaging for evaluation of nonspecific symptoms has led to increasing discovery of adrenal incidentalomas. Using CT scanning, the incidence of adrenal incidentalomas in the general population is 0.35–4.36%.

In evaluating such a mass, the major concerns to address are

1. Is the mass benign or malignant?
2. Does the mass secrete hormones, or is the mass nonfunctioning?

CAUSES

In one of the largest databases to date with 786 adrenal incidentalomas, the National Italian Study Group has confirmed that the most common finding (89%) on evaluation with hormone testing is a nonfunctioning mass (cortical adenoma, myelolipoma, cyst, ganglioneuroma, or other). Evaluation of the remaining masses revealed subclinical Cushing's syndrome (6.2%), pheochromocytoma (3.4%), aldosterone-secreting adenoma (0.89%), and a single virilizing tumor. Of note, most of the adrenocortical carcinomas found in this series were non–hormone secreting. Table 10-1 lists several common diagnoses associated with adrenal incidentalomas.

PRESENTATION

Although by definition patients with incidentalomas do not present with clinical evidence of hormone excess, a thorough history and physical exam for any signs and symptoms of hormonal dysfunction should be completed. Special effort should be made to elicit any subtle signs or symptoms suggestive of specific hormonal hyperfunction or malignancy. This search should include investigation for Cushing's syndrome (weight gain, moon facies, supraclavicular fat pads, thinned skin, easy bruising, proximal muscle weakness), pheochromocytoma (hypertension, paroxysms of pain, palpitations, perspiration, and/or pallor), aldosterone-secreting adenoma (hypertension or hypokalemia), and malignancy (weight loss, primary nonadrenal cancers, lymphoma, and virilizing signs or symptoms suggestive of adrenocortical carcinoma). A known history of malignancy makes metastasis to the adrenal gland more likely.

MANAGEMENT

Biochemical Testing

Biochemical testing should assess possible hormone secretion by the adrenal mass. Appropriate studies include

1. Serum potassium and plasma aldosterone concentration/plasma renin activity ratio (PAC/PRA) to address aldosterone excess

TABLE 10-1. DIFFERENTIAL DIAGNOSIS OF ADRENAL INCIDENTALOMA

Benign
>   Non–hormone secreting
>   >   Nonfunctioning adenoma
>   >   Lipoma/myelolipoma
>   >   Cyst
>   >   Ganglioneuroma
>   >   Hematoma
>   >   Infection (tuberculosis, fungal)
>   Hormone secreting
>   >   Pheochromocytoma
>   >   Aldosterone-secreting adenoma
>   >   Subclinical Cushing's syndrome

Malignant
>   Adrenocortical carcinoma
>   Metastatic neoplasm
>   Lymphoma
>   Malignant pheochromocytoma

2. Plasma metanephrines or 24-hour urine metanephrines and/or catecholamines to rule out subclinical pheochromocytoma
3. A 1-mg dexamethasone suppression test to rule out subclinical Cushing's syndrome
4. A dehydroepiandrosterone sulfate (DHEA-S) level should be drawn if virilizing signs or symptoms are present

Any positive results on these screening tests should prompt further evaluation. Please refer to chapters on Conn's Syndrome (Chap. 13), Cushing's Syndrome (Chap. 14), and Pheochromocytoma (Chap. 15) for more detailed discussion of these tests and their interpretation.

Radiologic Assessment

The probability of an adrenal mass being malignant **directly correlates with its size**. A number of lesion sizes ranging from 3 to 6 cm have been proposed as cut offs that should lead to surgical resection. A Mayo Clinic retrospective analysis of 342 adrenal masses removed over a 5-year period revealed that all adrenocortical carcinomas were ≥4 cm. In a larger retrospective series from Italy, a 4-cm cut off was 93% sensitive for adrenocortical carcinoma, but 76% of lesions >4 cm were benign.

   CT scan may be useful in establishing whether an adrenal mass is benign or malignant. A homogeneous adrenal mass <4 cm in size with smooth borders and an attenuation value <10 Hounsfield units strongly suggests a benign lesion. Diagnostic criteria are not as clear for lesions 4–6 cm in size, but, if they are hormonally inactive and have a benign appearance on CT scan, they can be monitored. Lesions >6 cm, regardless of appearance on CT scan, are more likely to be malignant and surgical referral is warranted. **MRI scanning** appears to be as effective as CT scan in distinguishing benign and malignant masses, with benign adenomas exhibiting signal drop on chemical shift imaging with intensity similar to T2-weighted images of the liver. Pheochromocytomas generally exhibit hyperintensity on T2-weighed imaging. Again, lesions >6 cm in size are more likely to be malignant even if they have a benign appearance on MRI and should prompt surgical referral.

Fine-Needle Aspiration/Tissue Biopsy

Generally, a thorough history and physical exam, biochemical testing, and radiologic assessment can establish the etiology of the adrenal incidentaloma. Biopsy of the adrenal mass is generally not advised as it is rarely helpful. The major exception is a patient with a known extraadrenal primary malignancy; in this case, biopsy may help distinguish recurrence/metastasis of cancer from a benign adenoma. However, biopsy should only be done if pheochromocytoma has been ruled out by biochemical testing, as biopsy of a pheochromocytoma can precipitate a hypertensive emergency.

Treatment

At the completion of the above clinical, biochemical, and radiologic evaluation, any mass that suggests primary adrenocortical malignancy by size or radiologic characteristics warrants **surgical removal** as long as the patient is a good surgical candidate. If, however, the mass suggests a metastasis or a primary nonadrenal cancer, such as lymphoma, generally no surgical removal is needed, but rather treatment of the primary cancer. Adrenal function is unlikely to be hindered by tumor invasion, because more than 70–80% of the gland function must be interrupted to pose any risk for adrenal crisis.

Hypersecreting adrenal incidentalomas found to be **pheochromocytomas** or **aldosterone-secreting adenomas** should be considered for surgical removal as well, based on criteria for their respective diagnoses. Resection of a pheochromocytoma requires preoperative α-adrenergic blockade and volume expansion with oral salt or IV saline. However, surgical treatment for subclinical Cushing's syndrome remains controversial.

It is important to determine whether or not there is excessive cortisol secretion prior to surgical excision of an adrenal mass. The diagnoses of a hormonally hypersecreting adrenal mass and adrenocortical carcinoma are not mutually exclusive. It is common for adrenocortical carcinomas to release excessive cortisol. If there is any suspicion of excessive cortisol secretion, one should be aware of the possibility of **adrenal crisis** during or after the surgery. It has been reported several times in the literature that even mild cortisol hypersecretion of one adrenal gland may atrophy the contralateral adrenal gland. When the hyperfunctioning adrenal gland is removed, the atrophied gland may not be able to compensate in the setting of postsurgical recovery. These patients should be covered with stress-dose steroids during surgery and receive a corticotropin stimulation test after surgery to diagnose any resulting adrenal insufficiency. Patients who fail postoperative testing may require months of glucocorticoid replacement before recovery of the hypothalamic-pituitary-adrenal axis. Thus, even if the size of the mass warrants its removal, the patient should still undergo a complete biochemical workup to rule out subclinical Cushing's syndrome or pheochromocytoma.

Follow-Up

After hormonal evaluation and close re-examination of the radiologic images, if the adrenal incidentaloma is found to be neither a primary adrenal carcinoma nor a hypersecreting adenoma it is reasonable to presume that the incidentaloma is benign. Schedules for follow-up by repeat radiologic imaging and biochemical analyses remain controversial. Most of these schedules recommend repeat imaging at 3 months and again during the following year. A significant increase in the size of the mass (e.g., >1 cm) should raise the possibility of malignancy and lead to surgical referral. Patients should also be evaluated yearly with a thorough history and physical exam for development of overt signs of hypersecretion or malignancy. Many practitioners continue to follow adrenal incidentalomas with radiographic imaging every few years. As the data to support such a practice are limited, the usefulness remains controversial.

KEY POINTS TO REMEMBER

- Size is important. Adrenal masses >4 cm are more likely to be malignant, and surgical resection should be considered.

- The great majority (approximately 89%) of adrenal incidentalomas are benign, nonfunctioning masses.
- A full biochemical workup should be completed before any surgery is done. Findings suggestive of pheochromocytoma would require preoperative medical preparation. Testing suggestive of Cushing's syndrome or subclinical Cushing's syndrome warrants intraoperative stress-dose steroid coverage and postoperative corticotropin stimulation testing.

REFERENCES AND SUGGESTED READINGS

Boland GW, et al. Characterization of adrenal masses using unenhanced CT: an analysis of the CT literature. *AJR Am J Roentgenol* 1998;171(1):201–204.

Bülow B, Ahrén B. Adrenal incidentaloma—experience of a standardized diagnostic programme in the Swedish prospective study. *J Int Med* 2002;252:239–246.

Dunnick NR, Korobkin M. Imaging of adrenal incidentalomas: current status. *AJR Am J Roentgenol* 2002;179:559–568.

Grumbach MM, Biller BMK, Braunstein GD, et al. Management of the clinically inapparent adrenal mass ("incidentaloma"). *Ann Intern Med* 2003;138:424–429.

Herrera MF, et al. Incidentally discovered adrenal tumors: an institutional perspective. *Surgery* 1991;110(6):1014–1021.

Kloos RT, et al. Incidentally discovered adrenal masses. *Endocrine Rev* 1995;16(4):460–484.

Mantero F, et al. Adrenal incidentaloma: an overview of hormonal data from the national Italian study group. *Horm Res* 1997;47:284–289.

Mantero F, et al. A survey on adrenal incidentaloma in Italy. *J Clin Endocrinol Metab* 2000;85(2):637–644.

McLeod MK, et al. Sub-clinical Cushing's syndrome in patients with adrenal gland incidentalomas: pitfalls in diagnosis and management. *Am Surg* 1990;56:398–403.

Young WF. Management approaches to adrenal incidentalomas: a view from Rochester, Minnesota. *Endocrinol Metab Clin North Am* 2000;29(1):159–185.

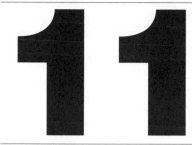

Adrenal Insufficiency

Grace S. Eng

INTRODUCTION

Adrenal insufficiency can present insidiously with nonspecific, vague symptoms. Patients may remain undiagnosed for quite some time until a significant physical stressor precipitates severe adrenal insufficiency—an endocrine emergency.

The adrenal axis is a complex balance of hormones from the hypothalamus, pituitary, and adrenal glands. A defect in any one of these locations can lead to hypofunction of the adrenals. Primary adrenal insufficiency corresponds to dysfunction at the level of the adrenal gland; whereas secondary adrenal insufficiency refers to loss of ACTH hormone from the pituitary. Tertiary adrenal insufficiency refers to loss of corticotropin-releasing hormone (CRH).

CAUSES

The causes of adrenal insufficiency are best grouped as primary (adrenal) vs secondary (central) losses. When Thomas Addison first described his eponymous syndrome in 1855, he described what is now known as primary adrenal insufficiency from any cause. At that time, the most common etiology was tuberculous infiltration. Over the years, autoimmune destruction of the adrenal gland has emerged as the leading cause of primary adrenal insufficiency in the United States. Consequently, the term Addison's disease often is used inappropriately to refer only to adrenal insufficiency of autoimmune origin. Autoimmune adrenalitis can stand alone or as part of the polyglandular autoimmune syndrome (both types I and II).

Worldwide, tuberculous infiltration remains the leading cause of **primary adrenal insufficiency**, especially where tuberculosis is still endemic. Other major etiologies to consider include adrenomyeloleukodystrophy (the most common cause in children), HIV-related opportunistic infections (most commonly CMV), bilateral adrenal hemorrhage associated with coagulopathies or sepsis, and metastatic cancer involving more than 80–90% of the total adrenal mass. Rarely, medications can precipitate adrenal insufficiency in a person with insufficient cortisol-producing reserve. Rifampin (Rifadin) and phenytoin (Dilantin) increase cortisol metabolism, whereas ketoconazole (Nizoral) decreases cortisol secretion (Table 11-1).

The loss of ACTH secretion, seen in **secondary adrenal insufficiency,** is most commonly caused by the long-term suppression of the pituitary by high levels of glucocorticoids. Decreased tonal ACTH stimulation of the adrenal glands results in adrenal atrophy over several weeks. Those at highest risk of developing secondary adrenal insufficiency from exogenous glucocorticoid use are patients who have received more than 10 mg of prednisone (Deltasone) daily. Furthermore, if the dose is taken at night, the normal circadian early morning surge of ACTH is suppressed, putting the patient at further risk of developing adrenal gland atrophy and subsequent adrenal insufficiency.

The other major causes of secondary insufficiency are processes that destroy the pituitary or hypothalamus (see Table 11-1). Lack of ACTH secretion is usually associated with the loss of the other pituitary hormones such as follicle-stimulating hormone (FSH), luteinizing hormone (LH), and thyroid-stimulating hormone (TSH). Isolated ACTH deficiency has been reported, but is rare.

TABLE 11-1. CAUSES OF ADRENAL INSUFFICIENCY

Primary

    Idiopathic/autoimmune

    Tuberculosis

    Adrenoleukodystrophy

    HIV-related opportunistic infections (CMV, *Mycobacterium avium*-intracellulare, *Cryptococcus*, histoplasmosis, *Pneumocystis carinii*, toxoplasmosis)

    Metastatic carcinoma (lung, breast)

    Adrenal hemorrhage (e.g., meningococcal sepsis with Waterhouse-Friderichsen syndrome)

    Sepsis

    Infarction [e.g., antiphospholipid syndrome, disseminated intravascular coagulopathy (DIC)]

    Medications [rifampin (Rifadin), phenytoin (Dilantin), ketoconazole (Nizoral)]

    Congenital adrenal hyperplasia

    Familial hypocortisolism

Secondary

    Prolonged use of exogenous steroids

    Infection (tuberculosis)

    Neurosarcoidosis

    Metastasis

    Infarction (e.g., peripartum Sheehan's syndrome)

    Hemorrhage/apoplexy

    Primary pituitary mass (pituitary adenoma, craniopharyngioma, Rathke's cyst)

    Stalk lesion

    Lymphocytic hypophysitis

    Trauma

    Isolated ACTH deficiency

Adapted from Oelkers W. Adrenal insufficiency. *N Engl J Med* 1996;335:1206–1212; Seidenwurm DJ, et al. Metastases to the adrenal glands and the development of Addison's disease. *Cancer* 1984;43:552–557; and Mayo J, et al. Adrenal function in the human immunodeficiency virus-infected patient. *JAMA* 2002;162:1095–1098.

PRESENTATION

Acute Adrenal Insufficiency

Acute adrenal insufficiency is characterized by severe hypotension, nausea, vomiting, and, often, abdominal pain if the etiology is acute infarction or hemorrhage. Although the symptoms are nonspecific, it is critical to recognize the clinical syndrome, as acute adrenal crisis is an endocrine emergency requiring prompt treatment.

Chronic Adrenal Insufficiency

Chronic adrenal insufficiency is more insidious in its onset. A significant illness can transform latent chronic adrenal insufficiency into a life-threatening adrenal crisis. Hence, early recognition and diagnosis is essential. The presentation is dependent on the level of the hypothalamic-pituitary-adrenal axis affected. In patients with primary adrenal insufficiency, destruction of the adrenal gland generally leads to the loss of all adrenal hormones, including cortisol and aldosterone. The resulting lack of feedback inhibition on the pituitary by cortisol leads to increased ACTH secretion. This series of defects leads to a constellation of symptoms that can include nausea, vomiting, anorexia, weight loss, and fatigue. The increased ACTH levels give rise to generalized hyperpigmentation of the skin and mucosa, one of the most distinctive features of primary adrenal insufficiency; it is thought that ACTH directly stimulates the melanocortin receptor and up-regulates melanin synthesis. The loss of aldosterone can lead to renal salt wasting and resultant salt craving. Laboratory analysis can also demonstrate hyponatremia and hyperkalemia. Furthermore, as autoimmune disease is the most common etiology of adrenal insufficiency in the United States, it is common for patients with autoimmune adrenalitis to have evidence of other autoimmune diseases such as hypo- or hyperthyroidism, type I diabetes, or vitiligo.

Secondary Adrenal Insufficiency

In secondary adrenal insufficiency, patients have a loss of pituitary ACTH. This defect rarely occurs alone and is usually associated with other pituitary hormone losses. Patients with pituitary ACTH loss present with many of the same symptoms as primary adrenal insufficiency, including general malaise, anorexia, GI complaints, and weight loss. Additionally, because of the loss of other pituitary hormones, they may experience amenorrhea and decreased libido (LH, FSH), cold intolerance (TSH), and, rarely, polyuria (posterior pituitary vasopressin). Patients with secondary adrenal insufficiency do not have the hyperpigmentation seen in primary adrenal disease, as there is no ACTH to activate the melanocortin receptors. Another distinction from primary adrenal insufficiency is that the loss of pituitary ACTH does not affect aldosterone secretion, because aldosterone is primarily regulated by the renin-angiotensin system. Therefore, patients with secondary adrenal insufficiency do not have hyperkalemia. They can, however, present with hyponatremia.

MANAGEMENT

Laboratory Diagnostic Testing

Laboratory studies are used to document whether there is inadequate cortisol secretion by the adrenals and whether the cause of adrenal insufficiency is due to lack of ACTH or not. The circadian rhythm of cortisol secretion results in peak values between 4 and 8 A.M. and nadir values in the evening. Basal morning serum cortisol levels <3 mcg/dL are strongly suggestive of adrenal insufficiency. Random serum cortisol levels at other times of day are not informative unless they are in the high normal range, which would be consistent with an intact HPA axis.

The **cosyntropin stimulation test** has become the most widely used dynamic test to assess adrenal function. Serum cortisol levels >18 mcg/dL (500 nmol/L) to 20 mcg/dL (550 nmol/L) obtained 30 or 60 minutes after IV or IM injection of 250 mcg synthetic cosyntropin rule out primary adrenal insufficiency. Most cases of secondary and tertiary adrenal insufficiency also result in a failed cosyntropin stimulation test. Because it takes several weeks for the adrenals to atrophy after acute disruption of ACTH secretion (e.g., after pituitary injury), the cosyntropin stimulation test may be normal if administered in recent-onset secondary adrenal insufficiency. Also, chronic partial secondary adrenal insufficiency may not be detected by the cosyntropin stimulation test. More recently, the low-dose cosyntropin stimulation test has been suggested as a more sensitive and specific test. This version of the stimulation test is performed in the same manner as the standard-dose cosyntropin stimulation test, but in the low-dose cosyntropin stimulation test, only 1 mcg of cosyntropin is used. The same criteria for a normal test apply. Head-to-head testing of the standard-dose and low-dose tests generally shows modest improvements in sensitivity and specificity with the low-dose test. Cosyntropin is available only in 250-mcg vials, making a dilution to 1 mcg less convenient. The appropriate dose of cosyntropin for the accurate diagnosis of adrenal insufficiency remains controversial.

If **adrenal crisis** is suspected, the patient should be covered with 4 mg IV dexamethasone every 6 hours until the cosyntropin stimulation test can be performed.

The cosyntropin stimulation test is fast, accurate, and safe for diagnosing adrenal insufficiency, but does not differentiate between primary and secondary disease. An ACTH level drawn at the same time as a basal cortisol level can be helpful in this regard. When the cortisol level is low, a disproportionately elevated ACTH level suggests primary adrenal insufficiency.

Most steroid replacements interfere with the assay for serum cortisol. A patient already receiving steroid replacement should be **switched to dexamethasone** (Decadron) on the day before the test, which does not crossreact with cortisol assay, to avoid false-negative results (e.g., 5 mg prednisone = 0.75 mg dexamethasone).

Both the standard and low-dose cosyntropin stimulation tests have been widely adopted for diagnosing adrenal insufficiency because of their high sensitivity and specificity as well as their ease and safety. Other tests include the **insulin tolerance test (ITT)** and the metyrapone stimulation test. Although the ITT has long been considered the gold standard, it is uncomfortable for the patient and requires close monitoring because the significant hypoglycemia resulting from the test is potentially dangerous. The ITT is contraindicated in patients with histories of seizure, susceptibility to seizure, or cardiovascular disease. Furthermore, the standard and low-dose cosyntropin stimulation tests have been shown to correlate well with the ITT. The **metyrapone stimulation test** is most useful in confirming secondary adrenal insufficiency. Its use is limited, as the clinical presentation and an ACTH level done with cosyntropin stimulation testing usually identifies the etiology of adrenal insufficiency. Additionally, the metyrapone stimulation test should not be performed in patients who have known severe cortisol deficiency, as the metyrapone can precipitate an adrenal crisis. Metyrapone is not readily available and must be obtained by special arrangement from the pharmacist.

Radiologic Evaluation

Radiologic imaging should only be performed once laboratory diagnosis of adrenal insufficiency and its source is made using one of the stimulation tests. The laboratory tests should identify whether the patient has primary or secondary adrenal insufficiency. If the patient's clinical presentation is highly suggestive of autoimmune adrenalitis, radiologic evaluation is not necessary. For patients with chemical diagnosis of primary adrenal insufficiency, CT of the adrenal glands is helpful in identifying inflammation suggestive of infection, hemorrhage, or malignancy. Patients with laboratory evaluation suggestive of secondary adrenal insufficiency should have a brain MRI with coned-down views of the pituitary, looking for a hypothalamic or pituitary mass.

Maintenance Treatment

Maintenance therapy involves glucocorticoid replacement at physiologic levels. Additionally, those with primary adrenal insufficiency should also be given mineralocorticoid replacement. Patients and their families should be counseled about the increased steroid needs during sick days. A medical alert bracelet that notes steroid dependence is also important.

Many maintenance treatment regimens have been suggested. **Chronic therapy** for patients with either primary or secondary adrenal insufficiency requires glucocorticoid replacement with 15–30 mg PO of hydrocortisone/day or its equivalent [prednisone (Deltasone), 5.0–7.5 mg PO total/day, or dexamethasone (Decadron), 0.75–1.25 mg PO total/day]. The glucocorticoids can be administered in 1–3 divided doses. It is best to give a **single dose in the morning** to mimic normal diurnal variation. If the patient thinks he or she could benefit from a split-dose regimen, usually the larger dose is given in the morning and the smaller dose in the afternoon. Treatment should be tailored to the patient's symptoms so as to avoid fatigue, weight loss, hyponatremia, and, in primary adrenal insufficiency, hyperpigmentation. However, one should also avoid the complications of excess glucocorticoid replacement, such as weight gain, osteoporosis, and immune compromise.

Mineralocorticoid replacement is also required for patients with primary adrenal insufficiency and is administered as 0.05–0.2 mg PO fludrocortisone (Florinef) daily.

The dose should be titrated to patients' symptoms of orthostasis as well as to normalize potassium levels and suppress renin levels to the high end of normal.

If a patient is diagnosed with both adrenal insufficiency and hypothyroidism at the same time, the patient must first have adequate glucocorticoid replacement before initiating thyroid hormone therapy so as to not precipitate adrenal crisis.

Stress Dosing

Patients undergoing physically significant stressors have increased glucocorticoid needs. Patients should be advised that development of febrile illness, nausea, or vomiting may warrant increases in their daily glucocorticoid requirements. In addition to aggressive hydration, we recommend **initially doubling the usual daily dose** and then **doubling the dose again** if symptoms of adrenal insufficiency, such as nausea, vomiting, or orthostasis, do not resolve. If at this point the patient's symptoms still do not resolve, a commercially available injectable dexamethasone kit can be prescribed for home use. If at any time there is uncertainty regarding the status or safety of the patient, the patient should be sent to the nearest hospital for IV steroids. When the acute illness has resolved, patients may return to their usual daily replacement doses within 1–2 days.

In acute adrenal insufficiency or adrenal crisis, rapid treatment is essential for survival of the patient. Volume replacement using normal saline or D5-normal saline is essential. The patients also require "stress-dose" steroids. If the diagnosis is unclear, the patient should be treated first with dexamethasone, 4 mg IV, then undergo cosyntropin-stimulation testing. Patients with a clearly identified history of adrenal insufficiency are usually treated with 50–100 mg of hydrocortisone IV every 6–8 hours until their condition has stabilized. In adrenal crisis, any signs or symptoms should resolve quickly, generally over the following 1–2 hours. Once the stressor has been alleviated, steroid doses can be tapered rapidly to the usual glucocorticoid daily dose.

Perioperative Dosing

Determining the appropriate coverage for surgical procedures is dependent on the complexity and duration of the procedure. Patients taking chronic steroids or carrying a diagnosis of known adrenal insufficiency will likely require additional coverage during their procedure. For patients undergoing local anesthesia for <1 hour, the patient's usual daily dose should suffice. For surgery limited to the limbs involving general anesthesia, patients should continue their usual daily steroid dose preoperatively and then receive the dose again via IV during the procedure. Patients undergoing surgery involving the thoracic or abdominal cavities should be given their baseline daily dose preoperatively and then receive the equivalent of hydrocortisone, 50 mg IV, every 6–8 hours during the procedure and for 2–3 days after surgery. The dose can be rapidly tapered to the patient's usual daily dose over the following 1–2 days. During the perioperative and postsurgical period, inadequate steroid coverage may be manifested by signs and symptoms of impending adrenal crisis such as hypotension, nausea, vomiting, or fever. If adrenal insufficiency is the cause of these signs and symptoms, they should resolve quickly once the patient is covered with adequate steroid doses.

KEY POINTS TO REMEMBER

- Signs and symptoms of adrenal insufficiency are subtle.
- The corticotropin-stimulation test is simple to perform. Draw a baseline serum ACTH and cortisol. Draw a second serum cortisol level precisely 30 minutes after administration of the 250 mcg of corticotropin IV or IM. A level <18–20 mcg/dL is highly sensitive for diagnosing adrenal insufficiency.
- If adrenal crisis is suspected, first treat the patient with 4 mg IV dexamethasone. The corticotropin stimulation test can then be performed safely and properly without delay in treating the patient.
- Adrenally insufficient patients should be informed that, while undergoing a physically stressful illness or procedure, they will likely have higher glucocorticoid needs.

REFERENCES AND SUGGESTED READINGS

Abdu TA, et al. Comparison of the low dose short synacthen test (1 µg), the conventional dose short synacthen test (250 µg), and the insulin tolerance test for assessment of the hypothalamo-pituitary-adrenal axis in patients with pituitary disease. *J Clin Endocrinol Metab* 1999;84:838–843.

Axelrod L. Perioperative management of patients treated with glucocorticoids. *Endocrinol Metab Clin North Am* 2003;32:367–383.

Coursin DB, Wood KE. Corticosteroid supplementation for adrenal insufficiency. *JAMA* 2002;287:236–240.

Dorin RI, et al. Diagnosis of adrenal insufficiency. *Ann Intern Med* 2003;139:194–204.

Grinspoon SK, Biller BK. Laboratory assessment of adrenal insufficiency. *J Clin Endocrinol Metab* 1994;79:923–931.

Guttman PH. Addison's disease. *Arch Pathol* 1930;10:742–935.

Mayo J, et al. Adrenal function in the human immunodeficiency virus-infected patient. *JAMA* 2002;162:1095–1098.

Neiman LK, Orth DN. Adrenal insufficiency. In: Rose BD, ed. *UpToDate*. Wellesley, MA: UpToDate, 2003.

Oelkers W. Adrenal insufficiency. *N Engl J Med* 1996;335:1206–1212.

Oelkers W. Hyponatremia and inappropriate secretion of vasopressin (antidiuretic hormone) in patients with hypopituitarism. *N Engl J Med* 1989;321:492–496.

Salem M, et al. Perioperative glucocorticoid coverage. A reassessment 42 years after emergence of a problem. *Ann Surg* 1994;219:416–425.

Seidenwurm DJ, et al. Metastases to the adrenal glands and the development of Addison's disease. *Cancer* 1984;43:552–557.

Thaler LM, Blevins LS. Adrenocorticotropin stimulation test in the evaluation of patients with suspected central adrenal insufficiency. *J Clin Endocrinol Metab* 1998;83:2726–2729.

Zelissen PM, et al. Associated autoimmunity in Addison's disease. *J Autoimmun* 1995; 8:121–130.

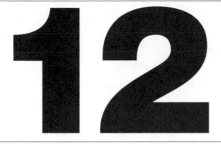

Adult Congenital Adrenal Hyperplasia

Dominic N. Reeds

INTRODUCTION

Congenital adrenal hyperplasia (CAH) consists of a group of diseases characterized by various genetic disorders in adrenal steroid biosynthetic enzymes. Reduced cortisol biosynthesis in CAH places patients at risk for acute adrenal crisis. In response to low cortisol levels, there is a compensatory increase in serum ACTH. These high ACTH levels induce hyperplasic changes of the dysfunctional adrenal tissue and increase production of virilizing steroids with little or no increase in cortisol production. Among the variety of genetic defects that result in CAH, only two result in virilization. 95% of the cases are from **21-hydroxylase deficiency** and 5% are due to 11-hydroxylase deficiency. The incidence of classic 21-hydroxylase deficiency is thought to be 1 per 14,000. The majority of cases of classic CAH are discovered during childhood; however, better understanding of the genetics and pathophysiology of CAH has led to frequent discoveries of its milder, nonclassic forms during adulthood. The overall incidence of CAH is not known but appears to be 1–6% in adolescents and adults with hyperandrogenism. 11-Hydroxylase deficiency occurs in 1 per 100,000 births. Therapy for all forms of CAH consists of a balance between sufficient glucocorticoid replacement to suppress the overproduction of androgens and to prevent adrenal crises, while avoiding complications related to glucocorticoid excess. Discussion of CAH in this chapter is limited to 21-hydroxylase deficiency.

PATHOGENESIS

Deficient cortisol production is the key aberration in CAH, and mastery of the adrenal steroid biosynthesis pathway is essential to understanding the pathogenesis of the disease and the rationale behind treatment (Fig. 12-1).

Differing mutations occurring within the gene encoding 21-hydroxylase affect the severity and expression of the disease. Mutations associated with large reductions in enzyme activity result in severe deficiencies of aldosterone and cortisol; whereas, mutations associated with milder reductions result in less servere hormone abnormalities and a nonclassic course. The reduction in cortisol levels stimulates ACTH release by the pituitary, in turn causing increased production of cortisol precursors, such as progesterone and 17-OH progesterone (17-OHP), which may be metabolized to androgen precursors (see Fig. 12-1).

Three-fourths of patients with classic CAH are "salt wasters," as they have no 21-hydroxylase activity and produce insufficient aldosterone to retain sodium. The remaining one-fourth of patients, who produce low but detectable enzyme activity, retain enough ability to produce aldosterone, and, although virilized, do not sodium waste, and so are known as "simple virilizers." Those who retain 20–60% of enzymatic activity typically present in adulthood with more subtle, nonclassic forms. All patients with classic 21-hydroxylase deficiency are at high risk for development of adrenal insufficiency without exogenous glucocorticoid administration, but acute adrenal crisis is uncommon in nonclassic forms.

PRESENTATION

History

Classic 21-hydroxylase deficiency presents at or within several weeks of birth with hypotension as a result of adrenal insufficiency and virilization. The symptoms of nonclassic 21-hydroxylase deficiency are subtle. It may mimic polycystic ovary syn-

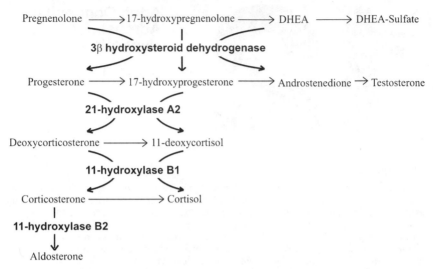

FIG. 12-1. The adrenal steroid biosynthesis pathway. DHEA, dehydroepiandrosterone.

drome, with symptoms of acne, hirsutism, and irregular menses. In male patients, complaints may be infertility and acne.

The differential diagnosis for nonclassic CAH in adults is limited but includes polycystic ovarian syndrome, virilizing adrenal or ovarian tumors, and exogenous anabolic steroid use.

Physical Exam

Hyperandrogenic features dominate the physical exam, with temporal hair loss, hirsutism, and acne. Patients with classic CAH may have reduced height due to androgen excess during puberty and from over-replacement of glucocorticoids. However, with more modern hormone replacement regimens, most patients attain their predicted adult height as adjusted for parental height.

MANAGEMENT

Laboratory Diagnosis

Classic 21-hydroxylase deficiency is characterized by significantly elevated levels of 17-OHP in infancy, with varying degrees of virilization that may not become apparent until later in childhood. Nonclassic CAH may have borderline or normal 17-OHP. Ideally, 8 A.M. 17-OHP levels should be drawn in the follicular phase in women. A 17-OHP of <2 ng/mL makes CAH unlikely, and a value >4 ng/mL has been reported to have 100% specificity and 90% sensitivity. Values between 2 and 4 ng/mL require ACTH stimulation by administering 250 mcg of synthetic ACTH IV and checking the plasma concentration levels of 17-OHP before and 60 minutes after the drug is given; values may be compared with standard curves, which are easily obtainable. If the post-ACTH cortisol level is <20 mcg/dL, the patient should be made aware of the need to take additional cortisol during times of physiologic stress. It should be noted that there are no reports of deaths from adrenal insufficiency as a result of nonclassic CAH in the medical literature. First-generation family members of affected patients should be screened for CAH due to the absence of clinical signs and potential harm that may result if a patient does not receive therapy.

Treatment

Treatment of adults with nonclassic 21-OH deficiency consists of administering the lowest dose of glucocorticoid replacement to suppress excess androgen production. **Dexamethasone** (Decadron) is often considered to be the most effective treatment in adults, although there is an increased risk of overtreatment. Hydrocortisone is the preferred treatment in children because of improved clinical outcomes with respect to final adult height. Typical glucocorticoid replacement doses are 0.25–0.75 mg PO daily of dexamethasone or 10–25 mg/m^2 PO daily of hydrocortisone in 2 or 3 divided doses. Nocturnal dosing of hydrocortisone appears to be most effective in suppressing ACTH. Adults with classic, salt-wasting CAH require glucocorticoid AND mineralocorticoid replacement. Generally, as little as 0.1 mg of fludrocortisone is sufficient.

Monitoring the effects of steroid replacement is crucial. 17-OHP levels are relatively resistant to suppression by glucocorticoids, and, thus, a normal 17-OHP level often represents overtreatment. 17-OHP levels should be maintained at the upper end of normal to mildly supranormal levels. Androstenedione levels are more sensitive to suppression and may be a better indicator of replacement dosing, with a goal of keeping the androstenedione levels in the upper one-third of normal range. Mineralocorticoid replacement may be monitored by following potassium levels. Elevated renin levels or hypotension may signify insufficient mineralocorticoid replacement.

Pregnancy in classic CAH should be managed by an endocrinologist. Dexamethasone is avoided during pregnancy because it readily crosses the placenta and is poorly degraded. An equivalent dose of prednisone or hydrocortisone, both of which are degraded by placental 3 beta-hydroxysteroid dehydrogenase, should be used. Women with nonclassic CAH generally do not require glucocorticoid therapy during pregnancy.

Adrenal crisis in patients with CAH is managed with glucocorticoid replacement as described in Chap. 11, Adrenal Insufficiency.

REFERENCES AND SUGGESTED READINGS

Augarten A, et al. Reversible male infertility in late onset congenital adrenal hyperplasia. *J Endocrinol Invest* 1991;14(3):237–240.

Bode HH, et al. Home monitoring of 17 hydroxyprogesterone levels in congenital adrenal hyperplasia with filter paper blood samples. *J Pediatr* 1999;134(2):185–189.

Carroll MC, Campbell RD, Porter RR. Mapping of steroid 21-hydroxylase genes adjacent to complement component C4 genes in HLA, the major histocompatibility complex in man. *Proc Natl Acad Sci U S A* 1985;82(2):521–525.

Culter GB, Laue L. Congenital adrenal hyperplasia due to 21-hydroxylase deficiency. *N Engl J Med* 1990;323(26):1806–1813.

Dewailly D. Nonclassic 21-hydroxylase deficiency. *Semin Reprod Med* 2002;20:243–248.

Horrocks PM, London DR. A comparison of three glucocorticoid suppressive regimes in adults with congenital adrenal hyperplasia. *Clin Endocrinol* 1982;17(6):547–556.

Horrocks PM, London DR. Effects of long term dexamethasone treatment in adult patients with congenital adrenal hyperplasia. *Clin Endocrinol* 1987;27(6):635–642.

Hughes IA. Management of congenital adrenal hyperplasia. *Arch Dis Child* 1988;63(11):1399–1404.

Kohn B, et al. Late-onset steroid 21-hydroxylase deficiency: a variant of classical congenital adrenal hyperplasia. *J Clin Endocrinol Metab* 1982;55(5):817–827.

Levine LS, et al. Genetic and hormonal characterization of cryptic 21-hydroxylase deficiency. *J Clin Endocrinol Metab* 1981;53(6):1193–1198.

Lopes LA, et al. Should we monitor more closely the dosage of 9 alpha-fluorohydrocortisone in salt-losing congenital adrenal hyperplasia? *J Ped Endocrinol* 1998;11(6):733–737.

Merke DP, Cutler GB. New approaches to the treatment of congenital adrenal hyperplasia. *JAMA* 1997;277(13):1073–1076.

Miller WL. Congenital adrenal hyperplasia in the adult patient. *Adv Intern Med* 1999;44:155–173.

New MI, et al. Growth and final height in classical and nonclassical 21-hydroxylase deficiency. *Acta Paediatr Jpn* 1988;30(suppl):79–88.

Pang SY, et al. Worldwide experience in newborn screening for classical congenital adrenal hyperplasia due to 21-hydroxylase deficiency. *Pediatrics* 1988;81(6):866–874.

Speiser PW. Congenital adrenal hyperplasia owing to 21-hydroxylase deficiency. *Endocrinol Metab Clin North Am* 2001;30(1):31–59.

Speiser PW, et al. Disease expression and molecular genotype in congenital adrenal hyperplasia due to 21-hydroxylase deficiency. *J Clin Invest* 1992;90(2):584–595.

White PC, Curnow KM, Pascoe L. Disorders of steroid 11-beta-hydroxylase isozymes. *Endocr Rev* 1994;15:421.

White PC, New MI, Dupont B. Congenital adrenal hyperplasia: part 1. *N Engl J Med* 1987;316:1519.

White PC, New MI, Dupont B. Congenital adrenal hyperplasia: part 2. *N Engl J Med* 1987;316:1580.

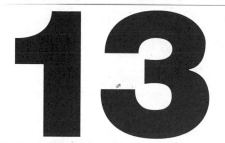

Conn's Syndrome

Jeannie Chen

INTRODUCTION

Primary aldosteronism is a syndrome of renin-independent aldosterone overproduction initially described by Jerome W. Conn in 1955. The condition is classically characterized by hypertension, hypokalemia, and metabolic alkalosis secondary to mineralocorticoid excess. Reported prevalence rates for primary aldosteronism vary from 0.05–2.20% to more recent reports of 5–15% of patients with hypertension. The trend toward higher prevalence rates likely reflects increased screening in hypertensive patients and variation in the diagnostic criteria. **Screening for primary aldosteronism** is indicated in individuals with hypertension and hypokalemia, refractory hypertension, spontaneous hypokalemia, severe hypokalemia in patients on modest doses of diuretics, or difficulty in maintaining normokalemia with K^+ supplements. The absence of hypertension or hypokalemia does not preclude screening.

CAUSES

Five subtypes of primary aldosteronism have been described:

- Aldosterone-producing adrenal adenomas (APAs) account for approximately 40% of cases. Hyperaldosteronism tends to be more severe, with more pronounced hypertension and hypokalemia.
- Idiopathic hyperaldosteronism (IHA) due to bilateral adrenal hyperplasia is present in 50–60% of cases. Aldosterone excess, in general, is milder.
- Unilateral primary adrenal hyperplasia (PAH) has similar biochemical features to APAs, but represents a rare form of hyperaldosteronism.
- Aldosterone-producing adrenocortical carcinomas are also a rare cause of primary aldosteronism.
- Familial hyperaldosteronism. Type I, or glucocorticoid-remediable aldosteronism (GRA), is inherited as an autosomal dominant trait. A chimeric gene is formed from an unequal crossing over of the 11 beta-hydroxylase gene regulatory elements with the coding region of the aldosterone synthase gene. In the chimeric gene, ACTH positively regulates the expression of aldosterone synthase and aldosterone production. This disorder represents <3% of cases of primary aldosteronism. Type II also has an autosomal dominant inheritance, but it is ACTH independent. Characteristics are similar to nonfamilial causes of primary aldosteronism. The genetic defect is unknown.

PRESENTATION

Patients with primary aldosteronism develop hypertension in their fourth to seventh decades, except for those with GRA, in which hypertension can be evident at birth or early childhood. There is a slight female predominance, except in GRA, in which males and females are affected equally. Patients with GRA have an increased prevalence of early cerebrovascular complications, especially hemorrhagic strokes from ruptured intracerebral aneurysms. The family history in patients with GRA may not consistently reveal hypertension, as environmental factors such as sodium intake may be mitigating factors.

Clinical Presentation

Patients may have few, if any, symptoms. Symptoms related to hypokalemia, such as muscle weakness and cramping, can occur. Other symptoms are nonspecific and may include headache, fatigue, palpitations, and polyuria.

There are no specific physical findings in primary aldosteronism. The majority of patients have hypertension, which may be mild to severe, but patients may be normotensive at diagnosis. Although excess sodium retention and volume expansion are thought to mediate the hypertension, edema is rare. Signs of end-organ damage, such as retinopathy, proteinuria, and left ventricular hypertrophy, relate to the severity and duration of hypertension.

Laboratory Findings

Laboratory findings may include hypokalemia, metabolic alkalosis, and mild hypernatremia. Hypokalemia may be spontaneous or become pronounced when patients are placed on diuretics. A subset of patients are normokalemic.

MANAGEMENT

Evaluation for primary aldosteronism consists of screening for the disorder followed by confirmatory testing. Once the diagnosis is secure, studies are undertaken to determine the subtype. The differential diagnosis for patients with hypertension and hypokalemia includes

- Primary aldosteronism
- Secondary aldosteronism
- States of real or apparent mineralocorticoid excess

A summary of these conditions is provided in Table 13-1. These disorders can be distinguished by measuring **plasma renin activity (PRA)** and **plasma aldosterone concentration (PAC)**. Low PRA separates primary from secondary hyperaldosteronism. Low PRA and low PAC characterize states of real or apparent mineralocorticoid excess.

Screening Tests

The **PAC/PRA ratio** (reported as ng/dL per ng/mL/hour) is a commonly used screening test. Ratios of >20 to >50 have been reported as supportive of primary aldosteronism. A PAC/PRA ratio >30 and PAC >20 ng/dL has been reported to yield 90% sensitivity and 91% specificity. Use of the ratio alone without consideration of the absolute value for PAC may be misleading. A subset of patients with essential hypertension may have elevated ratios by virtue of low PRA without concomitant elevation in PAC. The captopril test has also been used as a screening test. Other findings suggestive of primary aldosteronism include inappropriate kaliuresis (>30 mEq/day) in the presence of hypokalemia, PRA <1 ng/mL/hour, PAC >30 ng/dL, and 24-hour urine aldosterone excretion >15 mcg/day.

Any biochemical testing of the renin-angiotensin-aldosterone axis should occur in a sodium- and volume-replete state. In addition, serum K^+ levels should be normalized before testing. K^+ loading at the time of testing may increase aldosterone secretion. Patients should ideally be taken off medications that interfere with the renin-angiotensin-aldosterone axis if feasible. These medications include spironolactone (Aldactone), ACE inhibitors, beta blockers, diuretics, and angiotensin receptor blockers. Patients must be off these medications for at least 2–4 weeks and off spironolactone for at least 6–8 weeks before testing. Alpha blockers and calcium channel blockers do not have an appreciable effect on the renin-angiotensin-aldosterone axis.

TABLE 13-1. DIFFERENTIAL DIAGNOSIS FOR HYPERTENSION AND HYPOKALEMIA

Decreased PRA and increased PAC	Increased PRA and increased PAC	Decreased PRA and decreased PAC
Primary aldosteronism	Secondary aldosteronism	Real mineralocorticoid excess
APA	Renovascular disease	17 alpha-hydroxylase deficiency
IHA	Renin-secreting tumor	11 beta-hydroxylase deficiency
GRA	Malignant hyperten-	Deoxycorticosterone-secreting
PAH	sion	tumors
Adrenocortical car-	Chronic renal disease	Apparent mineralocorticoid
cinoma	Congestive heart fail-	excess
	ure[a]	11 beta-hydroxysteroid dehy-
	Cirrhosis[a]	drogenase deficiency
	Diuretic abuse[a]	Chronic licorice ingestion (gly-
	Volume depletion[a]	cyrrhizic and glycyrrhetinic
	Bartter's syndrome[a]	acid)
	Gitelman's syndrome[a]	Severe Cushing's syndrome
		Liddle's syndrome

APA, aldosterone-producing adrenal adenomas; GRA, glucocorticoid-remediable aldosteronism; IHA, idiopathic hyperaldosteronism; PAH, primary adrenal hyperplasia; PRA, plasma renin activity; PAC, plasma aldosterone concentration.
[a]May not present with hypertension.

Confirmatory Tests

Confirmation requires demonstration of nonsuppression of aldosterone by sodium loading. A 24-hour urine aldosterone level >10–14 mcg after 3–5 days of oral sodium loading confirms the diagnosis. Alternatively, plasma aldosterone levels can be measured after a 2-L saline infusion given over 4 hours if clinical status permits. Values >10 ng/dL confirm primary aldosteronism. The fludrocortisone suppression test is not commonly performed.

Determining Subtype

Treatment choice depends on the subtype, which is first addressed by CT or MRI of the adrenals. An adenoma ≥1 cm in 1 gland with an irrefutably normal contralateral gland is consistent with APA. If atypical features are found in either gland, other studies can be performed, including adrenal venous sampling for aldosterone and cortisol, postural stimulation (APA shows a paradoxical fall in PAC/PRA from a supine 8 A.M. sample and a sample obtained after 4 hours of upright posture), adrenal scintigraphy with I[131]-labeled cholesterol analogue 6 beta-[^{131}I]iodomethyl-19-norcholesterol (N-59), dexamethasone suppression testing (PAC suppresses to <4 ng/dL in GRA), and measurement of plasma 18-OH corticosterone (elevated in APA) or of urinary 18-hydroxycortisol and 18-oxocortisol (markedly elevated in GRA). GRA may be confirmed by genetic testing. The differential diagnosis of primary aldosteronism subtypes is summarized in Table 13-2.

Treatment

Unilateral total adrenalectomy is the treatment of choice in APA and PAH. Laparoscopic adrenalectomy is associated with shorter hospital stays and lower morbidity than an open approach. Adequate blood pressure control and correction of hypokalemia with spironolactone before surgery is recommended. Hypokalemia is corrected rapidly after adrenalectomy for APA. Hypertension, although improved, may persist for several months after surgery. End-organ damage, changes in vascular tone, neph-

TABLE 13-2. DIFFERENTIAL DIAGNOSIS OF PRIMARY ALDOSTERONISM SUBTYPES

	APA	IHA	GRA
Adrenal venous sampling	Lateralization	No lateralization	No lateralization
Postural stimulation test	Fall in PAC	Increase or no change in PAC	Fall in PAC
Adrenal scintigraphy	Lateralization	No lateralization	No lateralization
18-OH corticosterone	>100 ng/dL	<50 ng/dL	<50 ng/dL
18-hydroxycortisol; 18-oxocortisol	Mildly elevated	No change	Greatly elevated
Dexamethasone suppressibility	No	No	Yes

APA, aldosterone-producing adrenal adenomas; IHA, idiopathic hyperaldosteronism; GRA, glucocorticoid-remediable aldosteronism; PAC, plasma aldosterone concentration.

rosclerosis, or essential hypertension may contribute to persistent postoperative hypertension.

Medical management is reserved for patients with bilateral disease or patients with APA or PAH who refuse surgery or are poor surgical candidates. Patients require lifelong therapy. There is little risk for malignant transformation of aldosterone-secreting adenomas. Effective pharmacologic agents include

- Spironolactone (Aldactone) at doses of 200–400 mg PO daily in divided doses is rapidly effective in correcting hypokalemia, but its antihypertensive effects may not be apparent for several weeks. Antiandrogenic side effects, including gynecomastia and erectile dysfunction in men and menstrual irregularities in women, limit its tolerability.
- Amiloride (Midamor) is an effective alternative to spironolactone. Doses of 10–30 mg PO daily in divided doses can normalize serum K^+. Adjunctive therapy with other antihypertensives may be needed to control blood pressure. Side effects include dizziness, fatigue, and impotence.
- Triamterene (Dyrenium) at doses of 200–300 mg PO daily in divided doses is an alternative to spironolactone and amiloride. Side effects include dizziness and nausea.

K^+ supplements should not be given routinely with the above agents, as hyperkalemia may result. Other second-line agents that may be used include dihydropyridine calcium channel blockers, diuretics, ACE-inhibitors, and angiotensin II receptor antagonists. Eplerenone (Inspra), a new selective aldosterone receptor blocker, may prove to be an alternative to spirinolactone.

Patients with GRA may be treated with **glucocorticoids** at the lowest effective dose to avoid iatrogenic Cushing's syndrome. Alternatively, patients may be treated with a mineralocorticoid antagonist as monotherapy with similar results.

KEY POINTS TO REMEMBER

- Symptoms of Conn's syndrome, if present at all, may be related to hypokalemia (muscle weakness and cramping) or may be nonspecific (headache, fatigue, palpitations, and polyuria).
- The majority of patients with Conn's syndrome have hypertension.
- Laboratory findings may include hypokalemia, metabolic alkalosis, and mild hypernatremia.
- The PAC/PRA ratio can be used as a screening test for Conn's syndrome and, if abnormal, should be followed by a confirmatory test demonstrating nonsuppression of aldosterone by sodium loading.
- Unilateral total adrenalectomy is the treatment of choice in APA and PAH.

- Medical management is reserved for patients with bilateral disease or patients with APA or PAH who refuse surgery or are poor surgical candidates.

REFERENCES AND SUGGESTED READINGS

Blumenfeld JD, et al. Diagnosis and treatment of primary hyperaldosteronism. *Ann Intern Med* 1994;121:877–885.

Dluhy RG, Lifton RP. Glucocorticoid-remediable aldosteronism. *J Clin Endocrinol Metab* 1999;84:4341–4344.

Fontes RG, et al. Reassessment of the predictive value of the postural stimulation test in primary aldosteronism. *Am J Hyperten* 1991;4:786–791.

Gordon RD, et al. Primary aldosteronism and other forms of mineralocorticoid hypertension. In Swales J, ed. *Textbook of hypertension*. Oxford: Blackwell Scientific, 1994:865–892.

Hambling C, et al. Re-evaluation of the captopril test for the diagnosis of primary hyperaldosteronism. *Clin Endocrinol* 1992;36(5):499–503.

Lim PO, et al. A review of the medical treatment of primary aldosteronism. *J Hypertens* 2001;19:353–361.

Lim PO, et al. High prevalence of primary aldosteronism in the Tayside Hypertension Clinic population. *J Hum Hypertens* 2000;14:311–315.

Litchfield WR, Dluhy RG. Primary aldosteronism. *Endocrinol Metab Clin North Am* 1995;24:593–612.

Litchfield WR, et al. Evaluation of the dexamethasone suppression test for the diagnosis of glucocorticoid-remediable aldosteronism. *J Clin Endocrinol Metab* 1997;82:3570–3573.

Litchfield WR, et al. Intracranial aneurysm and hemorrhagic stroke in glucocorticoid-remediable aldosteronism. *Hypertension* 1998;31:445–450.

Jonsson JR, et al. A new genetic test for familial hyperaldosteronism type I aids in the detection of curable hypertension. *Biochem Biophys Res Commun* 1995;207:565–571.

Snow MH, et al. Normotensive primary aldosteronism. *BMJ* 1976;1:1125–1126.

Torpy DJ, et al. Familial hyperaldosteronism type II: description of a large kindred and exclusion of the aldosterone synthase (CYP11B2) gene. *J Clin Endocrinol Metab* 1998;83:3214–3218.

Ulick S, et al. The unique steroidogenesis of the aldosteronoma in the differential diagnosis of primary aldosteronism. *J Clin Endocrinol Metab* 1993;76:873–878.

Weinberger MH, Fineberg NS. The diagnosis of primary aldosteronism and separation of two major subtypes. *Arch Intern Med* 1993;153:2125–2129.

Young WF, et al. Primary aldosteronism: adrenal vein sampling. *Surgery* 1996;120:913–920.

Young WF, et al. Primary aldosteronism: diagnosis and treatment. *Mayo Clin Proc* 1990;65:96–110.

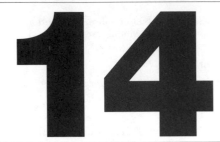

Cushing's Syndrome

Jeannie Chen

INTRODUCTION

Cushing's syndrome is a state of chronic glucocorticoid excess from either endogenous or exogenous sources. The most common cause of Cushing's syndrome is iatrogenic, exogenous steroid use. Cushing's disease, originally described by Harvey Cushing in 1932, results specifically from ACTH-secreting pituitary adenomas and is the most common cause of endogenous glucocorticoid excess. Due to the nonspecific nature of the symptoms and signs of Cushing's syndrome and to the limitations in available testing, the diagnosis of Cushing's syndrome is one of the most challenging in endocrinology.

CAUSES

Endogenous Cushing's syndrome is either ACTH-dependent or ACTH-independent. ACTH-dependent Cushing's disease represents 70% of all cases and has an incidence of 5–25 per 1 million per year, with females 3–8 times more likely to have the disease. **Ectopic** ACTH syndrome accounts for 12–15% of cases. Small cell lung cancer is the source of ectopic ACTH in more than one-half of the cases. ACTH-independent causes of Cushing's syndrome include adrenal adenoma and carcinoma, which represent 10% and 8% of cases, respectively. Other causes of Cushing's syndrome are rare and include both ACTH-dependent causes [ectopic corticotropin-releasing hormone (CRH) syndrome] and ACTH-independent causes (micronodular and macronodular adrenal hyperplasia and other adrenal hyperplasias associated with hormone or receptor excess).

Cushing's syndrome can be associated with indolent tumors and other states of hormone excess. One series documented Cushing's disease in 16% of patients with multiple endocrine neoplasia 1 (MEN1) and Zollinger-Ellison syndrome. Ectopic production of ACTH or CRH by tumors, such as pheochromocytoma, carcinoid, and other neuroendocrine tumors, can also cause Cushing's syndrome. One-half of the cases of bilateral micronodular adrenal hyperplasia occur in Carney's complex, an autosomal dominant syndrome associated with endocrine tumors such as pituitary adenomas and testicular tumors, cardiac myxomas, blue nevi, and schwannomas. Hypercortisolism from hyperplastic adrenal nodules can also occur in McCune-Albright syndrome, which is associated with multiple autonomous hyperfunctioning endocrinopathies, as well as café-au-lait spots and polyostotic fibrous dysplasia.

PRESENTATION

Patients with Cushing's syndrome present with varying degrees of glucocorticoid excess. Patients also may demonstrate variable degrees of androgen and mineralocorticoid excess. The frequency of various signs and symptoms in a series of patients with Cushing's syndrome is presented in Table 14-1. Symptoms of Cushing's syndrome that occur in the setting of malignancy may be overshadowed by manifestations of the malignancy. Patients with cyclical Cushing's syndrome may have intermittent symptoms. Cushing's syndrome during pregnancy can be difficult to diagnose as both con-

TABLE 14-1. FREQUENCY OF SIGNS AND SYMPTOMS IN PATIENTS WITH CUSHING'S SYNDROME (N = 302)

Sign/symptom	Frequency (%)
Truncal obesity	96
Facial fullness	82
Diabetes or glucose intolerance	80
Gonadal dysfunction	74
Hirsutism, acne	72
Hypertension	68
Muscle weakness	64
Skin atrophy and bruising	62
Mood disorders	58
Osteoporosis	38
Edema	18
Polydipsia, polyuria	10
Fungal infection	6

From Moscaro M, Barzon L, Fallo F, et al. Cushing's syndrome. *Lancet* 2001:357:783–791.

ditions may be complicated by excessive weight gain, striae, hypertension, edema, and glucose intolerance.

Findings on exam are nonspecific, variable, and dependent on the presence and severity of glucocorticoid, mineralocorticoid, and androgen excess. Findings suggestive of Cushing's syndrome include the following:

- Central obesity with enlarged fat pads (buffalo hump, moon facies, supraclavicular fat pads, exophthalmos)
- Wide, purple striae
- Hyperpigmentation (in ectopic ACTH syndrome)
- Skin atrophy
- Spontaneous ecchymoses
- Virilization (in adrenal carcinoma)
- Weight loss or anorexia (in ectopic ACTH syndrome associated with malignancy)
- Proximal myopathy/muscle wasting
- Growth failure in children
- Unexplained osteoporosis or osteopenia
- Hypokalemic alkalosis

Differential Diagnosis

Cushing's syndrome must be distinguished from pseudo-Cushing's states and from conditions associated with elevated cortisol without Cushing's syndrome.

Pseudo-Cushing's Syndrome

- Major depressive disorder
- Alcohol excess

Hypercortisolism without Cushing's Syndrome

- Obesity
- Anorexia nervosa/psychiatric illness

- Stress/trauma/acute illness
- States of elevated cortisol-binding protein (pregnancy, estrogen therapy, hyperthyroidism)
- Familial generalized glucocorticoid resistance

The metabolic syndrome may mimic Cushing's syndrome, with central obesity, hypertension, and glucose intolerance. Female patients with the metabolic syndrome may also have features of polycystic ovary syndrome and present with menstrual irregularities and hyperandrogenism (hirsutism, acne).

MANAGEMENT

Evaluation

The evaluation of Cushing's syndrome consists of biochemical confirmation and differentiation between ACTH-dependent and ACTH-independent causes. Due to the possibility of both pituitary and adrenal incidentalomas, it is essential for biochemical diagnosis to precede imaging studies. **Diagnostic tests** used in the evaluation for Cushing's syndrome are listed in Table 14-2. These tests are designed to detect excess cortisol secretion, the loss of the normal feedback of the hypothalamic-pituitary-adrenal (HPA) axis, and the loss of the normal diurnal rhythm of cortisol secretion.

The **1-mg overnight dexamethasone (Decadron) suppression test** is commonly used as a screening test. However, it has a high false-positive rate and requires confirmation by another method. The 24-hour **urine free cortisol** measurement is the best test for diagnosing Cushing's syndrome. Values 2- to 3-fold higher than the normal range obtained on at least two separate occasions strongly support the diagnosis of Cushing's syndrome. In the event of mild elevations of urine free cortisol or suspected cyclic Cushing's, multiple collections may be necessary. Use of the other confirmatory tests in Table 14-2 may aid in differentiating the subtle nuances between mild Cushing's, cyclic Cushing's, or pseudo-Cushing's syndrome. Each test has various drawbacks. Causes of false-positive and false-negative results are listed in Table 14-3.

Once endogenous Cushing's syndrome has been confirmed, further management is determined by measuring plasma ACTH levels to **differentiate ACTH-dependent from ACTH-independent causes**. Undetectable or low levels of ACTH (<5 mcg/dL) characterize a primary adrenal source. ACTH levels >15 mcg/dL usually indicate an ACTH-dependent cause. An ACTH level in the 5–15 mcg/dL range is indeterminate and should be repeated. There can be considerable overlap in ACTH levels between patients with Cushing's disease and ectopic ACTH syndrome, especially those with occult malignancy or bronchial carcinoid tumors. The distinction between the two is critical in determining subsequent treatment. Tests that help differentiate pituitary Cushing's disease from ectopic ACTH syndrome are listed in Table 14-4.

Treatment

ACTH-Independent Cushing's Syndrome

Adrenal imaging by either CT or MRI will demonstrate unilateral or bilateral disease. Patients with adrenal adenoma or carcinoma are treated with unilateral adrenalectomy. Bilateral adrenalectomy is recommended for patients with bilateral micronodular or macronodular disease. During and after unilateral adrenalectomy, patients should receive glucocorticoid replacement until the HPA axis recovers from the prolonged suppressive effects of glucocorticoid excess. Patients with bilateral adrenalectomy require lifelong glucocorticoid and mineralocorticoid replacement. In addition to adrenalectomy, patients with adrenal carcinomas typically require medications to control hypercortisolemia, which frequently recurs.

Cushing's Disease

Transsphenoidal adenomectomy is considered first-line therapy for patients with Cushing's disease. Patients with incomplete resection of the tumor may undergo

TABLE 14-2. DIAGNOSTIC TESTS IN THE EVALUATION OF CUSHING'S SYNDROME

Test	Protocol	Measurements	Interpretation	Sensitivity (%)	Specificity (%)
1 mg overnight DST	Dex, 1 mg PO at 11 P.M.	8 A.M. plasma cortisol.	Normal, <5 mcg/dL.	98	70–80
24-hr urine free cortisol	24-hr urine collection.	Cortisol, creatinine.	Values 2- to 3-fold higher than the upper limit of normal suggest Cushing's.	95–100	98
2-day low-dose urine DST	Dex, 0.5 mg PO q6h × 48 hrs (last dose 6 A.M.).	24-hr urine collection for cortisol, 17-OHCS, creatinine during last 24 hrs of dex administration.	Urine free cortisol >36 mcg/day or urine 17-OHCS >4 mg/day suggests Cushing's.	56–69	74–100
2-day low-dose serum DST	Dex, 0.5 mg PO q6h × 48 hrs (last dose 6 A.M.).	Plasma cortisol 2 hrs after last dose of dex.	Normal <1.4 mcg/dL.	90	100
CRH/dex	Same as LDDST with first dose dex given at noon and CRH, 1 mcg/kg IV at 8 A.M. after last dose of dex.	Plasma cortisol 15 mins after CRH injection.	Cortisol >1.4 mcg/dL suggests Cushing's.	100	100
Late-night salivary cortisol	11 P.M. sample.	Salivary cortisol.	Value <1.3 ng/mL excludes Cushing's.	92	100
Midnight plasma cortisol	Indwelling catheter. Hospitalization recommended	Midnight plasma cortisol.	Cortisol >7.5 mcg/dL suggests Cushing's.	96	100

CRH, corticotropin-releasing hormone; dex, dexamethasone; DST, dexamethasone suppression test; LDDST, low-dose dexamthasone suppression test; 17-OHCS, 17-hydroxycorticosteroid.

TABLE 14-3. CAUSES OF FALSE-POSITIVE AND FALSE-NEGATIVE RESULTS ON BIOCHEMICAL TESTING FOR CUSHING'S SYNDROME

	False-positive	False-negative
1 mg overnight DST	Error with timing of dex administration Meds increasing metabolism of dex Decreased absorption of dex Hypercortisolemia without Cushing's syndrome Pseudo-Cushing's syndrome	Chronic renal failure (glomerular filtration rate, <30 mL/min) Increased sensitivity of HPA axis to dex
24-hr urine free cortisol	High fluid intake Interference with carbamazepine (Carbatrol, Tegretol) with HPLC assay Hypercortisolemia without Cushing's syndrome Pseudo-Cushing's syndrome	Cyclic Cushing's Early Cushing's Chronic renal failure
2-day low-dose DST	As above	As above
Midnight plasma cortisol	Stress from hospitalization, blood draw Critically ill patients Patients with depression	Cyclic Cushing's
Late-night salivary cortisol	Same as for midnight serum cortisol	Cyclic Cushing's

dex, dexamethasone; DST, dexamethasone suppression test; HPA, hypothalamic-pituitary-adrenal; HPLC, high-performance liquid chromatography.

repeat surgery or pituitary irradiation with either conventional radiation or stereotactic radiation with the ^{60}Co gamma knife. Pituitary irradiation may not control the hypercortisolemia for months to years, and patients require medical therapy until the full effects of the radiation are seen. Bilateral adrenalectomy may need to be performed in patients with refractory disease. Nelson's syndrome occurs in up to 25% of patients with Cushing's disease who are treated with bilateral adrenalectomy. In this syndrome, the pituitary enlarges and the patient develops hyperpigmentation associated with high ACTH levels. Pituitary irradiation before bilateral adrenalectomy may prevent Nelson's syndrome. Surgical cure with transsphenoidal adenomectomy can be assessed with postoperative morning cortisol and ACTH levels, which are undetectable with successful complete resection of the tumor. During and after transsphenoidal resection of the adenoma, patients require glucocorticoid replacement until recovery of the HPA axis.

Ectopic ACTH and CRH Syndrome
Tumors that can be localized by imaging studies should be removed surgically. Imaging studies include CT, MRI, and somatostatin receptor scintigraphy. Areas that may be imaged for the presence of tumor include the chest, abdomen, pelvis, or neck. If the source is an occult tumor or if there is metastatic disease, medical treatment is required. Tumors expressing somatostatin receptors may be responsive to somatostatin analogues. Bilateral adrenalectomy may be performed in refractory cases.

Medical Therapy
The following adrenal enzyme inhibitors may be used to treat hypercortisolemia.

TABLE 14-4. DIFFERENTIATING PITUITARY CUSHING'S DISEASE FROM ECTOPIC ACTH SYNDROME

Test	Protocol	Interpretation	Sensitivity (%)	Specificity (%)
2-day HDDST	Collect 24-hr urine for 17-OH or urine free cortisol and creatinine; give dex, 2 mg PO q6h × 48 hrs; re-collect urine during last 24 hrs of dex administration.	Pituitary Cushing's will have suppression of urine 17-OH by >64% or a >90% reduction in urine free cortisol.	83	100
8 mg dex	Measure plasma cortisol at 8 A.M.; give dex, 8 mg PO at 11 P.M.; redraw plasma cortisol next morning at 8 A.M.	Pituitary Cushing's will have suppression of cortisol by 50% compared to baseline.	92	100
CRH	CRH, 1 mcg/kg IV bolus at 8 A.M. (given through indwelling catheter placed 2 hrs before bolus); draw plasma ACTH at –5, –1 min before CRH and +15, +30 mins after CRH.	Increase of ACTH (mean of +15 and +30 mins values) by 35% over baseline (mean of –5 and –1 min) suggests pituitary Cushing's.	93	100
IPSS	Simultaneous bilateral inferior petrosal sampling and peripheral sampling for ACTH before and after CRH, 100 mcg IV.	Pituitary Cushing's if basal petrosal:peripheral ≥2 or post-CRH petrosal:peripheral ≥3.	95–100	100

CRH, corticotropin-releasing hormone; dex, dexamethasone; HDDST, high-dose dexamethasone suppression test; IPSS, inferior petrosal sinus sampling.

Mitotane

Mitotane (Lysodren) inhibits cholesterol side chain cleavage and 11 beta-hydroxylase. Mitotane induces permanent destruction of adrenocortical cells and, therefore, can be used to achieve medical adrenalectomy as an alternative to surgical adrenalectomy. Glucocorticoid replacement is started at initiation of mitotane treatment. Mineralocorticoid treatment may eventually be required. Side effects are generally dose dependent and include GI symptoms, weakness, lethargy, leukopenia, gynecomastia, and hypercholesterolemia. Doses start at 0.5 mg PO at bedtime and are increased to 1–12 mg PO daily in divided doses q6h.

Ketoconazole

Ketoconazole (Nizoral), an antifungal, inhibits C17-20 lyase, 11 beta-hydroxylase, and cholesterol side chain cleavage. Its cortisol-reducing effects are dose dependent and can be seen rapidly. The major side effect is liver toxicity. Other side effects include gynecomastia, impotence, and GI symptoms. Doses range from 200–1200 mg PO daily in 2–3 divided doses.

Metyrapone

Metyrapone (Metopirone) inhibits 11 beta-hydroxylase. Major side effects include increased androgens, hypertension, and hypokalemia through increased 11-deoxycorticosterone. Doses range from 250 mg to 1 g PO given q6h. Lower doses of 500–750 mg PO daily can be used when given in combination with ketoconazole and/or aminoglutethimide (Cytadren).

Aminoglutethimide

Aminoglutethimide (Cytadren) is an anticonvulsant that inhibits cholesterol side chain cleavage. Doses range from 500–2000 mg PO daily in divided doses. Side effects include GI upset, lethargy, ataxia, hypothyroidism, headache, bone marrow suppression, and skin rash. It is not as effective as monotherapy compared to ketoconazole or metyrapone and thus is frequently used in combination with other agents.

Ketoconazole is usually the first-line medication, with metyrapone and then aminoglutethimide added if necessary. Patients treated with these medications should have plasma cortisol and 24-hour urine free cortisol levels monitored and doses titrated to keep cortisol levels in the normal range. Glucocorticoid replacement is added as cortisol levels approach the normal range.

Other Beneficial Agents

- Mifepristone (RU486): This antiprogestational agent is a cortisol receptor antagonist at high doses.
- Octreotide (Sandostatin): May be useful for ectopic ACTH syndrome.
- Etomidate (Amidate): The only IV drug that can reduce cortisol levels. May be useful in hospitalized patients for acute management when used in nonhypnotic doses as a continuous infusion.
- Bromocriptine (Parlodel): Has only a modest effect in Cushing's disease.

Cushing's Syndrome during Pregnancy

Rare cases of Cushing's syndrome during pregnancy have been reported. Pregnant patients may be effectively treated with transsphenoidal surgery and/or radiation for Cushing's disease. Bilateral adrenalectomy can also be performed. Metyrapone and aminoglutethimide may be used during pregnancy, but mitotane and ketoconazole, which are teratogenic, are contraindicated.

PROGNOSIS

Untreated, Cushing's syndrome is associated with increased morbidity and mortality. In addition to morbidity from signs and symptoms listed in Table 14-1, patients are hypercoagulable and may develop thromboembolic complications. Cure rates after transsphenoidal surgery for Cushing's disease range from 80–90%, depending on the various criteria used to define a cure. Postoperative random plasma cortisol levels of 1.8–5 mcg/dL have been used to designate a cure in various series of studies. An additional 45–80% of the patients undergoing pituitary irradiation after unsuccessful pituitary surgery experience remission. Patients requiring a second pituitary surgery have a remission rate of 43–71%.

Patients with adrenal adenomas and benign ACTH-secreting tumors that can be completely resected can be cured. The prognosis is worse for patients with adrenal carcinomas or malignant ACTH-secreting tumors. These patients are rarely cured, but the hypercortisolemia can be controlled with medications or bilateral adrenalectomy. These patients usually succumb to the underlying malignancy rather than to the effects of hypercortisolemia.

KEY POINTS TO REMEMBER

* The most common cause of Cushing's syndrome is iatrogenic, exogenous steroid use.
* Findings suggestive of Cushing's syndrome include central obesity, striae, hyperpigmentation, skin atrophy, spontaneous ecchymoses, virilization, weight loss, anorexia, proximal myopathy/muscle wasting, unexplained osteoporosis, and hypokalemic alkalosis.
* The evaluation of Cushing's syndrome consists of biochemical confirmation and differentiation between ACTH-dependent and ACTH-independent causes.
* The 24-hour urine free cortisol measurement is the best test for diagnosing Cushing's syndrome.
* Plasma ACTH levels differentiate ACTH-dependent from ACTH-independent causes.
* Patients with adrenal adenoma or carcinoma are treated with unilateral adrenalectomy.
* Transsphenoidal adenomectomy is considered first-line therapy for patients with Cushing's disease.
* ACTH-secreting tumors that can be localized by imaging studies should be removed surgically. Occult tumors and metastatic disease require medical treatment.

REFERENCES AND SUGGESTED READINGS

Aron DC, et al. Cushing's syndrome and pregnancy. *Am J Obstet Gynecol* 1990;162: 244–252.

Boscaro M, et al. Cushing's syndrome. *Lancet* 2001;357:783–791.

Casonato A, et al. Abnormalities of von Willebrand factor are also part of the prothrombotic state of Cushing's syndrome. *Blood Coag Fibrinol* 1999;10:145–151.

Flack MR, et al. Urine free cortisol in the high-dose dexamethasone suppression test for the differential diagnosis of the Cushing syndrome. *Ann Intern Med* 1986;116:211–217.

Invitti C, et al. Diagnosis and management of Cushing's syndrome: results of an Italian multicentre study. *J Clin Endocrinol Metab* 1999;4:440–448.

Jenkins, et al. The long-term outcome after adrenalectomy and prophylactic pituitary radiotherapy in adrenoACTH-dependent Cushing's syndrome. *J Clin Endocrinol Metab* 1995;80:165–171.

Koerten JM, et al. Cushing's syndrome in pregnancy: a case report and literature review. *Am J Obstet Gynecol* 1986;154:626–628.

Maton PN, et al. Cushing's syndrome in patients with Zollinger-Ellison syndrome. *N Engl J Med* 1986;315:1–5.

Meier CA, Biller BM. Clinical and biochemical evaluation of Cushing's syndrome. *Endo Metab Clin North Am* 1997;26:741–763.

Newell-Price J, et al. The diagnosis and differential diagnosis of Cushing's syndrome and pseudo-Cushing's states. *Endo Rev* 1998;19:647–672.

Nieman LK, et al. A simplified morning ovine ACTH-releasing hormone stimulation test for the differential diagnosis of adrenoACTH-dependent Cushing's syndrome. *J Clin Endocrinol Metab* 1993;77:1308–1312.

Orth DN. Cushing's syndrome. *N Engl J Med* 1995;332:791–803.

Orth DN, Kovacs WJ. The adrenal cortex. In: Wilson JD, et al., eds. *Williams textbook of endocrinology*, 9th ed. Philadelphia: W.B. Saunders, 1998:565–595.

Papanicolaou DA, et al. A single midnight serum cortisol measurement distinguishes Cushing's syndrome from pseudo-Cushing states. *J Clin Endocrinol Metab* 1998; 83:1163–1167.

Raff H, et al. Late-night salivary cortisol as a screening test for Cushing's syndrome. *J Clin Endocrinol Metab* 1998;83:2681–2686.

Sonino N, et al. Risk factors and long-term outcome in pituitary-dependent Cushing's disease. *J Clin Endocrinol Metab* 1999;81:2647–2652.

Tyrrell JB, et al. An overnight high-dose dexamethasone suppression test for rapid differential diagnosis of Cushing's syndrome. *Ann Intern Med* 1986;104:180–186.

Yanovski JA, et al. ACTH-releasing hormone stimulation following low-dose dexamethasone administration: a new test to distinguish Cushing's syndrome from pseudo-Cushing's states. *JAMA* 1993;269:2232–2238.

15

Pheochromocytoma

Michael Jakoby

INTRODUCTION

Pheochromocytoma is a catecholamine-producing tumor of neurochromaffin cells. It occurs from infancy to old age, with peak incidence in the third and fourth decades of life. It is a rare tumor and accounts for <0.2% of cases of hypertension. However, pheochromocytoma may be fatal if undiagnosed and untreated.

Most pheochromocytomas arise in the adrenal medulla, but extraadrenal pheochromocytomas may occur in anatomic regions that contain sympathetic ganglia. Extraadrenal pheochromocytomas are called **paragangliomas**. Sporadic pheochromocytomas are usually solitary, unilateral, and intraadrenal tumors. Familial pheochromocytomas are also typically intraadrenal, but they are often multicentric and bilateral (≥70%).

Pheochromocytoma may occur in the context of autosomal dominant hereditary syndromes. Hereditary disorders associated with pheochromocytoma are multiple endocrine neoplasia 2 (MEN2), von Hippel-Lindau syndrome, and neurofibromatosis type 1. The frequency of familial pheochromocytoma in two large series was approximately 20%. Genetic screening is recommended for patients diagnosed with pheochromocytoma before age 20 years, bilateral adrenal tumors, multiple paragangliomas, or who have a family history of pheochromocytoma or paraganglioma.

Pheochromocytomas are malignant in 10–15% of cases as defined by local invasion or distant metastases. Biochemical behavior and histologic appearance do not predict malignant potential. Malignant pheochromocytomas tend to be indolent and metastasize to bone, liver, lymph nodes, and lung.

CAUSES

Differential Diagnosis

- Essential hypertension
- Anxiety disorder (during therapy with tricyclic antidepressant drugs)
- Clonidine withdrawal
- MAOI pressor crisis [tranylcypromine (Parnate), phenelzine (Nardil), isocarboxazid]
- Cocaine abuse
- Amphetamine abuse
- Over-the-counter decongestants
- Myocardial infarction
- Aortic dissection
- Thyrotoxicosis (hyperthyroidism does not elevate diastolic blood pressure)
- Incidental adrenal adenoma
- Neuroblastoma/ganglioneuroblastoma (malignant tumors of the adrenals and sympathetic chain, hypertension is uncommon, usually occur in childhood)
- Ganglioneuroma (benign tumors of the sympathetic chain, usually found in the posterior mediastinum, clinical features similar to paragangliomas)
- Diencephalic epilepsy

PRESENTATION

History

Patients with pheochromocytoma often experience a characteristic paroxysm or crisis caused by release of catecholamines. The classic symptomatic triad includes

- Headache
- Sweating
- Palpitations

Blood pressure is elevated, often to alarming levels, when measured during a paroxysm. Frequent symptoms are summarized in Table 15-1.
Characteristics of paroxysms include

- Usually last 30–40 minutes
- May be precipitated by displacement of abdominal contents (e.g., lifting, bending, palpation)
- Usually occur with enough frequency over the course of 1–2 days to observe an event and measure blood pressure
- Tend to increase in frequency and severity over time

Despite the association of pheochromocytoma with paroxysms, in one large series, episodic symptoms only occurred in slightly more than one-half of patients.

Physical Exam

Hypertension is the most common feature of pheochromocytoma and occurs in >90% of patients. It is usually sustained and may resemble essential hypertension in the absence of paroxysms. Only 25–40% of patients experience truly episodic hypertension. Hypertension is often severe, refractory to conventional therapy, and associated with signs of end-organ damage such as proteinuria or retinopathy.
Findings on physical exam may include

- Resting hypertension (often severe)
- Postural hypotension
- Resting tachycardia
- Fever
- Perspiration

TABLE 15-1. SYMPTOMS OCCURRING IN AT LEAST 20% OF PHEOCHROMOCYTOMA PATIENTS

Symptom	Frequency (%)
Headache	80
Perspiration	71
Palpitations	64
Pallor	42
Nausea	42
Tremor	31
Weakness/fatigue	28
Anxiety	22
Epigastric pain	22

Data from Thomas JE, Rooke ED, Kvale WF. The neurologist's experience with pheocromocytoma. A review of 100 cases. *JAMA* 1966;197(10):754–758.

- Pallor (especially of the face and chest)
- Tremor
- Abdominal mass
- Hypertension and paroxysmal symptoms after abdominal palpation
- Hypertensive retinopathy (grade 1 or 2 in approximately 40% of patients; grade 3 or 4 in approximately 50% of patients)
- Retinal angiomas (von Hippel-Lindau syndrome)
- Hyperplastic corneal nerves (slit lamp exam, MEN2B)
- Mucosal neuromas (MEN2B)
- Marfanoid body habitus (MEN2B)
- Thyroid nodule (MEN2A or 2B)
- Café-au-lait spots (neurofibromatosis)

MANAGEMENT

Diagnostic Evaluation

There are two components to the diagnosis of pheochromocytoma: biochemical confirmation and localization of the tumor. Medications and factors that may complicate evaluation are summarized in Table 15-2.

Biochemical Diagnosis

Pheochromocytoma is diagnosed by demonstrating **elevated levels of catecholamines** (epinephrine and norepinephrine) or **catecholamine metabolites** in plasma or urine. Metanephrines (metanephrine and normetanephrine) and vanillylmandelic acid (VMA) are the diagnostic catecholamine metabolites. Diagnostic studies include

- Plasma catecholamines
- Plasma metanephrines
- 24-hour urine catecholamines, metanephrines, and VMA

Plasma catecholamines should be measured after a patient has been resting supine with a venous catheter in place for at least 30 minutes. Measurements of **24-hour urine catecholamines** and **metanephrines** are generally superior to urine VMA and plasma catecholamines, and they are the most commonly ordered tests. National Institutes of Health investigators have found measurement of plasma free metanephrines the superior modality to screen for both hereditary

TABLE 15-2. CAUSES OF FALSE-POSITIVE CATECHOLAMINES AND METANEPHRINES TESTING

Phenoxybenzamine (Dibenzyline)

Tricyclic antidepressants

Antipsychotics

Beta-blockers

Acetaminophen[a] (Tylenol)

Levodopa (Sinemet)

Ethanol

Withdrawal of clonidine (Catapres) or other antihypertensive agents

Major physiological stress (myocardial infarction, stroke, sleep apnea)

[a]Plasma unconjugated metanephrines measured by high-performance liquid chromatography are unaffected by acetaminophen.
Adapted from Young WF, Kaplan NM. Diagnosis and treatment of pheochromocytoma in adults. In: Rose BD, ed. *UpToDate*. Wellesley, MA: UpToDate, 2003.

TABLE 15-3. PERFORMANCE CHARACTERISTICS OF BIOCHEMICAL ASSAYS
FOR PHEOCHROMOCYTOMA

Test	Sensitivity (%)	Specificity (%)	Sensitivity at 100% specificity (%)
NIH series[a]			
Plasma			
Metanephrines	99	89	82
Catecholamines	85	80	38
Urine			
Metanephrines	76	94	53
Catecholamines	83	88	64
Vanillylmandelic acid	63	94	43
Mayo series[b]			
Plasma metanephrines	97	85	—
24-hr urine metanephrines and catecholamines	90	98	—

[a]Adapted from Pacak K, Linenan WM, Eisenhofer G, et al. Recent advances in genetics, diagnosis, localization, and treatment of pheochromocytoma. *Ann Intern Med* 2001;134:315.
[b]Adapted from Sawka AM, Jaeschke R, Singh RJ, et al. A comparison of biochemical tests for pheochromocytoma: measurement of fractionated plasma metanephrines compared with the combination of 24-hour urinary metanephrines and catecholamines. *J Clin Endocrinol Metab* 2003;88:553.

and sporadic pheochromocytoma. However, Mayo Clinic investigators recommend 24-hour urine metanephrines and catecholamines as an initial screen in the evaluation of sporadic pheochromocytoma due to greater specificity. Performance characteristics of individual tests in both series are summarized in Table 15-3. Biochemical parameters typically are elevated more than 2-fold when a pheochromocytoma is present.

Assays for catecholamines and their metabolites have made pharmacological tests for pheochromocytoma largely unnecessary. The clonidine suppression test and glucagon stimulation test are two that are occasionally helpful.

The **clonidine suppression test** may be useful when plasma catecholamines are elevated but nondiagnostic; a decrease in plasma norepinephrine by >50% is expected, whereas consistently elevated levels suggest pheochromocytoma. False-positive results can occur in patients taking tricyclic antidepressants, beta-blockers, or diuretics. A more than 3-fold rise in plasma norepinephrine after administration of glucagon diagnoses pheochromocytoma with high specificity, but the test has low sensitivity. Premedication with an alpha-adrenergic blocker is necessary to limit the potential pressor response to norepinephrine.

Several medications or diagnostic agents may precipitate a **hypertensive crisis** in the setting of pheochromocytoma (Table 15-4). These should be avoided until pheochromocytoma has been excluded, resected, or the patient has been pre-medicated with an alpha-adrenergic antagonist.

Anatomic Localization

Radiologic evaluation should be initiated only after biochemical diagnosis of pheochromocytoma is confirmed. Tumors are usually located by one or more of the following modalities:

- CT
- MRI
- ^{131}I-metaiodobenzylguanidine (MIBG) scan

TABLE 15-4. MEDICATIONS AND DIAGNOSTIC AGENTS THAT MAY PRECIPITATE HYPERTENSIVE CRISES

Drugs
  Beta-blockers
  MAOIs
  Tricyclic antidepressants
  Phenothiazines
  Metoclopramide (Reglan)
  Opiates
  Atropine
  Glucagon
  Droperidol (Inapsine)
  Sympathomimetic amines
Diagnostic reagents
  Radiographic contrast
  Cosyntropin (Cortrosyn)

- ^{111}In-pentetreotide scan (OctreoScan)
- PET

Because approximately 95% of pheochromocytomas are intraabdominal, an abdominal CT or MRI scan is usually obtained first. Both CT and MRI have high sensitivity (95–100%) but relatively low specificity (approximately 70%) due to detection of adrenal "incidentalomas." Hyperintensity on T2-weighted MRI images may distinguish pheochromocytoma from other adrenal tumors.

If the CT or MRI scan does not detect an intraadrenal tumor, then evaluation for extraadrenal pheochromocytoma should be undertaken with either whole-body CT or MRI imaging or nuclear scintigraphy. MIBG is a substrate for norepinephrine transport that is concentrated in pheochromocytomas. MIBG scans have lower sensitivity (80–90%) but higher specificity (95–100%) than either CT or MRI. An OctreoScan may detect tumors in unusual locations when other modalities have failed, and PET scanning may be useful in identifying metastases. Locations of paragangliomas are summarized in Table 15-5.

TABLE 15-5. LOCATIONS OF PARAGANGLIOMAS

Location	Frequency (%)
Head and neck	3
Thorax	10
Abdomen	
Superior paraaortic ganglia	46
Inferior paraaortic ganglia	29
Bladder	10
Pelvis	2

Adapted from Whalen RK, Althausen AF, Daniels GH. Extra-adrenal pheochromocytoma. *J Urol* 1992;47:1.

Treatment

Surgical resection is the definitive therapy for pheochromocytoma. However, patients must undergo appropriate medical preparation to control the effects of excessive adrenergic stimulation and prevent intraoperative hypertensive crisis. An endocrinologist or other physician experienced in the management of pheochromocytoma should supervise preoperative therapy.

- **Blood pressure control.** Perioperative alpha-adrenergic blockade with phenoxybenzamine (Dibenzyline), is a widely used approach. A starting dose of 10 mg PO qd or bid is titrated until the patient's blood pressure and symptoms are controlled and orthostasis occurs. Volume expansion (e.g., with oral salt supplements or IV fluids) helps minimize hypotension.
- **Heart rate control.** Tachycardia may require treatment with a beta-blocker, but therapy should be withheld until alpha-adrenergic blockade is achieved to prevent a paradoxical rise in blood pressure.

Preoperative treatment with a calcium channel blocker has also been demonstrated to be effective. Metyrosine (Demser) (1–2 g PO daily), an agent that inhibits catecholamine biosynthesis, may be added to phenoxybenzamine therapy and is useful for long-term management of inoperable patients.

Pheochromocytomas have traditionally been resected through a transabdominal approach, but refinements in radiologic localization have permitted an increase in laparoscopic resections through a flank incision. Intraoperative hypertension and cardiac arrhythmias usually occur during anesthesia induction, intubation, or tumor manipulation. Risk factors for **operative complications** include

- Large tumor
- High urine catecholamine and metanephrine levels
- Prolonged surgery and anesthesia

After tumor resection, patients may experience mild hypotension (blood pressure approximately 90/60 mm Hg). Severe hypotension can be avoided with aggressive fluid replacement. Approximately 10–15% of patients experience postoperative hypoglycemia that can be managed by short-term infusion of glucose.

Surgical debulking and chronic medical therapy are used to control symptoms in the setting of **malignant pheochromocytoma**. Radiation therapy may be useful for treatment of symptomatic bone metastases. Combination chemotherapy with cyclophosphamide, vincristine, and dacarbazine or high-dose ^{131}I-MIBG may result in partial responses but is generally of limited value.

Pheochromocytoma is a rare but potentially lethal cause of hypertension during **pregnancy**. Diagnosis is usually confirmed by elevation of urinary catecholamines and metanephrines, and anatomic localization by MRI. Nuclear scintigraphy and stimulation tests are considered unsafe. Women should be prepared for surgery with alpha-adrenergic blockade followed by beta-blockade as necessary for tachycardia. If the diagnosis of pheochromocytoma is made before 24 weeks, gestation, surgical resection is usually performed. After 24 weeks, gestation, medical management is continued until fetal maturation, at which time a combined Cesarean delivery and tumor resection is performed.

Prognosis

Long-term follow-up is indicated in all patients. Catecholamines and metanephrines should be rechecked approximately 1 week after surgery to assess the adequacy of tumor resection by monitoring for a return to the laboratory reference range. If levels are normal, patients should be screened annually for 5 years and biannually thereafter or if symptoms suspicious for pheochromocytoma recur. Patients with familial tumor syndromes, bilateral tumors, or paragangliomas should be monitored annually. In one large series, pheochromocytoma recurred as a benign or malignant tumor in 14% of patients with an apparently benign tumor at the time of surgical resection. Hypertension-free survival in patients without recurrence was 74% at 5 years and 45% at 10 years. Survival does not appear to be affected by the site of the tumor. Patients with malignant pheochromocytoma have a 5-year survival of approximately 40%.

KEY POINTS TO REMEMBER

- Pheochromocytomas are catecholamine hypersecreting tumors of neurochromaffin cells in the adrenal medulla. Neurochromaffin tumors arising in sympathetic ganglia are called paragangliomas.
- Pheochromocytomas cause hypertension, often severe. Patients may experience a classic triad of paroxysmal symptoms that includes severe headache, diaphoresis, and palpitations.
- Pheochromocytoma is diagnosed by measuring elevations of plasma or urine catecholamines and their metabolites, normetanephrine and metanephrine (collectively called metanephrines).
- Tumors are typically located by MRI or CT imaging. Pheochromocytomas have a characteristic bright appearance on T2-weighted MRI images. Nuclear scintigraphy is sometimes required when MRI or CT does not identify a tumor.
- Surgery is the only cure for pheochromocytomas and paragangliomas. Patients must be prepared for surgery by alpha-adrenergic blockade or combined alpha- and beta-adrenergic blockade to avoid hypertensive crises during resection.

REFERENCES AND SUGGESTED READINGS

Dluhy RG, Lawrence JE, Williams GH. Endocrine hypertension. In: Larsen PR, Kronenberg HM, Melmed S, et al., eds. *Williams textbook of endocrinology*, 10th ed. Philadelphia: WB Saunders, 2003:552–585.

Eisenhofer G, Lenders JW, Linehan WM, et al. Plasma normetanephrine and metanephrine for detecting pheochromocytoma in von Hippel-Lindau disease and multiple endocrine neoplasia type 2. *N Engl J Med* 1999;340:1872.

Eisenhofer G, Lenders JW, Pacak K. Biochemical diagnosis of pheochromocytoma. *Front Horm Res* 2004;31:76.

Gimm O, Koch CA, Januszewicz A, et al. The genetic basis of pheochromocytoma. *Front Horm Res* 2004;31:45.

Goldstein RE, O'Neill JA Jr, Holcomb GW III, et al. Clinical experience over 48 years with pheochromocytoma. *Ann Surg* 1999;229:755.

Ilias S, Pacak K. Current approaches and recommended algorithm for the diagnostic localization of pheochomocytoma. *J Clin Endocrinol Metab* 2004;89:479.

Kinney MA, Warner ME, vaHeerden JA, et al. Perianesthetic risks and outcomes of pheochromocytoma and paraganglioma resections. *Anesth Analg* 2000;91:1118.

Neumann HP, Berger DP, Sigmund G, et al. Pheochromocytomas, multiple endocrine neoplasia type 2, and von Hippel-Lindau disease. *N Engl J Med* 1993;329:1531.

Pacak K, Linehan WM, Eisenhofer G, et al. Recent advances in genetics, diagnosis, localization, and treatment of pheochromocytoma. *Ann Intern Med* 2001;134:315.

Plouin PF, Chatellier G, Fofol I, et al. Tumor recurrence and hypertension persistence after successful pheochomocytoma surgery. *Hypertension* 1997;29:1133.

Roden M, Raffesberg W, Raber W, et al. Quantification of unconjugated metanephrines in human plasma without interference by acetaminophen. *Clin Chem* 2001;47(6):1061–1067.

Roman S. Pheochromocytoma and functional paraganglioma. *Curr Opin Oncol* 2004;16:8.

Sawka AM, Jaeschke R, Singh RJ, et al. A comparison of biochemical tests for pheochromocytoma: measurement of fractionated plasma metanephrines compared with the combination of 24-hour urinary metanephrines and catecholamines. *J Clin Endocrinol Metab* 2003;88:553.

Thomas JE, Rooke ED, Kvale WF. The neurologist's experience with pheochromocytoma. A review of 100 cases. *JAMA* 1966;197(10):754–758.

Ulchaker JC, Goldfarb DA, Bravo EL, et al. Successful outcomes in pheochromocytoma surgery in the modern era. *J Urol* 1999;161:764.

Young WF, Kaplan NM. Diagnosis and treatment of pheochromocytoma in adults. In: Rose BD, ed. *UpToDate*. Wellesley, MA: UpToDate, 2003.

IV

Gonadal Disorders

16

Amenorrhea

Bharathi Raju and
Subramaniam Pennathur

INTRODUCTION

Beginning in puberty, pulsatile gonadotropin-releasing hormone (GnRH) production stimulates secretion and release of luteinizing hormone (LH) and follicle-stimulating hormone (FSH) from the pituitary gland. FSH, in turn, stimulates ovarian follicles to develop. The follicle with the most FSH receptors becomes the dominant follicle, whereas the remaining follicles eventually undergo atresia. The thecal cells surrounding the follicles produce androgens, which are aromatized to **estradiol** by neighboring granulosa cells. As the follicles develop, estradiol levels increase. The increasing level of estradiol provides negative feedback to the pituitary to suppress FSH. As FSH concentrations decrease, most of the follicles undergo atresia, whereas the dominant follicle persists.

LH concentration increases under the influence of estradiol. Granulosa cells express LH receptors, and the increasing level of LH stimulates them to produce **progesterone**. The combination of estradiol and progesterone promotes a midcycle surge in LH. Approximately 36 hours after the LH surge, the oocyte is released from the dominant follicle at the surface of the ovary. The granulosa cells continue to produce progesterone for approximately 14 days after ovulation, but then involute unless pregnancy is established, in which case chorionic gonadotropin maintains the corpus luteum. The decline in estradiol and progesterone results in sloughing of the endometrium and the onset of menses.

Disturbance of this cycle at any level—the hypothalamus, pituitary, uterus, or ovary—can lead to disruption of the normal menstrual cycle, including cessation of menses.

Puberty is characterized by onset of regular menstrual cycles and development of secondary sexual features. The average time between the onset of thelarche (breast development) and menarche (onset of menses) is 2 years. The age of menarche is variable depending on genetic and socioeconomic factors. The mean age of menarche in the United States is approximately 12 years.

An average adult **menstrual cycle** lasts approximately 28 days and usually has little cycle variability between the ages of 20 and 40 years. There is considerably more variation in a woman's menstrual cycle for the first 5–7 years after menarche and for the last 10 years before menopause.

The mean age of **menopause** in the United States is 51 years but may occur earlier in women who smoke, have never had children, or have a family history of early menopause. Cessation of menses before age 40 years is generally considered to be premature menopause. The 2–8 years before menopause are often characterized by irregular menses and breakthrough bleeding, as the normal ovulatory cycle is interspersed with anovulatory cycles of varying length.

Definition

Amenorrhea is defined as the absence of menses. Amenorrhea is further subdivide into primary or secondary amenorrhea.

Primary amenorrhea is defined as the absence of menarche by age 14 years in g without other signs of secondary sexual development, or by age 16 years in the r ence of otherwise normal secondary sexual development.

Secondary amenorrhea is defined as the absence of menses for >3 cycles or for 6 months in women who have previously experienced spontaneous menses.

CAUSES

Primary Amenorrhea

Primary amenorrhea usually results from an anatomic or genetic abnormality (Table 16-1), although most causes of secondary amenorrhea may also present as primary amenorrhea.

The most common cause of primary amenorrhea is chromosomal abnormalities causing **gonadal dysgenesis** (45%). Congenital anatomic lesions of reproductive organs account for approximately 20% of primary amenorrhea. Menses cannot occur without an intact reproductive tract, including the uterus, cervix, and vagina. An imperforate hymen can lead to obstruction of menstrual blood flow and lack of menses, and patients present with complaints of amenorrhea and cyclical abdominal pain.

Abnormal müllerian development secondary to various syndromes, such as androgen insensitivity syndrome and vanishing testes syndrome, can lead to primary amenorrhea. Patients with complete androgen insensitivity syndrome (also referred to as testicular feminization) are characterized by 46XY karyotype and appear as phenotypically normal women, including breast development, but have absence of the uterus, fallopian tubes, and the upper two-thirds of the vagina. The syndrome is caused by a defect in the androgen receptor that results in resistance to the actions of testosterone. The external genitalia appear to be female, although the testes can often be palpated in the labia or inguinal region.

Enzyme deficiencies causing abnormalities in steroidogenesis, such as 5 alpha-reductase deficiency or 17 alpha-hydroxylase deficiency, may be apparent at birth but are often more obvious when the patient manifests delayed pubertal development.

The most common ovarian causes of primary amenorrhea are **polycystic ovary syndrome (PCOS)** (see Chap. 20, Polycystic Ovary Syndrome) and **Turner's syndrome**. Turner's syndrome is due to absence of one of the X chromosomes (45XO). The patients

TABLE 16-1. CAUSES OF PRIMARY AMENORRHEA

Congenital anatomic lesions

    Complete or partial agenesis of the müllerian structures (uterus, fallopian tubes, upper one-third of vagina) due to various syndromes such as androgen insensitivity syndrome or vanishing testes syndrome

    Enzyme deficiencies causing abnormalities in steroidogenesis (5 alpha-reductase deficiency or 17 alpha-hydroxylase deficiency)

    Outflow obstruction (imperforate hymen or transverse vaginal septum)

Physiologic

    Physiologic delay of puberty

    Pregnancy

Ovarian etiologies

    Turner's syndrome (45XO)

    Polycystic ovary syndrome

Gonadotropin deficiency

    Idiopathic hypogonadotrophic hypogonadism or Kallmann's syndrome

    Damage to hypothalamus or pituitary from trauma, mass effect (adenoma, craniopharyngioma), infarction (Sheehan's syndrome), infiltrative or inflammatory diseases (sarcoidosis, lymphocytic hypophysitis)

    Functional hypothalamic amenorrhea (exercise, eating disorders, stress)

have normal development of external female genitalia, uterus, and fallopian tubes until puberty when there is failure of sexual maturation due to lack of estrogen.

There are multiple **hypothalamic causes** of primary amenorrhea, including functional hypothalamic amenorrhea, tumors, infiltrative lesions, and infections. Congenital GnRH deficiency due to idiopathic hypogonadotropic hypogonadism (IHH) or Kallmann's syndrome causes amenorrhea due to deficiency or absence of GnRH secretion. Kallmann's syndrome is associated with anosmia, which distinguishes it from IHH. Functional amenorrhea is due to abnormal GnRH secretion, resulting in subsequent low GnRH pulsations, decreased serum LH, absent LH surge, anovulation, and low serum estradiol. Anorexia nervosa, stress, and exercise are some of the common causes of functional hypothalamic amenorrhea. Infiltrative diseases and tumors, such as craniopharyngioma, germinoma, and histiocytosis, can cause either primary or secondary amenorrhea, depending on the age at which they present.

Hyperprolactinemia, whether from a pituitary adenoma or secondary source, can cause primary or secondary amenorrhea and may be associated with galactorrhea.

Physiologic causes, such as pregnancy or physiologic delay of puberty, should always be considered in the evaluation of primary amenorrhea.

Secondary Amenorrhea

Pregnancy is the most common cause of secondary amenorrhea. After pregnancy, ovarian disease (40%) and hypothalamic dysfunction (35%) are also common causes. Certainly, if the woman is of a typical age and/or manifests the usual associated symptoms (e.g., hot flashes, vaginal dryness), physiologic menopause should be considered.

Hyperandrogenism from any source can lead to ovarian failure and amenorrhea due to chronic anovulation. The most common example of this is PCOS and is covered in Chap. 20, Polycystic Ovary Syndrome. Other, less common, ovarian etiologies include ovarian tumors, premature ovarian failure (idiopathic, autoimmune, radiation, chemotherapy), and mosaic Turner's syndrome. Adrenal carcinoma may also present with signs and symptoms of hyperandrogenism and virilization.

All of the **hypothalamic lesions** that cause primary amenorrhea except congenital GnRH deficiency can also cause secondary amenorrhea. Of all of the hypothalamic etiologies, the most common cause of secondary amenorrhea is functional hypothalamic amenorrhea. Other less common hypothalamic causes are listed in Table 16-2.

Prolactin-secreting pituitary tumors are also a fairly common cause of secondary amenorrhea, comprising almost 20% of cases. Other, less common, pituitary causes of secondary amenorrhea are listed in Table 16-2.

Primary **hypothyroidism** can cause amenorrhea via thyrotroph and/or lactotroph hyperplasia and hyperprolactinemia.

PRESENTATION

Evaluation of Amenorrhea

History
A careful history includes

* Age of menarche
* Frequency and length of previous menstrual cycles
* Number of pregnancies and any complications
* Family history of pubertal development (e.g., physiologic delay of puberty)
* Symptoms of estrogen deficiency (e.g., hot flashes, vaginal dryness, decreased libido)
* Symptoms of endocrine diseases (e.g., hypothyroidism, galactorrhea)
* Symptoms of mass effect (e.g., headache, visual disturbance)
* Weight changes
* Dietary habits
* Exercise regimen
* Medication or drug use
* Gynecologic surgery/instrumentation or infection

TABLE 16-2. CAUSES OF SECONDARY AMENORRHEA

Physiologic
  Pregnancy
  Menopause
Ovarian etiologies
  Polycystic ovary syndrome
  Premature ovarian failure
  Mosaic Turner's syndrome
Uterine etiologies
  Asherman's syndrome (acquired scarring of the endometrial lining)
Pituitary etiologies
  PRL-secreting pituitary tumor
  Other nonlactotrophic pituitary adenomas
  Empty sella syndrome
  Pituitary infarction (Sheehan's syndrome)
  Infiltrative lesions (lymphocytic hypophysitis)
  Radiation
Hypothalamic etiologies
  Functional hypothalamic amenorrhea (exercise, anorexia, stress)
  Infiltrative diseases of the hypothalamus (sarcoidosis, lymphoma, Langerhans' cell histiocytosis, hemochromatosis)
Endocrine disorders
  Primary hypothyroidism
  Hyperprolactinemia from cause other than PRL-secreting pituitary tumor (e.g., medication induced)
  Late-onset congenital adrenal hyperplasia

PRL, prolactin.

Physical Exam
Physical exam should include weight, height, breast exam, and pelvic exam. Be alert for signs of galactorrhea, hirsutism, and virilization (male pattern balding, deepening voice, clitoral enlargement). Note the stage of pubertal development in adolescents.

Patients with **hirsutism** should have a free serum testosterone level checked, because a mildly elevated testosterone level in this setting is most commonly associated with PCOS (see Chap. 18, Hirsutism). A 17-hydroxyprogesterone level can also be measured if late-onset congenital adrenal hyperplasia is suspected (see Chap. 12, Adult Congenital Adrenal Hyperplasia).

Signs of **virilization** on physical exam should always prompt further evaluation for an androgen-secreting tumor. Testosterone and dehydroepiandrosterone sulfate (DHEA-S) should be measured, and, if elevated (total testosterone, >200 ng/dL; DHEA-S, >600 mcg/dL), appropriate imaging should be ordered.

Absence of müllerian structures on exam can be confirmed with ultrasound and should prompt further evaluation with a karyotype analysis and serum testosterone level.

Laboratory Evaluation
Rule out preganancy by checking **beta-human chorionic gonadotropin (hCG)**. If the beta-hCG is negative, other basic lab tests should include **thyroid-stimulating hormone (TSH), prolactin (PRL) level, and FSH**.

• An elevated FSH level suggests a gonadal cause, whereas a low FSH level points to a central cause.
• Further evaluation and management for women with hyperprolactinemia is discussed in Chap. 2, Prolactinoma.
• Evaluation and treatment for patients with primary hypothyroidism is covered in Chap. 9, Hypothyroidism.

ELEVATED FSH LEVELS. If the FSH level is elevated, this suggests a **primary ovarian etiology.** In the setting of primary amenorrhea, a karyotype analysis should be performed to rule out a chromosomal abnormality such as Turner's syndrome.

In the setting of secondary amenorrhea, a karyotype analysis should also be performed to rule out mosaic Turner's syndrome unless there is a clear etiology for premature ovarian failure such as prior radiation, prior chemotherapy, or the patient is of an appropriate age and has associated symptoms to diagnose physiologic menopause.

NORMAL OR LOW FSH LEVELS. Inappropriately normal or low FSH levels suggest the possibility of hypogonadotropic hypogonadism, and a cranial MRI is indicated to rule out a hypothalamic or pituitary lesion unless other conditions are present that explain low gonadotropin levels (e.g., hypothyroidism).

In women who have normal hormone levels and a history of uterine infection or instrumentation, the possibility of outflow obstruction (Asherman's syndrome) should be addressed with a progestin challenge (medroxyprogesterone, 10 mg PO daily × 10 days). Withdrawal bleeding in response to progestin rules out a uterine outflow tract obstruction. In the context of an elevated LH level and hirsutism, withdrawal bleeding after progestin challenge suggests PCOS. Failure to respond to the progestin challenge with bleeding suggests either inadequate estrogen production to support endometrial proliferation or outflow tract obstruction. To differentiate these possibilities, the challenge is repeated with a combination of estrogen and progesterone (estradiol, 0.625 mg PO daily × 35 days, with medroxyprogesterone, 10 mg PO daily for days 26–35). Failure to bleed in response to this combination regimen strongly suggests outflow obstruction and should lead to anatomic investigation by hysterosalpingogram or hysteroscopy. Some patients with hypogonadotropic hypogonadism fail to bleed in response to the combination challenge.

TREATMENT

Treatment for amenorrhea is directed at correcting the underlying etiology and, if possible and desired, achieving fertility.

Patients with a congenital or genetic cause for their primary amenorrhea should be counseled about the underlying cause and their potential for achieving sexual maturation and reproduction. Restoration of fertility is not possible for patients with gonadal failure, so therapy should be directed at helping the patient to achieve sexual maturation and induction of menses. Induction of puberty should be pursued under the direction of a specialist because the timing of menarche can greatly effect epiphyseal closure and final height. Patients with congenital anatomic abnormalities may require surgical correction. Patients with Y chromosomal material and residual testes should have their testes excised after puberty due to the increased risk of testicular cancer after age 25 years.

Correcting the precipitating factors for functional hypothalamic disorders usually restores the normal menstrual cycle. Ovulation and fertility can often be restored in patients with hypothalamic amenorrhea through administration of pulsatile GnRH therapy. GnRH is injected every 1–2 hours by a programmable pump to simulate endogenous GnRH secretion. Treatment with pulsatile GnRH achieves fertility in approximately 90% of women after 6 cycles and carries a low risk of multiple pregnancies.

Patients with anovulation due to pituitary disease do not respond to GnRH therapy and require therapy with exogenous gonadotropins if fertility is desired. Pure recombinant FSH and LH can be used in an effort to achieve fertility, but this should only be done under the direction of an experienced specialist, and patients should be warned that the chances of having a multiple pregnancy with this method are high.

Patients with either hypothalamic or pituitary disease who do not desire fertility and patients with secondary ovarian failure can simply be treated with hormone replacement therapy until the age of menopause, at which time continuing hormone replacement becomes controversial and will need to be addressed on an individual basis. The goals for these women are to avoid the risk of endometrial hyperplasia by inducing a withdrawal bleed at least once every 3 months, and to alleviate the symptoms and sequelae of a chronic low-estrogen state, including loss of bone mineral density.

Specific therapy for PCOS is discussed in Chap. 20, Polycystic Ovary Syndrome, and is aimed at controlling hirsutism, resuming menstruation, achieving fertility, and avoiding long-term sequelae of PCOS (endometrial hyperplasia, dyslipidemia, and glucose intolerance). Management for patients with hyperprolactinemia or prolactinoma is discussed in Chap. 2, Prolactinoma.

KEY POINTS TO REMEMBER

- Amenorrhea is a symptom, not a diagnosis, and requires investigation into the underlying cause.
- The first step in the evaluation of either primary or secondary amenorrhea should be to rule out pregnancy.
- A careful history and physical exam can often narrow down the differential diagnosis for amenorrhea.
- Signs of virilization should always prompt an evaluation for an androgen-secreting tumor.
- If the underlying cause of amenorrhea cannot be reversed, treatment should be aimed at alleviating the symptoms of chronic hypoestrogenemia, avoiding the long-term sequelae of hypoestrogenemia, and, if possible and desired, achieving fertility.

REFERENCES AND SUGGESTED READINGS

Baird DT. Amenorrhea. *Lancet* 1997;350:275–279.

Barbieri RL. Causes of and diagnostic approach to secondary amenorrhea. In: Rose BD, ed. *UpToDate*. Wellesley, MA: UpToDate, 2003.

Casper RF. Diagnosis and clinical manifestations of menopause. In: Rose BD, ed. *UpToDate*. Wellesley, MA: UpToDate, 2003.

Crowley WF Jr, Jameson JL Jr. Clinical counterpoint: gonadotropin-releasing hormone deficiency: perspectives from clinical investigation. *Endocr Rev* 1992;13:635.

Groff TR, Shulkin BL, Utiger RD, et al. Amenorrhea, galactorrhea, hyperprolactinemia, and suprasellar pituitary enlargement as presenting features of primary hypothyroidism. *Obstet Gynecol* 1984;63:86S.

Marshall JC, et al. Hypothalamic dysfunction. *Molec Cell Endocrinol* 2001;183:29–32.

Martin KA, Taylor AE. The normal menstrual cycle. In: *UpToDate*. Rose BD, ed. Wellesley, MA: UpToDate, 2003.

McIver B, Romanski SA, Nippoldt TB. Evaluation and management of amenorrhea. *Mayo Clin Proc* 1997;72:1161–1169.

Santoro N, Filicori M, Crowley WF. Hypogonadotropic disorders in men and women: diagnosis and therapy with pulsatile gonadotropin-releasing hormone. *Endocr Rev* 1986;7:11.

Taylor AE, Barbieri RL. Causes of and diagnostic approach to primary amenorrhea. In: Rose BD, ed. *UpToDate*. Wellesley, MA: UpToDate, 2003.

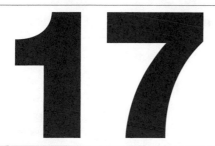

Gynecomastia

Subramaniam Pennathur

INTRODUCTION

Enlargement of the male breast is termed **gynecomastia**. Histologically, there is proliferation of glandular tissue of the breast. Often, this can be part of normal physiologic response, but several pathologic states can result in gynecomastia. True gynecomastia needs to be differentiated from **pseudogynecomastia**, which occurs in obese men and is characterized by adipose tissue deposition without proliferation of glandular tissue.

CAUSES

The key causes of gynecomastia are summarized in Table 17-1. Breast growth in men is primarily mediated by estrogen. Many disorders that result in gynecomastia are characterized by an imbalance between circulating androgens and estrogens. Mechanisms include excess production of estrogen or a deficient production of androgens. There could also be an elevation of estrogenic precursors or androgen resistance. The role of prolactin (PRL) in the pathogenesis of gynecomastia is minimal, and patients with hyperprolactinemia typically do not develop gynecomastia. PRL can indirectly cause gynecomastia by suppressing gonadal function, thus altering the androgen to estrogen ratio. This effect, however, is less common.

Physiologic Gynecomastia

Newborns can develop physiologic gynecomastia due to high levels of circulating estrogen during pregnancy. This typically regresses a few weeks after birth. Pubertal gynecomastia typically occurs in adolescents around puberty (median age, 14 years). It can be asymmetric, often tender, and regresses within a few years. Gynecomastia of aging can occur in otherwise healthy older men (50–80 years), and drug therapy may be a contributing factor.

Pathologic Gynecomastia

Pathologic gynecomastia can occur through several different mechanisms.

Decreased Production/Effect of Androgens

Primary hypogonadism (reviewed in Chap. 19, Male Hypogonadism) can be due to a congenital abnormality, such as Klinefelter's syndrome, or enzymatic defects in the testosterone biosynthesis pathway. Other causes include trauma, infection, or androgen resistance. The net effect is an alteration of the androgen to estrogen ratio and gynecomastia. Primary hypogonadism is more likely to be associated with gynecomastia than the secondary form, probably due to the effect of the supranormal serum luteinizing hormone (LH) and follicle-stimulating hormone (FSH) concentrations on testicular aromatase activity. Secondary hypogonadism can also be associated with gynecomastia, but less frequently.

TABLE 17-1. CAUSES OF GYNECOMASTIA

Physiologic causes

  Newborn

  Pubertal

  Aging

Pathologic causes

  Decreased production/action of androgens: Klinefelter's syndrome, defects in testosterone synthesis, androgen resistance, trauma, viral orchitis

  Increased estrogen production: testicular tumors, carcinomas producing hCG, true hermaphroditism, feminizing adrenal carcinomas

  Drugs: antiandrogens [spironolactone (Aldactone), finasteride (Propecia)], estrogens and their analogues, gonadotropins, calcium blockers, ACE inhibitors, tricyclic antidepressants, diazepam, omeprazole (Prilosec), cimetidine (Tagamet), ranitidine (Zantac), alkylating agents, antiretroviral agents, androgens, phenytoin (Dilantin), phenothiazines, ketoconazole, and anabolic steroids

  Systemic illness: cirrhosis, renal failure, thyrotoxicosis, malnutrition

  Refeeding after starvation

  Idiopathic

hCG, human chorionic gonadotropin.
Adapted from Wilson JD. Endocrine disorders of the breast. In: Braunwald E, et al., eds. *Harrison's principles of internal medicine*, 15th ed. New York: McGraw-Hill, 2002:2170–2172.

Increased Production of Estrogen

Germ cell tumors of the testes or bronchogenic carcinomas can secrete human chorionic gonadotropin (hCG), which can stimulate estrogen production, leading to gynecomastia. Patients with true hermaphroditism can have increased estrogen production from ovarian elements in their gonads. Leydig and Sertoli cell tumors of the testes and feminizing adrenocortical carcinomas can also lead to increased estrogen secretion.

Drugs

Drugs can cause gynecomastia via several mechanisms. Estrogen and its analogues and gonadotropins directly increase estrogenic activity in the plasma. Antiandrogens, such as spironolactone (Aldactone), can block androgen receptors, thereby altering the androgen to estrogen ratio. Some drugs, such as alkylating agents and ketoconazole (Nizoral), can suppress testosterone biosynthesis. Finally, the mechanisms through which certain drugs induce gynecomastia remain to be determined. Examples in this category include tricyclic antidepressants, diazepam (Valium), and antiretroviral agents.

Systemic Illnesses

Roughly two-thirds of patients with cirrhosis have gynecomastia. There is an increased production of androstenedione from the adrenals in patients with cirrhosis as well as enhanced aromatization to estrone and estradiol. Serum testosterone levels are lower in patients with advanced renal failure who are on dialysis, and up to 50% of these patients may have gynecomastia. Gynecomastia is also associated with malnutrition, refeeding syndrome, and thyrotoxicosis.

MANAGEMENT

Diagnostic Evaluation

A careful history and physical exam should be performed in all patients and will reveal the etiology in most patients. The history should focus on timing of the gynecomastia, presence of pain, history of pubertal development, and symptoms of systemic illnesses such as liver disease, renal disease, or thyrotoxicosis. A careful drug history is very important and should be obtained in all patients.

When performing the physical exam, it is important to first differentiate between gynecomastia and pseudogynecomastia by exam of the areolar tissue; true gynecomastia is characterized by a symmetric ridge of glandular tissue. If the patient is a peripubertal boy with a normal physical and genital exam, reevaluation at 6 months is appropriate as this likely represents pubertal physiologic gynecomastia. Further testing can be carried out if there is no improvement in 6 months. Physical exam should focus on the testes. If the testicular volume is diminished, a karyotype analysis would be appropriate. A workup of testicular tumor is warranted if the exam reveals asymmetric testes.

If the patient has symptoms or signs of liver disease, renal disease, hypogonadism, or thyrotoxicosis, further laboratory diagnosis of these specific etiologies should be pursued.

If the gynecomastia is of recent onset, painful, or tender, an extensive evaluation is warranted. If there is a firm or hard breast mass, a biopsy should be performed to rule out breast cancer. Gynecomastia associated with features of androgen deficiency should be investigated. If, however, the gynecomastia is asymptomatic and discovered on routine exam in a patient with no underlying disease or drug intake, a more conservative approach with periodic follow-up is appropriate.

Laboratory Evaluation

- Plasma **LH** and **testosterone**. An elevated LH and low testosterone is consistent with primary hypogonadism. If LH and testosterone levels are low, it is consistent with secondary hypogonadism, provided PRL levels are normal. If PRL is elevated in this setting, it implies that hyperprolactinemia is the cause of the consequent hypogonadism. An increase in both LH and testosterone is consistent with androgen resistance.
- An elevated **beta-hCG** level is consistent with an hCG-secreting neoplasm. Further evaluation should include testicular ultrasound to rule out testicular germ cell tumors. CT scanning may localize an extragonadal germ cell tumor or bronchogenic carcinoma.
- An elevated **estradiol** level should be investigated with a testicular ultrasound to rule out a Leydig or Sertoli cell tumor. If the ultrasound is normal, an adrenal CT or MRI is indicated to rule out an adrenal neoplasm. 24-Hour urinary 17-ketosteroids levels are elevated in adrenocortical carcinoma. If the adrenal imaging studies are negative, workup should focus on causes of increased extraglandular aromatase activity.
- If none of the above workup is revealing, a diagnosis of **idiopathic gynecomastia** may be entertained.

Treatment

When an underlying cause for the gynecomastia is identified, **correction of the cause** typically corrects the problem. For example, hormonal replacement therapy in hypogonadal men improves gynecomastia. Withdrawal of the offending drug can correct gynecomastia in some cases. However, if the gynecomastia is long-standing and the glandular proliferation has been replaced by fibrosis, correction of the primary disorder may not lead to resolution. **Surgery** is the best available therapy in such instances and when the primary cause cannot be corrected. Surgical correction is also indicated in patients who have continued growth and tenderness of the breast, when malignancy is suspected, or for cosmetic problems. In addition to avoidance of an offending agent, several strategies can be helpful in reducing incidence of drug-induced gynecomastia. A 3-month trial of **antiestrogens**, such as tamoxifen (Nolvadex), in patients with painful gynecomastia may cause partial or complete remission and is a reasonable therapeutic option before referring patients for surgery.

KEY POINTS TO REMEMBER

- Gynecomastia is caused by an imbalance between circulating levels of androgens and estrogens.
- A careful drug history should be obtained in all patients presenting with gynecomastia.
- A thorough physical exam includes careful palpation of the breast tissue looking for tenderness or masses, evaluation for testicular volume and masses, and evaluation for systemic illness such as cirrhosis, renal failure, and thyrotoxicosis.
- Further laboratory evaluation may include plasma LH, testosterone, beta-hCG, and estradiol levels.
- Testicular ultrasound and adrenal CT or MRI may be needed to rule out neoplasm.
- A diagnosis of idiopathic gynecomastia should only be entertained after other causes have been ruled out.
- Correction of the underlying cause usually results in resolution of the gynecomastia.

REFERENCES AND SUGGESTED READINGS

Braunstein GD. Gynecomastia. *N Engl J Med* 1993;328:490.

Braunstein GD, Glassman H. Gynecomastia. In: Bardin CW, ed. *Current therapy in endocrinology and metabolism*, 6th ed. Philadelphia: Mosby, 1997.

Carlson HE. Gynecomastia. *N Engl J Med* 1980;303:795.

Freeman RM, Lawton RL, Fearing MO. Gynecomastia: an endocrinologic complication of hemodialysis. *Ann Intern Med* 1968;69:67.

Gordon GG, Olivo J, Fereidoon R, et al. Conversion of androgens to estrogen in cirrhosis of the liver. *J Clin Endocrinol Metab* 1975;40:1018.

Parker LN, Gray DR, Lai MK, et al. Treatment of gynecomastia with tamoxifen: a double-blind crossover study. *Metabolism* 1986;35:705.

Staiman VR, Lowe FC. Tamoxifen for flutamide/finasteride-induced gynecomastia. *Urology* 1997;50:929.

Waterfall NB, Glaser MG. A study of the effects of radiation on prevention of gynecomastia due to estrogen therapy. *Clin Oncol* 1979;5:257.

Wilson JD. Endocrine disorders of the breast. In: Braunwald E, et al., eds. *Harrison's principles of internal medicine*, 15th ed. New York: McGraw-Hill, 2002:2170–2172.

18

Hirsutism

Subramaniam Pennathur

INTRODUCTION

Hirsutism is defined as excessive male-pattern, androgen-dependent terminal hair (pigmented, long, and coarse) growth in women. In men, terminal hair is normally seen on the face, chest, back, and abdomen. Although the true prevalence of hirsutism remains unclear, roughly 10% of women of reproductive age have hirsutism. The most common causes of hirsutism are polycystic ovary syndrome (PCOS) and idiopathic hirsutism. Hirsutism can often be mild, reflecting a variant of normal hair growth. However, it may also represent a more serious underlying disorder. Hirsutism is commonly associated with other cutaneous manifestations such as acne and male-pattern balding. **Virilization** is characterized by deepening of the voice, increased muscle mass, clitoromegaly, and breast atrophy. Although hirsutism occasionally warrants further workup, virilization must be investigated for ominous causes such as adrenal or ovarian neoplasms.

Genetic factors, race, and ethnicity of the patient should be considered in determining the definition of "normal" hair growth. Women of Mediterranean origin tend to have greater hair growth, whereas Native American and Asian women tend to have less hair. Dark-haired individuals tend, in general, to have more hair than blonde women. Family history is also an important factor in discerning what is normal for a particular individual. Any change in pattern or quality of hair growth irrespective of ethnicity is an important consideration.

CAUSES

Causes of hirsutism are listed in Table 18-1. Although **androgen excess** (usually testosterone) underlies most cases of hirsutism, there is not a good correlation between androgen levels and the degree of hirsutism. This is due to variability of end-organ sensitivity and local factors and rate of conversion of testosterone to dihydrotestosterone (DHT). Soft, nonpigmented vellus hair (called lanugo hair in infants) is androgen-independent and does not represent true hirsutism. Similarly **hypertrichosis**, a condition in which there is an increase in total body hair (androgen-independent vellus hair in nonsexual areas) can be associated with some metabolic disorders and adverse effects of some drugs and does not represent true hirsutism.

Polycystic Ovary Syndrome

PCOS is the most common cause of hyperandrogenism in women of the reproductive age group. The minimum criteria for this diagnosis proposed by the National Institutes of Health consensus conference include menstrual irregularity and clinical or biochemical evidence of hyperandrogenism. The onset of menstrual abnormality is usually in the peripubertal period. The clinical features, diagnosis, and management of PCOS are discussed in Chap. 20, Polycystic Ovary Syndrome.

Idiopathic Hirsutism

Idiopathic hirsutism refers to hirsute women with no other clinical abnormality and no identifiable underlying disorder. Menstrual cycles are normal in these women. It

TABLE 18-1. CAUSES OF HIRSUTISM

Common causes
    Polycystic ovary syndrome (PCOS)
    Idiopathic
Other causes (less common)
    Ovarian
        Ovarian neoplasms
        Insulin resistance syndromes
    Adrenal
        Classic and nonclassic congenital adrenal hyperplasia
        Adrenal neoplasms
        Premature adrenarche
    Drugs
        Oral contraceptives containing androgenic progestins
        Cyclosporine (Gengraf), minoxidil, diazoxide, androgens, phenytoin (Dilantin)
    Other endocrine disorders
        Hyperprolactinemia, Cushing's syndrome
    Miscellaneous
        Increased peripheral androgen production obesity
        Pregnancy

Adapted from Ehrmann DA. Hirsutism and virilization. In: Braunwald E, et al., eds. *Harrison's principles of internal medicine*, 15th ed. New York: McGraw-Hill, 2001:297–301.

may represent a milder form of PCOS, but the absence of irregular menses distinguishes this disorder from PCOS.

Ovarian Causes

An androgen-secreting tumor of the ovary usually occurs later in life and progresses rapidly. Sertoli-Leydig cell tumors, hilus cell tumors, and granulose-theca cell tumors can cause hyperandrogenism. Serum testosterone levels are significantly elevated and are usually >150 ng/dL. Marked hyperinsulinemia occurring with insulin resistance syndromes can promote ovarian hyperandrogenism.

Adrenal Causes

Adrenal neoplasms are rare causes of hirsutism. Rare adenomas can secrete testosterone. However, most are carcinomas that secrete dehydroepiandrosterone sulfate (DHEA-S). Some adrenal tumors secrete both androgen and cortisol, so signs of Cushing's syndrome and androgen excess can be present in the same patient. A high level of DHEA-S suggests the diagnosis of adrenal carcinoma. Excess androgen production is also a feature of congenital adrenal hyperplasia (CAH). The nonclassic form of CAH, which is usually due to 21-hydroxylase deficiency, results in excess production of 17-hydroxyprogesterone and androstenedione, which in turn result in hirsutism and, sometimes, menstrual irregularity.

Other Causes

Some women with hyperprolactinemia can have hirsutism. Drugs listed in Table 18-1 can cause hirsutism. Therefore, a careful drug history should be obtained in all patients evaluated for hirsutism.

PRESENTATION

History

Key features in history that are helpful in assessment include the age and time of onset of symptoms, rate of progression, associated features, such as acne or frontal balding, and symptoms of virilization. Rapid progression and signs of virilization usually are ominous and may indicate ovarian or adrenal neoplasms.

Irregular menses usually indicates an ovarian cause of hyperandrogenism. Galactorrhea may indicate hyperprolactinemia. Weight gain, striae, hypertension, and easy bruising can suggest Cushing's syndrome. A careful drug history should be obtained from all patients.

Physical Exam

Physical exam should include measurement of height, weight, calculation of BMI, and blood pressure. An objective assessment of hair distribution and quality of hair should be noted. A simple scoring scale, such as the modified scale of Ferriman and Gallwey in which a scoring system of 0–4 is used for each of 9 androgen-dependent sites, can be used. (See Ehrmann DA. Hirsutism and virilization. In: Braunwald E, et al., eds. *Harrison's principles of internal medicine*, 15th ed. New York: McGraw-Hill, 2001:299, Fig. 53-1 for a specific example of this scoring system.) Additional cutaneous evidence of androgen excess, such as acne, should be noted. The examiner should carefully assess the patient for any signs of virilization.

MANAGEMENT

Most women with hirsutism have the idiopathic form or PCOS. Nonetheless, it is important to exclude rare and more serious causes such as ovarian or adrenal neoplasms. Some important clinical features that suggest these other causes include

- Virilization
- Progressive worsening of symptoms and a more abrupt onset
- Onset later in life (third decade or higher)—PCOS typically manifests around puberty
- Marked elevations of DHEA-S and free testosterone

Laboratory Data

Several different androgens can be secreted in excess levels in hirsute women. DHEA-S usually represents an adrenal origin. Androstenedione and testosterone can be derived from either ovarian or adrenal sources. Testosterone is the most important circulating androgen and is converted to DHT by 5 alpha-reductase. DHT has a higher affinity for the androgen receptor. The local production of DHT in the pilosebaceous unit (type 1 receptor) mediates effects of androgens.

Women with normal ovulatory menses and mild hirsutism can be followed without any further testing. More extensive testing is indicated if moderate to severe hirsutism occurs or there are red flags to suspect a more serious disorder.

The following laboratory tests can be used in the evaluation of hirsutism.

Serum Testosterone

Serum testosterone can be measured either as total or free testosterone. Free testosterone (biologically active) is typically higher in women with excess androgenic states because of an androgen-induced decrease in sex hormone binding globulin concentrations. However, clinically, total testosterone typically provides an adequate estimate of androgen excess state. Serum total testosterone is often high (>150 ng/dL) in androgen secreting tumors. PCOS and the idiopathic form typically have lower levels.

Dehydroepiandrosterone Sulfate

Women with androgen-secreting adrenal tumors typically have DHEA-S levels >800 mcg/dL. This test is usually indicated when signs of virilization are present and the symptoms are more abrupt in nature.

Serum Prolactin
A normal serum prolactin level excludes hyperprolactinemia.

17-Hydroxyprogesterone
ACTH-stimulated 17-hydroxyprogesterone level <1000 ng/dL usually excludes late-onset CAH.

Cushing's Syndrome
Tests to rule out Cushing's syndrome may be warranted in the appropriate clinical setting (reviewed in Chap. 14, Cushing's Syndrome).

Further radiologic studies, such as transvaginal ultrasound, CT, and MRI, are indicated if a tumor is suspected because of markedly elevated androgen levels.

Treatment

The treatment of women with hirsutism should be individualized to the patient. Reassurance may be sufficient in a woman with mild hirsutism and normal ovulatory menses. More specific therapy is indicated for more severe forms or if the patient requests therapy. Treatment of the underlying cause is important for secondary forms of hirsutism. Response to pharmacologic therapy is slow and may take several months. Typically, biochemical abnormalities resolve before clinical improvement. Pregnancy should be excluded in all patients before initiation of oral contraceptives and antiandrogens. Continued contraception should be counseled for all patients taking antiandrogens, as these drugs are teratogenic. Women who desire pregnancy should not be started on pharmacotherapy for hirsutism. The treatment specific for PCOS is discussed in Chap. 20, Polycystic Ovary Syndrome.

Nonpharmacologic Treatment
Obese women should be encouraged to lose weight with caloric restriction and exercise. Weight loss can lower androgen levels and improve hirsutism. Hirsutism can also be treated by removal of hair by bleaching, waxing, shaving, depilatories, electrolysis, or laser treatment. Laser treatments are expensive, but remove hair permanently. Topical eflornithine (Vaniqa) applied twice daily has been used for removal of facial hair; however, it must be used indefinitely to prevent hair regrowth.

Oral Contraceptives
Combination estrogen-progestin oral contraceptives are the best first-line agents in patients who do not desire pregnancy. They are effective in decreasing hirsutism in roughly 60–80% of patients. Treatment should be initiated by a combination preparation that contains ethinyl estradiol in conjunction with a progestin with little androgenic activity. Mechanisms of action include increasing sex hormone–binding globulin levels and lowering of free testosterone, suppression of luteinizing hormone (LH) release and decreased ovarian androgen production, and decreased adrenal androgen production.

Antiandrogens
Antiandrogens are more effective when added to oral contraceptives than when used alone. Spironolactone (Aldactone) (100 mg PO daily) can decrease the effect of androgens by blocking the androgen receptor. When used in combination with an oral contraceptive, both androgen levels and action are decreased. It can be an effective agent to treat hirsutism. Finasteride (Propecia) (5 mg PO daily), which blocks conversion of testosterone to DHT, can also be used to treat hirsutism. Flutamide (Eulexin) (250 mg PO bid) may also be effective. Because of the teratogenic potential of antiandrogens, they must be used only when women are treated with effective contraception.

Gonadotropin-Releasing Hormone Agonists
Gonadotropin-releasing hormone (GnRH) agonists inhibit ovarian androgen production by inhibiting gonadotropins. The ensuing estrogen deficiency can be treated with a com-

bination estrogen-progestin pill. The GnRH agonist–oral contraceptive combination is less effective and more expensive than antiandrogen-contraceptive combination.

KEY POINTS TO REMEMBER

* The most common causes of hirsutism are PCOS and idiopathic hirsutism.
* Rapid progression and signs of virilization are ominous and may indicate ovarian or adrenal neoplasms.
* Women who desire pregnancy should not be started on pharmacotherapy for hirsutism.
* Combination estrogen-progestin oral contraceptives are the best first-line agents in patients who do not desire pregnancy.
* Antiandrogens are more effective when added to oral contraceptives than when used alone.

REFERENCES AND SUGGESTED READINGS

Azziz R, Dewailly D, Owerbach D. Nonclassic adrenal hyperplasia: current concepts. *J Clin Endocrinol Metab* 1994;78:810.

Derksen J, Nagesser SK, Meinders AE, et al. Identification of virilizing adrenal tumors in hirsute women. *N Engl J Med* 1994;331:968.

Ehrmann DA. Hirsutism and virilization. In: Braunwald E, et al., eds. *Harrison's principles of internal medicine*, 15th ed. New York: McGraw-Hill, 2001:297–301.

Ehrmann DA, Barnes RB, Rosenfield RL. Hyperandrogenism, hirsutism and polycystic ovary syndrome. In: DeGroot LJ, Jameson JL, eds. *Endocrinology*, 4th ed. Philadelphia: WB Saunders, 2001:2122–2137.

Hatch R, Rosenfield RL, Kim MH, Tredway D. Hirsutism: implications, etiology, and management. *Am J Obstet Gynecol* 1981;140:815.

Kirschner MA, Samojlik E, Silber D. A comparison of androgen production and clearance in hirsute and obese women. *J Steroid Biochem* 1983;19:607

Matteri RK, Stanczyk FZ, Gentzschein EE, et al. Androgen sulfate and glucuronide conjugates in nonhirsute and hirsute women with polycystic ovarian syndrome. *Am J Obstet Gynecol* 1989;161:1704.

Pazos F, Escobar-Morreale HF, Balsa J. Prospective randomized study comparing the long-acting gonadotropin-releasing hormone agonist triptorelin, flutamide, and cyproterone acetate, used in combination with an oral contraceptive, in the treatment of hirsutism. *Fertil Steril* 1999;71:122.

Taylor AE, Barbieri RL. Treatment of hirsutism. In: Rose BD, ed. *UpToDate*. Wellesley, MA: UpToDate, 2003.

Zawadzki JK, Dunaif A. Diagnostic criteria for polycystic ovary syndrome: towards a rational approach. In: Dunaif A, ed. *Polycystic ovary syndrome, current issues in endocrinology and metabolism*, 4th ed. Boston: Blackwell Scientific Publications, 1992.

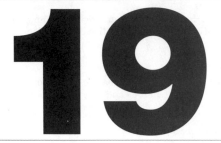

Male Hypogonadism

Bharathi Raju and
Subramaniam Pennathur

INTRODUCTION

Male hypogonadism refers to the impairment of either testosterone or sperm production by the testis. It can be classified into primary or secondary hypogonadism. In primary hypogonadism, the abnormality is due to the failure of the testis (hypergonadotropic hypogonadism), and the secondary form is due to defects at the hypothalamic-pituitary level (hypogonadotrophic hypogonadism). Rarely, hypogonadism can be due to defects at the receptor level, such as androgen resistance syndromes, which are characterized by resistance to the effects of testosterone.

Overview of the Male Gonadal Function

An overview of the male gonadal axis is outlined in Fig. 19-1. The gonadotropins, luteinizing hormone (LH) and follicle-stimulating hormone (FSH), are secreted by the anterior pituitary gland and control testosterone production by Leydig cells and spermatozoa production by seminiferous tubules. LH and FSH are, in turn, under the control of gonadotropin-releasing hormone (GnRH), which is produced in the hypothalamus and secreted into pituitary portal vessels. GnRH, LH, and FSH secretion are controlled by the negative feedback from testis by testosterone and inhibin B.

Testosterone is the major product of Leydig cells. LH stimulates the testis in a pulsatile manner, resulting from the pulsatile GnRH secretion by the hypothalamus. An adult testis produces approximately 7 mg of testosterone daily.

FSH and LH control seminiferous tubule **production of sperm**. The action of LH is through local secretion of testosterone. Both FSH and testosterone are required to stimulate spermatogenesis quantitatively. LH secretion is negatively regulated by testosterone, estradiol, and dihydrotestosterone (DHT). FSH is under the negative influence of inhibin B and testosterone. They are stimulated in a pulsatile fashion by GnRH (see Fig. 19-1).

60–70% of **testosterone** is transported in plasma bound to sex hormone–binding globulin (SHBG), 2% is free, and the remainder is bound to albumin. Both free testosterone and albumin-bound testosterone are bioavailable. Circulating SHBG levels (and, thereby, total testosterone) can be increased by thyroxine (T_4) or decreased by androgens and glucocorticoids. Liver diseases, protein-losing states, obesity, and genetic SHBG deficiency can also affect SHBG levels. Testosterone levels are high in the morning and nadir in the afternoon. This diurnal rhythm is lost in older men.

Approximately 6–8% of testosterone is converted to more potent **DHT** by 5 alpha-reductase in prostate, testis, liver, kidney, and skin. A small proportion (0.2%) of testosterone is converted to estradiol by aromatase. The actions of testosterone are the combined effects of testosterone, plus its active androgenic (DHT) and estrogenic (estradiol) metabolites. The testosterone-receptor complex is responsible for gonadotropin regulation, stimulation of spermatogenesis, and virilization of the wolffian ducts, whereas the DHT-receptor complex mediates virilization of the external genitalia during embryogenesis and most of the virilization that occurs at male puberty. Estradiol inhibits gonadotropin secretion and promotes epiphyseal maturation in the adolescent male.

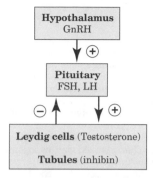

FIG. 19-1. The male gonadal axis. FSH, follicle-stimulating hormone; GnRH, gonadotropin-releasing hormone; LH, luteinizing hormone.

CAUSES

Primary Hypogonadism

Primary hypogonadism is more common than the secondary form and is more likely to be associated with a decrease in sperm production than in testosterone production. In addition, primary hypogonadism is more likely to be associated with gynecomastia, probably due to the effect of the supranormal serum LH and FSH concentrations on testicular aromatase activity. This can result in increased formation of estradiol and elevated levels of estradiol relative to testosterone.

Developmental Defects

Klinefelter's syndrome is the most common congenital defect causing male hypogonadism (1 in 500 males). Clinical features include small, firm testis; varying degrees of impaired sexual development; azoospermia; gynecomastia; and elevated gonadotrophins. The underlying defect is the presence of an extra X chromosome, 47XXY being the most common. Diagnosis is confirmed by karyotype analysis.

A congenital decrease in testosterone synthesis and secretion can result from mutations of the genes that encode the enzymes necessary for testosterone biosynthesis. These mutations may result in decreased testosterone secretion, beginning in the first trimester of pregnancy, and incomplete virilization.

Acquired Diseases

Mumps is the most common infection affecting the testis leading to infertility and reduced testosterone.

Radiation affects both spermatogenesis and testosterone production. Impaired testosterone production is due to reduced blood flow to testis. The extent of damage to Leydig cells is directly related to dose of radiation and, inversely, to age.

Drugs, such as ketoconazole (Nizoral), spironolactone (Aldactone), and cyproterone, interfere with testosterone synthesis. Enzyme-inducing drugs, such as phenytoin (Dilantin) and carbamazepine (Carbatrol), can lower the bioavailable testosterone, raise SHBG and LH levels, and decrease metabolic clearance. Ethanol ingestion can reduce testosterone levels by inhibiting the synthesis of testosterone and by impairing the hypothalamic-pituitary axis. Cyclophosphamide and other alkylating agents can induce infertility. Spironolactone, cyproterone, cimetidine (Tagamet), and omeprazole (Prilosec) compete for the androgen receptor and can cause gynecomastia and impotence.

Systemic illnesses, such as renal failure (testicular failure, hyperprolactinemia), liver failure (both testicular failure and inhibition of hypothalamic-pituitary axis), sickle cell disease, chronic illness, thyrotoxicosis, and immune disorders, can lead to hypogonadism.

Secondary Hypogonadism

Congenital Disorders

Congenital abnormalities causing decreased gonadotrophins are rare. Idiopathic hypogonadotropic hypogonadism is a heterogeneous disorder due to isolated GnRH deficiency. Affected individuals are males presenting as teenagers due to deficient sexual maturation. They have normal male phenotype at birth because maternal human chorionic gonadotropin (hCG) stimulates normal sexual differentiation in the first trimester. However, they have impaired phallic development characterized by microphallus at birth due to lack of testosterone production in the final trimester. Clinical features include delayed bone age, osteopenia, eunuchoid body proportions, gynecomastia, and delayed puberty. They have low testosterone and low LH. Pulsatile GnRH treatment induces full pubertal development.

Kallmann's syndrome is characterized by hypogonadotropic hypogonadism and hyposmia with or without other nongonadal anomalies. Some patients with the X-linked form have a deletion of the KAL gene located on short arm of the X chromosome, which prevents migration of GnRH neurons to the brain from the olfactory placode during embryogenesis.

Hemochromatosis can cause selective gonadotropin deficiency due to deposition of iron in the pituitary cells.

Acquired Disorders

Any disease that affects the hypothalamic-pituitary axis by one of the following mechanisms leads to hypogonadotropic hypogonadism.

- Involvement of the hypothalamus, which impairs GnRH secretion
- Disease of the pituitary stalk, which interferes with the ability of GnRH to reach the pituitary gland
- Involvement of the pituitary gland, which directly diminishes LH and FSH secretion

Gonadotropin deficiency may result from a space-occupying lesion of sella either by destroying the pituitary gland or by interrupting the nerve fibers bringing GnRH to the hypophyseal circulation. Patients present with headaches, visual disturbances, and variable manifestations of hypopituitarism. ACTH-producing tumors can cause impotence, decreased libido, and infertility. Testosterone levels are low, and GnRH-stimulated LH concentrations are suppressed. Prolactinoma affects the pulsatile GnRH secretion and subsequently causes hypogonadism. Men have low testosterone levels and attenuated pulsatile LH secretion. Treatment with dopamine agonists can normalize prolactin (PRL) levels and restore sexual function.

Langerhans' cell histiocytosis and sarcoidosis may involve the hypothalamus and pituitary gland, causing hypogonadism. Leydig cell tumors and adrenal tumors produce estradiol, leading to gynecomastia and gonadotropin deficiency. hCG secreted by choriocarcinoma can increase estradiol levels and suppress gonadotropins. Trauma severing the pituitary stalk, critical illness, chronic narcotic administration, exogenous steroids, and pituitary apoplexy are some other causes of hypogonadism.

PRESENTATION

Clinical features depend on whether the impairment involves spermatogenesis or testosterone secretion, or both. It also depends on the time of onset of the defect. Impaired spermatogenesis leads to reduced sperm count and testicular size.

Reduced testosterone production during the first trimester of pregnancy leads to incomplete virilization. If the defect occurs during the third trimester, it leads to micropenis and a decrease in testosterone in the prepubertal period, resulting in incomplete pubertal development. Postpubertal defects lead to decreased libido, muscle mass, hair growth, energy, mood, hematocrit, and bone mass.

History

History should include developmental milestones, with emphasis on sexual development, current symptoms, and information pertaining to possible causes. History of ambiguous genitalia, micropenis, cryptorchidism, failed or delayed puberty, or decrease in libido, sexual function, and/or energy gives clues regarding time of onset of the hypogonadism. Inquiry should be made into the rapidity of onset and progression of the symptoms, presence or absence of early morning erections, and changes in voice, muscle strength, or hair growth. History of headache, visual problems, symptoms suggestive of kidney or liver disease, depression, thyroid disease, drug abuse, chemotherapy, radiation therapy, anosmia, ethanol abuse, and medication history can yield important clues regarding the etiology of the disease.

Physical Exam

A complete physical exam should be done to look for the presence of eunuchoid proportions, developmental anomalies, visual problems, hair distribution, and gynecomastia. Exam of the external genitalia should include measuring testicular size (normal, 4–7 cm) and volume (normal, 15–30 mL) and Tanner stage for adolescents.

Physical findings are not always present in adults, as some secondary sexual characteristics, such as reduced muscle mass, may take years to develop. In such instances, appropriate laboratory evaluation may be helpful.

MANAGEMENT

Diagnosis

Diagnosis is based on a thorough history, physical exam, and laboratory data. The general scheme for assessment of hypogonadism is outlined in Fig. 19-2. Initial laboratory evaluation should include testosterone levels, FSH, and LH. Presence of low testosterone with elevated FSH and LH denotes primary hypogonadism. Presence of low testosterone and low or normal FSH and LH indicates secondary hypogonadism. Measuring free testosterone becomes important when an abnormality affecting SHBG levels is suspected. Obesity reduces the SHBG binding with testosterone, and aging increases binding (elevating SHBG levels). Diurnal variations in the levels of testosterone need to be considered when interpreting results.

Semen analysis is the best means of analyzing sperm count. Subnormal sperm count and a normal serum testosterone concentration associated with a supranormal serum FSH and normal LH concentration indicates that the seminiferous tubules have been damaged, whereas testosterone production by the Leydig cells is still normal.

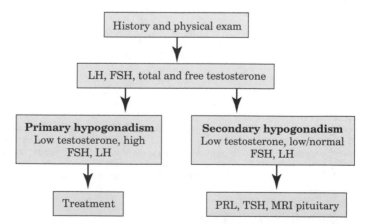

FIG. 19-2. Algorithm for assessment of hypogonadism. FSH, follicle-stimulating hormone; LH, luteinizing hormone; PRL, prolactin; TSH, thyroid-stimulating hormone.

Depending on the initial evaluation, PRL level, thyroid-stimulating hormone (TSH), free T_4, and MRI of the pituitary gland may be needed. Hyperprolactinemia can suppress gonadotrophins. Primary hypothyroidism can cause hyperprolactinemia and hypogonadism [due to elevated thyrotropin-releasing hormone (TRH)]. Further testing for infiltrative disorders and hemochromatosis should be considered in the appropriate clinical setting.

Treatment

The treatment of hypogonadism consists of replacing testosterone. Testosterone can be replaced by IM injections, 200 mg IM every 2 weeks; by transdermal testosterone (Androderm), 5-mg patch every day; or by testosterone gel (Androgel), 2.5–5 g applied topically to upper arm every day. Patients with secondary hypogonadism desiring fertility are treated with pulsatile GnRH or gonadotropins with hCG with or without FSH. Transdermal testosterone patches can be associated with skin rash and itching and may require application of corticosteroid cream.

Monitoring

Normalizing testosterone levels leads to improvement in symptoms and normal virilization in men. Improvements in muscle mass and bone density can be seen. Serum testosterone measurements are helpful to assess the adequacy of treatment. They should be measured midway between injections in patients receiving injectable testosterone. Dosage should be adjusted to maintain testosterone levels in the mid-normal range (600–750 ng/dL). In postpubertal men, it is reasonable to treat with the minimum amount of testosterone that alleviates symptoms of decreased libido, impaired sexual function, and energy levels. In patients treated with testosterone patch or gel, serum levels of testosterone can be measured at any time and should be in the normal range (400–900 ng/dL). In patients with primary hypogonadism, normalization of serum LH can be used as a surrogate marker to determine the adequacy of therapy. Patients receiving testosterone should be monitored for benign prostatic hyperplasia, prostate cancer, erythrocytosis, and the development or worsening of sleep apnea. Digital rectal exam (DRE) and measurement of prostate specific antigen (PSA) should be performed in men > age 50 years before initiation of testosterone therapy and annually thereafter. The patient should be promptly referred for a prostate biopsy if a nodule is palpated by DRE or if the PSA is elevated and discontinuation of therapy may be warranted. The hemoglobin and hematocrit should be monitored yearly to screen for the development of erythrocytosis.

KEY POINTS TO REMEMBER

- Male hypogonadism is divided into primary (due to the failure of the testis) and secondary (due to defects at the hypothalamic-pituitary level) causes.
- Primary hypogonadism is associated with a low testosterone level but high FSH and LH levels.
- Secondary hypogonadism is associated with a low testosterone level, as well as low or normal FSH and LH levels.
- Reduced testosterone production during the prepubertal period results in micropenis and incomplete pubertal development.
- Reduced testosterone production during the postpubertal period leads to decreased libido, muscle mass, hair growth, energy, mood, libido, hematocrit, and bone mass.
- Treatment for both causes of hypogonadism consists of testosterone replacement, with the goal of achieving normal serum testosterone levels and alleviating symptoms.
- DRE and PSA testing should be performed before initiating testosterone therapy and annually thereafter.

REFERENCES AND SUGGESTED READINGS

Christensen AK. Leydig cells. In: Hamilton DW, Greep RO, eds. *Handbook of physiology*. Baltimore: Williams & Wilkins, 1975:57–94.

Finkel DM, et al. Stimulation of spermatogenesis by gonadotropins in men with hypogonadotropic hypogonadism. *N Engl J Med* 1985;313:651-55.

Finkelstein JS, et al. Osteoporosis in men with idiopathic hypogonadotropic hypogonadism. *Ann Intern Med* 1987;106:354–361.

Gabrilove JL, et al. Feminizing adrenocortical tumors in the male: a review of 52 cases. *Medicine (Baltimore)* 1965;44:37–79.

Kuhn JM, et al. Evaluation of diagnostic criteria for Leydig cell tumors in adult men revealed by gynecomastia. *Clin Endocrinol* 1987;26:407–416.

Luton JP, et al. Reversible gonadotropin deficiency in male Cushing's disease. *J Clin Endocrinol Metab* 1977;45:488–495.

MacAdams MR et al. Reduction of serum testosterone levels during chronic glucocorticoid therapy. *Ann Intern Med* 1986;104:648–651.

Maya-Nunez G, et al. A recurrent missense mutation in the KAL gene in patients with X-linked Kallmann's syndrome. *J Clin Endocrinol Metab* 1998;83:1650–1653.

Payne AH, et al. *The Leydig cells.* Vienna, IL: Cache River Press, 1996.

Russell DW, Wilson JD. Steroid 5 alpha-reductase: two genes/two enzymes. *Annu Rev Biochem* 1994;63:25–61.

Sherins RJ, et al. Studies on the role of sex steroids in the feedback control of FSH concentrations in men. *J Clin Endocrinol Metab* 1973;36:886–893.

Snyder PJ. Clinical features, diagnosis and treatment of male hypogonadism in adults. In: Rose BD, ed. *UpToDate.* Wellesley, MA: UpToDate, 2003.

Spratt DI, et al. Long-term administration of gonadotropin-releasing hormone in men with idiopathic hypogonadotropic hypogonadism: a model for studies of the hormone's physiological effects. *Ann Intern Med* 1986;105:848–855.

Stepanas AV, et al. Endocrine studies in testicular tumor patients with and without gynecomastia: a report of 45 cases. *Cancer* 1978;41:369–376.

Von Schoultz B, Carlstrom K. On the regulation of sex-hormone binding globulin: a challenge of an old dogma and outlines of an alternative mechanism. *J Steroid Biochem Mol Biol* 1989;32:327–334.

Wu FCW, et al. Patterns of pulsatile luteinizing hormone and follicle-stimulating hormone secretion in prepubertal (midchildhood) boys and girls and patients with idiopathic hypogonadotrophic hypogonadism (Kallmann's syndrome): a study using an ultrasensitive time-resolved immunofluorometric assay. *J Clin Endocrinol Metab* 1991;72:1229–1237.

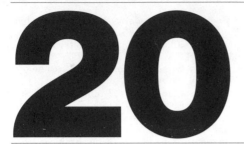

Polycystic Ovary Syndrome

Subramaniam Pennathur

INTRODUCTION

Definition

Although polycystic ovary syndrome (PCOS) was first described in 1935 by Stein and Levinthal, there has been considerable controversy regarding the diagnostic criteria required for the diagnosis. In 1990, the NIH Conference on PCOS proposed the following minimal criteria:

- Chronic anovulation
- Clinical (acne, hirsutism) or biochemical (elevated androgen level) evidence of hyperandrogenism, coupled with exclusion of other causes of female hyperandrogenism, such as androgen-secreting tumors, hyperprolactinemia, and nonclassic adrenal hyperplasia

Recently, revised criteria have been proposed by the Rotterdam PCOS Consensus Workshop Group. According to these revised criteria, 2 out of 3 of the following *and exclusion of other causes* are sufficient for establishing the diagnosis of PCOS:

- Oligo- and/or anovulation
- Clinical and/or biochemical evidence of hyperandrogenism
- Polycystic ovaries

For precise ultrasound criteria of polycystic ovaries, the reader is referred to the consensus report.

Prevalence

PCOS affects 5–10% of women of reproductive age, making it the most common endocrinopathy in women of this age group. There may be an increased association of PCOS in women with type 2 diabetes and in women who are taking antiepileptic agents, although the data are inconclusive.

PRESENTATION

Clinical Presentation

The key clinical features and presentation of PCOS are summarized in Table 20-1. PCOS can be seen in association with the metabolic syndrome (syndrome X, dysmetabolic syndrome). The Rotterdam Consensus report suggests that obese women with PCOS be screened for the metabolic syndrome.

Androgen Excess State

Androgen excess can result in hirsutism, acne, and androgenic alopecia (male-pattern balding). Hirsutism is characterized by excess terminal pigmented hair in a male pattern of distribution and commonly occurs on the chin, upper lip, periareolar area, and the lower abdomen. Alopecia is rare. Signs of virilization, such as deepening of voice,

TABLE 20-1. 2003 ROTTERDAM DIAGNOSTIC CRITERIA FOR POLYCYSTIC
OVARY SYNDROME

Major criteria (2 of 3 required for diagnosis)

Clinical signs of hyperandrogenism

Acne

Alopecia

Hirsutism

Menstrual irregularities associated with chronic oligo- or anovulation

Polycystic ovaries

Other causes of hyperandrogenemia must be excluded

Associated features (not required for diagnosis)

Hypothalamic-pituitary abnormalities (elevated LH/FSH ratio >2.5)

Insulin resistance and obesity

FSH, follicle-stimulating hormone; LH, luteinizing hormone.
Adapted from The Rotterdam ESHRE/ASRM-sponsored PCOS consensus workshop group. Revised
2003 consensus on diagnostic criteria and long-term health risks related to polycystic ovary syndrome (PCOS). *Human Reprod* 2004;19:41–47.

increased muscle mass, and clitoromegaly, are rarely seen with PCOS and, if present, should prompt evaluation for an androgen-secreting tumor.

Menstrual Irregularities

Menstrual dysfunction is a defining characteristic of PCOS and may be manifest in several different forms. It is usually associated with chronic oligo- or anovulation. Women with PCOS usually have adequate estrogen but are deficient in progesterone. This results in endometrial hyperplasia and dysfunctional uterine bleeding due to chronic estrogenic stimulation. Endometrial cancer can occur in young women with PCOS. Less commonly, endometrial atrophy and amenorrhea are presenting features. Women with PCOS may ovulate intermittently and, therefore, take longer to conceive. If pregnancy does occur, there is an increased risk for pregnancy-induced hypertension and gestational diabetes. A subset of women with PCOS have persistent anovulation and infertility.

Hypothalamic-Pituitary Abnormalities

The ratio between luteinizing hormone (LH) and follicle-stimulating hormone (FSH) is usually elevated in PCOS to >2.5. Women with PCOS tend to have an increased frequency and amplitude of normal LH pulses. In contrast, levels of FSH remain unchanged or low-normal, thereby increasing the ratio between the two hormones. This inappropriate secretion of pituitary gonadotropins likely results from elevated gonadotropin-releasing hormone (GnRH) secretion from the hypothalamus. It remains to be determined whether this defect in the GnRH pulse generation is a primary or a secondary abnormality. Some women with PCOS may also have mildly elevated prolactin (PRL) levels.

Ovarian Defects

There is an increased ovarian production of androstenedione by stromal and thecal cells in response to increased LH levels. The androstenedione can be converted to testosterone in the ovaries as well as in the peripheral tissues. Estradiol levels are typically normal to low, but estrone levels are significantly elevated. This is due to conversion of androstenedione to estrone in adipose tissue and further stimulates LH and suppresses FSH. Roughly 80% of women with PCOS have classic, multiple, small, peripheral ovarian follicles by transvaginal ultrasound.

Obesity and Insulin Resistance

Central visceral obesity is present in approximately one-half of women with PCOS. Hyperinsulinemia and insulin resistance can be present even in the absence of obesity. It is unclear how hyperinsulinemia and hyperandrogenism are connected. Although hyperinsulinemia can lead to ovarian hyperandrogenism, the reverse has not been established. Reducing insulin resistance by weight loss or pharmacologic means [metformin (Glucophage), thiazolidinediones] can be associated with lower androgen levels, suggesting an important role for insulin resistance in the pathogenesis of this disorder.

MANAGEMENT

Diagnosis

PCOS is diagnosed by clinical criteria (see Table 20-1). The onset of menstrual abnormality is usually in the peripubertal period and menarche can be delayed. Infertility may be a presenting complaint.

Laboratory Evaluation

The following biochemical abnormalities are associated with PCOS:

- Roughly 80% of the women with PCOS have an elevated serum androgen level with increases in both total and free testosterone levels. Because of androgen-induced inhibition of hepatic sex hormone–binding globulin, the elevation of free testosterone is more prominent.
- Elevated LH and normal FSH, resulting in an elevated LH/FSH ratio (>2.5).
- Serum estrone levels can be increased (with normal serum estradiol levels).
- Impaired glucose tolerance, and even frank type 2 diabetes mellitus due to the high level of insulin resistance in women with PCOS.

The **diagnosis of PCOS is one of exclusion**, and so all patients who meet the NIH criteria should undergo the following laboratory screening to exclude hyperprolactinemia, androgen-secreting tumors (adrenal or ovarian), and late-onset congenital adrenal hyperplasia (CAH).

- Serum PRL: Mild elevations in PRL can be seen in PCOS, but a normal serum PRL excludes hyperprolactinemia.
- Dehydroepiandrosterone sulfate (DHEA-S) and serum testosterone: Women with androgen-secreting tumors typically have abrupt onset of hirsutism, some signs of virilization, and amenorrhea. In patients with adrenal tumors, testosterone is often high (>150 ng/dL), DHEA-S is typically >600 mcg/dL, and serum LH is usally suppressed (unlike in patients with PCOS).
- A cosyntropin (ACTH)-stimulated 17-hydroxyprogesterone <1000 ng/dL usually excludes late-onset CAH.

Treatment

The treatment of women with PCOS should be individualized to the patient. There are several treatment options for each of the manifestations of PCOS. Most manifestations can be reversed by improving insulin resistance either by weight loss or by pharmacologic therapy. Typically, response to therapy is slow, with clinical changes lagging behind biochemical improvement by several months. Pregnancy should be excluded before initiation of pharmacologic therapy with oral contraceptives and antiandrogens.

Nonpharmacologic Treatment

Obese women with PCOS should be encouraged to lose weight with dietary caloric restriction and exercise. Improved insulin sensitivity can result in improvement in several manifestations of PCOS, including reestablishment of ovulatory cycles and lowering of androgen levels. Hirsutism can be treated by removal of hair by bleaching, waxing, shaving, depilatories, electrolysis, or laser treatment.

Pharmacologic Treatment

ORAL CONTRACEPTIVES. Oral contraceptives are the best first-line agents in patients who do not desire pregnancy. They allow the resumption of normal menses and prevent the chronic, unopposed, estrogenic stimulation of the endometrium. They also lower androgen levels. Hirsutism and acne respond well to estrogen therapy. Pregnancy should be excluded before initiating treatment. Typically, treatment should be initiated by a combination preparation that contains ethinyl estradiol in conjunction with a progestin with low androgenic activity such as norethindrone, ethynodiol diacetate, or a third-generation progestin (Norgestimate, Desogestrel, Drospirenone). In women who do not desire (or cannot take) oral contraceptive therapy, oral intermittent progestin therapy with a 7- to 10-day course of medroxyprogesterone acetate (Provera) once every 1–3 months can be considered. Although this therapy can offer endometrial protection, it does not reduce the effects of hyperandrogenism such as hirsutism and acne.

ANTIANDROGENS. Antiandrogens can be used in conjunction with oral contraceptives to derive further benefit. Spironolactone (Aldactone) (100 mg PO daily) decreases the effect of androgens by blocking the androgen receptor. When used alone, it has minimal effects on free testosterone levels. When used in combination with an oral contraceptive, both androgen levels and action are decreased. Spironolactone is an effective agent in the treatment of hirsutism. Finasteride (Propecia), which blocks conversion of testosterone to dihydrotestosterone, can also be used to treat hirsutism. Because of the teratogenic potential of antiandrogens, they must be used only when women are treated with effective contraception.

INSULIN SENSITIZERS. Several agents, such as metformin, troglitazone (Rezulin), and D-chiro-inositol can be effective in improving insulin sensitivity and lowering hyperinsulinemia. They can reduce androgen production and restore normal menses in women with PCOS. Metformin is the best-studied drug in this class of agents. Metformin increased insulin sensitivity, lowered androgen levels, and increased the likelihood of ovulatory cycles (either alone or in combination with clomiphene) in women with PCOS. Effective doses of metformin are between 1500 and 2000 mg/day. Troglitazone has been removed from the market due to risk of serious hepatotoxicity, but newer thiazolidinediones, such as pioglitazone (Actos) and rosiglitazone (Avandia), are being evaluated in PCOS.

SPECIAL CONSIDERATIONS

Long-Term Risks

The prevalence of impaired glucose tolerance and type 2 diabetes are increased in women with PCOS. This association is seen in both obese and nonobese women with PCOS. Women with a family history of type 2 diabetes are at even greater risk for development of diabetes. Some studies have demonstrated that women with PCOS tend to have a lower HDL and higher levels of triglycerides and LDL consistent with insulin resistance syndrome, although the data are conflicting. Whether women with PCOS and the metabolic syndrome are at increased cardiovascular risk remains for future investigation. Unopposed estrogenic stimulation of the uterus may increase the likelihood of endometrial carcinoma. Sleep apnea also occurs at a higher incidence in women with PCOS.

Infertility

When fertility is desired, oral contraceptives and antiandrogens cannot be used. It is important to complete a basic infertility evaluation of the couple, including a semen analysis of the man, to rule out other contributing factors. Weight loss and insulin sensitizers, such as metformin, may induce ovulatory cycles and permit pregnancy. Clomiphene citrate (Clomid) and exogenous gonadotropins may also be used to induce ovulation. An increased incidence of spontaneous miscarriage is associated with PCOS. Treatment with metformin may reduce the rate of miscarriage.

KEY POINTS TO REMEMBER

- Minimum criteria to diagnose PCOS are 2 of 3 of the following: oligo- or anovulation, clinical or biochemical evidence of hyperandrogenism, or polycystic ovaries. Other treatable conditions associated with hyperandrogenism should be excluded (hyperprolactinemia, androgen-producing tumors, late-onset CAH).
- PCOS is the most common endocrinopathy in women of reproductive age.
- The chronic estrogenic stimulation seen in PCOS results in endometrial hyperplasia and dysfunctional uterine bleeding and may lead to endometrial carcinoma.
- Other metabolic conditions associated with PCOS may include the metabolic syndrome, glucose intolerance or type 2 diabetes, dyslipidemia, sleep apnea, and infertility.
- The mainstay of treatment for PCOS includes a combination oral contraceptive preparation that contains ethinyl estradiol in conjunction with a progestin with low androgenic activity. An antiandrogen may be added for additional benefit in controlling hirsutism.
- Insulin sensitizers are promising therapies that can reduce insulin and androgen levels and increase ovulatory cycles.

REFERENCES AND SUGGESTED READINGS

Azziz R, Dewailly D, Owerbach D. Nonclassic adrenal hyperplasia: current concepts. *J Clin Endocrinol Metab* 1994;78:810.

Coulam CB, Anneger JF, Kranz JS. Chronic anovulation syndrome and associated neoplasia. *Obstet Gynecol* 1983;61:403.

Derksen J, Nagesser SK, Meinders AE, et al. Identification of virilizing adrenal tumors in hirsute women. *N Engl J Med* 1994;331:968.

Dunaif A. Hyperandrogenic anovulation (PCOS): a unique disorder of insulin action associated with increased risk of non-insulin dependent diabetes. *Am J Med* 1995;98(1A):33S–39S.

Dunaif A, Scott D, Finegood D, et al. The insulin-sensitizing agent troglitazone improves the metabolic and reproductive abnormalities in the polycystic ovary syndrome. *J Clin Endocrinol Metab* 1996;81:3299.

Dunaif A, Segal KR, Futterweit W, et al. Profound peripheral insulin resistance, independent of obesity, in polycystic ovary syndrome. *Diabetes* 1989;38:1165.

Marx TL, Mehta AE. Polycystic ovary syndrome: pathogenesis and treatment over the short and long term. *Cleveland Clinic Journal of Medicine* 2003;70(1):31–33, 36–41, 45.

Nestler JE, Jakubowicz DJ, Evans WS, et al. Effects of metformin on spontaneous and clomiphene-induced ovulation in the polycystic ovary syndrome. *N Engl J Med* 1998;338:1876.

Nestler JE, Jakubowicz DJ, Reamer P, et al. Ovulatory and metabolic effects of D-chiro-inositol in the polycystic ovary syndrome. *N Engl J Med* 1999;340:1314.

Pasquali R, Antenucci D, Casimirri F, et al. Clinical and hormonal characteristics of obese amenorrheic hyperandrogenic women before and after weight loss. *J Clin Endocrinol Metab* 1989;68:173.

The Rotterdam ESHRE/ASRM-sponsored PCOS consensus workshop group. Revised 2003 consensus on diagnostic criteria and long-term health risks related to polycystic ovary syndrome (PCOS). *Human Reprod* 2004;19:41–47.

Stein I, Leventhal M. Amenorrhea associated with bilateral polycystic ovaries. *Am J Obstet Gynecol* 1935;29:181.

Zawadzki JK, Dunaif A. Diagnostic criteria for polycystic ovary syndrome: towards a rational approach. In: A. Dunaif A, et al., eds. *Polycystic ovary syndrome: current issues in endocrinology and metabolism*, 4th ed. Boston: Blackwell Scientific Publications, 1992.

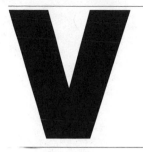

Disorders of Bone and Mineral Metabolism

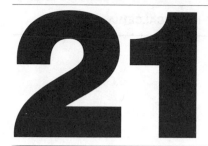

Hypercalcemia

Paul A. Kovach

INTRODUCTION

Hypercalcemia is remarkably common; the prevalence among a population varies from 0.2% to 4%. Primary hyperparathyroidism (PHP) and malignancy account for approximately 90% of cases. Among patients with asymptomatic hypercalcemia, PHP is the cause in approximately 90%. Hypercalcemia of malignancy is often found on evaluation of symptoms of the underlying disease and is more likely to present acutely than is hyperparathyroidism. The chronicity of the disease is often a clue to the underlying process—the longer the patient has been noted to be hypercalcemic, the less likely a malignancy becomes.

CAUSES

See Table 21-1.

Parathyroid-Related Hypercalcemia

Discussed in more detail in Chap. 22, Hyperparathyroidism, elevations in parathyroid hormone (PTH) cause an increase in serum calcium by three separate mechanisms.

1. Elevated calcitriol leads to an increase in gut intake of calcium.
2. There is an increase in resorption of calcium from bone.
3. There is an increase in renal reabsorption of filtered calcium.

Typically, hyperparathyroidism is due to a parathyroid adenoma; however, 4-gland hyperplasia and carcinoma are also seen. This may be seen as part of a familial multiple endocrine neoplasia (MEN) syndrome. Additionally, the less common familial hypocalciuric hypercalcemia is caused by a calcium sensor defect that causes an increase in the set point for serum calcium homeostasis.

Malignancy-Associated Hypercalcemia

Hypercalcemia is a common complication in late-stage malignancies; its prevalence in patients hospitalized with a malignancy is anywhere from 3% to 30%. There are multiple different mechanisms by which hypercalcemia may develop, although virtually all involve an increase in resorption of calcium from the bone and a decrease in renal calcium excretion. The frequency of hypercalcemia in various malignancies is found in Table 21-2.

The syndrome of humoral hypercalcemia of malignancy (HHM) is related to secretion of **PTH-related peptide** (PTHrP). PTHrP is a peptide with similar biologic activity and amino terminus homology to PTH. The syndrome is often seen in patients with squamous carcinomas and adenocarcinomas. The typical clinical picture involves elevated serum calcium in proportion to the elevation of PTHrP, much like the clinical picture of PHP. Unlike PHP, patients with HHM exhibit decreased levels of serum calcitriol and have impaired gut uptake of calcium as well as a decrease in serum chloride and a metabolic acidosis. Because the immediate effect of infusion of PTH and PTHrP in humans has sim-

TABLE 21-1. DIFFERENTIAL DIAGNOSIS OF HYPERCALCEMIA

Parathyroid related
  Primary hyperparathyroidism
  Tertiary hyperparathyroidism
  Familial hypocalciuric hypercalcemia
  MEN syndromes
  Lithium therapy
Malignancy related
  Secretion of parathyroid hormone–related peptide
  Osteoclastic activation
  Secretion of vitamin D
  Unknown mechanisms
Vitamin D related
  Granulomatous disease
  Infectious (mycobacterial, fungal, etc.)
  Noninfectious (sarcoidosis, eosinophilic granuloma, Wegener's granulomatosis, etc.)
  Vitamin D intoxication
  Williams syndrome
Miscellaneous endocrine
  Hyperthyroidism
  Pheochromocytoma
  Adrenal insufficiency
  Islet cell tumors
Miscellaneous
  Immobilization
  Milk-alkali syndrome
  Other medications/intoxications

MEN, multiple endocrine neoplasia.

ilar effects on serum calcium, serum $1,25(OH)_2$ vitamin D, and renal tubular calcium reabsorption, it is unclear why a clinical difference exists between the two syndromes.

Solid tumors that produce widespread bony metastases may also cause hypercalcemia. The prototypical example of this is breast carcinoma. It was previously thought that the elevation of calcium seen in these patients was most likely due to osteolysis by the tumor; however, there is growing evidence that this is mediated by osteoclasts. It is thought that in at least some of these cases, PTHrP produced locally acts to induce osteoclastic bone resorption. The PTHrP acts in a paracrine fashion, and serum levels may remain undetectable.

Hypercalcemia is noted in approximately 20–40% of patients with myeloma. The mechanism of hypercalcemia in myeloma involves an increase in osteoclast activation by virtue of cytokines secreted by the myeloma cells within the marrow. As opposed to breast cancer, in which markers of osteoblast activity are increased, the effects in myeloma are almost entirely osteolytic. Virtually all patients with myeloma have bony involvement of their disease; the patients who are most predisposed to developing hypercalcemia are those with an impaired glomerular filtration rate.

Patients with several different types of lymphomas are also predisposed to hypercalcemia. This is often associated with an increase in calcitriol, at least in T-cell lym-

TABLE 21-2. FREQUENCY OF HYPERCALCEMIA IN VARIOUS MALIGNANCIES

More common
   Breast cancer with bone metastases
   Squamous cell cancers (particularly lung)
   Multiple myeloma
   T- and B-cell lymphomas
   Hodgkin's disease
   Pancreatic islet cell tumors
   Cholangiocarcinoma
Common
   Adenocarcinomas (lung, renal, pancreatic, ovarian)
Uncommon
   Breast cancer without bone metastases
   Small cell lung cancer
   Colon cancer
   Uterine cancer
   Occult malignancy

phomas associated with human T-cell leukemia virus type I; the production of PTHrP has also been documented. Other hematologic malignancies, such as chronic lymphocytic leukemia, acute leukemias, and chronic myelogenous leukemia in transformation, have been associated with hypercalcemia, though this occurs infrequently enough that another cause for the increase in serum calcium should be sought.

Vitamin D–Related Hypercalcemia

Continuous ingestion of 50–100 times the recommended daily allowance of 200 IU of vitamin D is required to produce hypercalcemia in the normal person. This is typically seen in patients who are taking prescription doses of vitamin D such as that used with hypoparathyroidism or renal osteodystrophy. Less commonly, it is seen in patients who overdose on over-the-counter vitamin D preparations or multivitamins. The mechanism is thought to be related to excess conversion of calcidiol to calcitriol by 1-alpha hydroxylase, although calcidiol has metabolic activity as well. Because the vitamin is highly fat soluble, intoxication may persist for weeks.

Any granulomatous disease may cause hypercalcemia; it is seen in approximately 10% of those with sarcoidosis. Other potential granulomatous disorders that have been associated with hypercalcemia include noninfectious causes such as Wegener's granulomatosis, berylliosis, and eosinophilic granuloma. Infectious causes of granulomatous disorders include mycobacterial disease, such as tuberculosis or leprosy; fungal disorders, such as histoplasmosis, candidiasis, and coccidioidomycosis; and other atypical infections such as Bartonella. The underlying mechanism of this is an increase in production of calcitriol by macrophages. This production of vitamin D is insensitive to feedback regulation and is sensitive to modulators of the inflammatory response such as IFN-gamma.

Other Endocrine Causes of Hypercalcemia

Thyroid Disease

Hypercalcemia as a result of thyroid disease is typically mild but can be seen in as many as 20% of patients and is likely caused by an increase in osteoclastic bone resorption. Levels of $1,25(OH)_2$ vitamin D and PTH should be suppressed. This typically resolves with treatment of the underlying thyroid disorder, and beta-blockers may be of some benefit in the acute setting. If the hypercalcemia remains after correction of the hyperthyroid state, workup for other causes of hypercalcemia should be pursued.

Pheochromocytoma
Hypercalcemia is an infrequent complication of pheochromocytoma. This can be associated with MEN2A. If this is excluded [i.e., the patient has a depressed intact PTH (iPTH)], the tumor itself may be secreting PTHrP. Pheochromocytoma should be considered in all patients with hyperparathyroidism and hypertension.

Adrenal Insufficiency
Hypercalcemia may also be associated with adrenal insufficiency. This has typically been described with primary adrenal failure, though there are case reports in secondary adrenal failure as well. This is often thought to be due to a decrease in intravascular volume and relative hemoconcentration of serum albumin and bound calcium, though the exact pathophysiology is not well described.

Islet Cell Tumors of the Pancreas
Islet cell tumors of the pancreas have been associated with hypercalcemia. In some cases, this is associated with a MEN syndrome; in other cases, the tumors have been found to secrete PTHrP. Tumors that secrete vasoactive intestinal peptide have been found to cause hypercalcemia through unknown mechanisms. This is often associated with the WDHA syndrome—*w*atery *d*iarrhea, *h*ypokalemia, and *a*chlorhydria.

Miscellaneous Causes of Hypercalcemia

Immobilization
Immobilization typically causes hypercalciuria with bone reabsorption that is not associated with hypercalcemia. However, among certain patients with rapid bone turnover, hypercalcemia may develop. This may be seen in the young, in patients with underlying bone disease, and in patients in the early stages of a malignancy. It is thought to be due to increased osteoclast and decreased osteoblast activity. Laboratory findings include hypercalciuria and increased urinary hydroxyproline excretion. iPTH and $1,25(OH)_2$ vitamin D levels should be suppressed. Bone biopsy shows decreased bone formation and increased resorption. Resumption of normal physical activity typically corrects the hypercalcemia. If this is impossible, other medications, including corticosteroids, bisphosphonates, and calcitonin (Miacalcin), may be effective.

Milk-Alkali Syndrome
Patients with markedly increased calcium intake (in the range of 5–15 g/day) may develop hypercalcemia in what is termed the milk-alkali syndrome. This was initially described in the 1930s when the primary treatment for peptic ulcer disease was milk and bicarbonate. Today, it is typically seen in patients taking excessive amounts of calcium-containing antacids or dietary supplements. Less often, it is seen with excessive dietary intake of dairy products. It is typically characterized by an elevated serum calcium and bicarbonate and suppressed PTH.

Vitamin A
Excessive intake of vitamin A is thought to increase bone resorption of calcium. It is typically seen in those on fad diets (ingesting 10–20 times the recommended daily allowance), though it may also be seen in patients on therapy with retinoic acid derivatives for acne or malignancies.

Medications
Multiple other medications have been associated with hypercalcemia. The most common offenders are thiazide diuretics. Additional medications that have been implicated include estrogens used in the treatment of breast cancer with bony metastases, growth hormones, foscarnet (Foscavir), and methylxanthines such as theophylline (Uniphyl).

PRESENTATION

The initial workup of hypercalcemia is fairly straightforward. A careful history should be obtained, assessing for potential symptoms of hypercalcemia and looking for any potential medications, ingestions, or exposures that could explain the disease. A basic biochemical workup, including complete metabolic panel, ionized calcium, magnesium, and phosphorous, should be obtained. An assay for serum iPTH is also helpful.

The **symptoms of hypercalcemia** correlate with the time course of the illness as well as the overall level of calcium. In general, levels <12 mg/dL are asymptomatic; levels >15 mg/dL cause severe symptoms such as coma and cardiac arrest. The old saying "stones, bones, (psychiatric) moans, and (abdominal) groans" holds true and is a useful tool for remembering the most common symptoms.

Renal

Patients often have polyuria and polydipsia, as excess calcium blunts the renal response to antidiuretic hormone. Patients may also present with flank pain due to nephrolithiasis of calcium carbonate, citrate, oxalate, or phosphate stones. This is typically seen in patients with hyperparathyroidism but may also be seen in those with other causes for hypercalcemia.

Skeletal

Skeletal presentation depends on the underlying pathophysiology. Hyperparathyroid patients may have osteoporosis or osteitis fibrosa cystica. Patients with an underlying malignancy may present with bony pain due to metastases or pathologic fractures. Additionally, patients may develop metastatic calcification of the heart and soft tissues.

Neurologic

There is a wide range of neuropsychiatric presentations. Patients with chronic, mild hypercalcemia may have subtle symptoms of fatigue and difficulty with concentration. With more severe hypercalcemia, patients may present with weakness, confusion, and, eventually, coma. Additionally, patients may note headache, emotional lability, and irritability.

Gastrointestinal

Patients may complain of nausea, vomiting, constipation, and anorexia. Additionally, there may be some association with pancreatitis and peptic ulcer disease.

Cardiac

Patients may be noted to have a shortened QT_c interval on ECG, though this finding is not particularly sensitive or specific and should not be used in place of determinations of serum calcium to diagnose hypercalcemia. Additional ECG abnormalities include bradycardia and first-degree atrioventricular block. Various T-wave abnormalities that include notching, inversion, and a decrease in T-wave amplitude have also been noted.

TREATMENT

Serum Calcium Levels <12 mg/dL

Elevation of calcium to a level <12 mg/dL is most often asymptomatic and does not require urgent therapy, although patients should be monitered closely for development of symptoms or worsening hypercalcemia.

Serum Calcium Levels >12 mg/dL

With levels >12 mg/dL, emergent treatment may become necessary depending on the symptomatology of the patient. Most of the acute management of hypercalcemia focuses on **increasing the urinary excretion of calcium**. Patients should be hydrated with normal saline aggressively over 24–48 hours. This should lower the serum calcium level by 1–3 mg/dL, although the level will likely not normalize. If volume overload becomes an issue, addition of a loop diuretic may be helpful. It is important to note that aggressive diuresis in a volume-depleted patient may worsen the hypercalcemia by exacerbating the volume loss. **Thiazide diuretics are contraindicated**, as they increase renal reabsorption of calcium. Patients who are oliguric or anuric or those with severe symptomatology may require urgent hemodialysis against a low calcium bath.

Long-Term Management of Hypercalcemia

Further therapy to alleviate hypercalcemia focuses on the underlying cause of the disorder. **Bisphosphonates** are useful in patients with increased bony resorption of calcium. These act by binding to hydroxyapatite and inhibiting osteoclastic bone resorption. Multiple different bisphosphonates are available; newer members of the family are considerably more potent than older members. The previous standard of therapy for moderate hypercalcemia was pamidronate (Aredia) given as a 60-mg IV infusion over 4 hours every month. A newer bisphosphonate, zoledronate (Zometa), can be given as a 4-mg infusion over 15 minutes. Zoledronate has proven to be superior to pamidronate in the treatment of HHM in two randomized controlled trials.

Additional medications have proven to have some role in the treatment of hypercalcemia. Calcitonin, available as a nasal spray or injection, acts to inhibit osteoclasts and increase renal excretion of calcium. In hypercalcemia, it is typically used in doses of 4 IU/kg IM or subcutaneously (SC) every 12 hours. It has a relatively mild, transient effect on decreasing the level of calcium when used alone; when used in combination with a bisphosphonate, the reduction in serum calcium is more profound than when either drug is used alone. Corticosteroids are the definitive therapy for hypercalcemia due to adrenal insufficiency and may have some role in hypercalcemia due to increased levels of vitamins A or D. Corticosteroids act by decreasing gut uptake of calcium and are typically used in doses of hydrocortisone, 200 mg PO daily for 3–5 days. Ketoconazole (Nizoral) may also be effective in hypercalcemia due to increased vitamin D; it acts as an inhibitor of cytochrome P-450 hydroxylation of calcidiol to calcitriol.

Management of Hypercalcemia in Patients with Granulomatous Diseases

In patients with hypercalcemia due to sarcoidosis or other granulomatous disease, urine excretion of calcium should be checked yearly. If elevated, treatment with steroids (40–60 mg PO of prednisone or equivalent) should be effective in decreasing the production of calcitriol over a period of a few days. Hydroxychloroquine (Plaquenil) and ketoconazole are also potentially effective. Patients should be urged to avoid dietary vitamin D and excessive sunlight exposure.

KEY POINTS TO REMEMBER

- Presentation of hypercalcemia is best summarized by the classic memory aid "stones, bones, moans, and groans."
- Differential diagnosis is broad, although most cases are due to hyperparathyroidism or malignancy.
- Hypercalcemia of malignancy is related to secretion of PTHrP
- Acute management is with aggressive intravenous volume expansion; additional medications may be helpful.

REFERENCES AND SUGGESTED READINGS

Adams JS. Hypercalcemia due to granuloma-forming disorders. In: Favus MJ, ed. *Primer on the metabolic bone diseases and disorders of mineral metabolism,* 4th ed. Philadelphia: Lippincott Williams & Wilkins, 1999:212–214.

Major P, Lortholary A, Hon J, et al. Zoledronic acid is superior to pamidronate in the treatment of hypercalcemia of malignancy: a pooled analysis of two randomized controlled clinical trials. *J Clin Oncol* 2001;19(2):558–567.

Mundy GR, Guise TA. Hypercalcemia of malignancy. *Am J Med* 1997;103:134–145.

Roberts MM, Stewart AF. Humoral hypercalcemia of malignancy. In: Favus MJ, ed. *Primer on the metabolic bone diseases and disorders of mineral metabolism,* 4th ed. Philadelphia: Lippincott Williams & Wilkins, 1999:203–207.

Shane E. Hypercalcemia: pathogenesis, clinical manifestations, differential diagnosis, and management. In: Favus MJ, ed. *Primer on the metabolic bone diseases and disorders of mineral metabolism,* 4th ed. Philadelphia: Lippincott Williams & Wilkins, 1999:183–187.

Young C, et al. Hypercalcemia in sarcoidosis. *Lancet* 1999;353:374.

22

Hyperparathyroidism

Paul A. Kovach

INTRODUCTION

Hyperparathyroidism is one of the most common causes of hypercalcemia. With the development of automated serum chemistry analyzers in the mid-1970s, asymptomatic hypercalcemia became a common incidental finding and the prevalence of **primary hyperparathyroidism** (PHP) increased. Women with the disease outnumber men 3:1, and the disease most commonly presents in the sixth decade of life. An increased prevalence of PHP is seen in patients with thyroid disease and breast cancer. The effect of PHP on mortality is controversial, and previous reports have suggested that PHP is associated with an increased mortality from malignancy and coronary artery disease. A more recent review suggests that survival is not affected in patients with mild PHP, although mortality does increase with increasing levels of serum calcium.

Parathyroid hormone (PTH) is typically secreted by the parathyroid gland as an 84–amino acid peptide. The level of expression is decreased by elevations in the level of vitamin D. Additionally, a fall in the level of serum calcium acts within seconds to increase release of serum PTH. This is modulated through a transmembrane G protein–coupled calcium receptor on the parathyroid cell. The PTH-1 receptor is also a G protein–coupled receptor found on the kidneys, intestine, and on osteoblasts.

PTH causes an **increase in serum calcium** through 3 mechanisms:

- Prolonged secretion of PTH leads to an increase in the number and activity of osteoclasts. This leads to the release of calcium, phosphate, and breakdown products of collagen. Paradoxically, PTH, when given intermittently, is an effective treatment for osteoporosis.
- In the kidney, PTH acts to increase calcium and decrease phosphate resorption. Though the majority of calcium is resorbed in the proximal convoluted tubule, reabsorption of calcium in the distal convoluted tubule is the PTH-dependent process.
- Finally, PTH acts to increase mitochondrial 1 alpha-hydroxylase in cells in the proximal tubule. This acts over hours to increase the level of calcitriol, which leads to increased absorption of calcium by the small intestine.

The PTH molecule is metabolized by the liver and kidneys into amino, mid, and carboxy terminal fragments. Of these, only the amino terminal fragment has biologic activity. Because these fragments are excreted by the kidneys, a nearly 100-fold buildup of the metabolites of PTH in the circulation will be seen in **chronic kidney disease** (CKD). Older PTH assays were sensitive to all areas of the molecule, and as such were markedly elevated in CKD regardless of what the actual level of active PTH was. Newer, intact PTH assays have been formulated that are sensitive to only the biologically active form of the molecule, and they should be used when trying to assess PTH levels in patients with CKD.

CAUSES

Primary Hyperparathyroidism

PHP is the inappropriate secretion of PTH from one or more parathyroid glands. It is caused by a **benign adenoma of a single parathyroid gland** in approximately 80% of cases. Inactivation of a variety of tumor suppressor genes can be found in parathyroid adenomas, and approximately 20% show mutations of both copies of the multiple endocrine neoplasia 1 (MEN1) gene. 4-Gland hyperplasia is seen in approximately 15–20% of cases. Parathyroid carcinoma is quite rare and is found in only 0.5% of cases. Carcinomas can be difficult to distinguish pathologically from adenomas; gene studies may aid in this diagnosis in the future.

Familial hyperparathyroidism is most commonly associated with **MEN1**, also termed Werner's syndrome. Described in Chap. 31, Multiple Endocrine Neoplasia, MEN1 is a defect in a tumor suppressor gene inherited in an autosomal-dominant fashion. It is most commonly associated with parathyroid hyperplasia, pancreatic tumors, and pituitary adenomas, although it may also be associated with other tumors. The tumor suppressor gene, menin, encodes a 610–amino acid protein and is linked to chromosome 11. Multiple different mutations of this gene have been described. The hypercalcemia associated with it shows an equal distribution between sexes and typically presents around age 25 years. It is seen in approximately 95% of those with MEN1. Although it may be associated with a single parathyroid adenoma, much more commonly it involves multiglandular hyperplasia.

Hyperparathyroidism is a well-described component of **MEN2A**. The MEN2 syndromes are characterized chiefly by medullary thyroid cancer, which occurs with complete penetrance. Approximately 25–35% of patients develop asymmetric parathyroid hyperplasia in MEN2A. The syndromes are inherited in an autosomal-dominant fashion and are associated with defects in the RET proto-oncogene, which codes for a transmembrane tyrosine kinase.

Familial hypocalciuric hypercalcemia (FHH) is inherited in an autosomal-dominant fashion and is caused by a mutation of the calcium-sensing receptor that causes the set point for calcium to be abnormally high. Its prevalence is estimated at 1 in 78,000.

Secondary Hyperparathyroidism

In virtually all patients with CKD, hyperparathyroidism occurs. An explanation of this is the "trade-off" hypothesis. It is thought that with a fall in glomerular filtration rate, there is an increase in phosphorous concentration and a decrease in calcium. This leads to a physiologic increase in the levels of PTH to maintain calcium and phosphorus homeostasis. Additionally, as renal mass is lost, renal production of calcitriol decreases, causing decreased gut uptake of calcium. The physiologic response to this is an increase in PTH, which stimulates bone resorption of calcium. Because this is not a primary defect in the parathyroid gland and is instead a result of the **underlying renal injury**, it is termed secondary hyperparathyroidism.

Some patients will develop refractory secondary hyperparathyroidism. The parathyroid tissue becomes autonomously functioning, and secretion of PTH is no longer under physiologic control. If this autonomously elevated PTH occurs in the setting of hypercalcemia, **tertiary hyperparathyroidism** is said to be present.

PRESENTATION

Although hyperparathyroidism most often is found incidentally, it may present with typical **symptoms of hypercalcemia**. Nephrolithiasis is the most common presenting symptom, occurring in approximately 20% of those with mild disease. A decrease in glomerular filtration rate can be expected in <10% of patients—this is typically mild. Patients may present with skeletal complications. Overt osteitis fibrosa cystica is seen in <5% of patients and presents radiographically with a "salt-and-pepper" appearance of the skull, bone cysts, and brown tumors of the long bones. The effect of PHP on overall bone metabolism is complex; it has been shown that there is decreased density of cortical bone, typically measured at the distal radius, and increased density in more cancellous bone, measured at the lumbar spine. Nevertheless, pathologic fractures, particularly in the elderly, are thought to be a risk of the disease. Neuromuscular symptoms include a myopathy as well as vague feelings of fatigue and weakness. The latter are often noted in retrospect on surgical correction of hyperparathyroidism. Occasionally, a patient presents with life-threatening hypercalcemia from a parathyroid crisis, though this can be expected to occur in <2% of patients with the disease.

Uremic bone disease, also termed **renal osteodystrophy**, is the usual presentation—and most feared complication—of secondary hyperparathyroidism. As with PHP, uremic bone disease typically manifests itself as osteitis fibrosis cystica; however, it can also manifest as osteomalacia and dialysis-related amyloidosis. Patients with a chronically elevated calcium-phosphate product are also at an increased risk of calciphylaxis—a painful ischemic necrosis of the skin and soft tissues.

The **diagnostic workup** of hyperparathyroidism is fairly straightforward and is discussed in more detail in Chap. 21, Hypercalcemia. In the setting of elevated ionized calcium, intact PTH (iPTH) would be expected to be low to low-normal. If it is normal or elevated, the patient is hyperparathyroid. Secondary causes of hyperparathyroidism should be ruled out—the patient should have a serum creatinine and BUN determination, and should be questioned about lithium and thiazide usage. In asymptomatic patients, it may be useful to determine bone density as this may sway the decision as to whether to pursue surgery.

Differentiating patients with PHP from patients with FHH may be problematic. The **presentation of FHH** is typically benign, and rates of nephrolithiasis are no different than those in the general population. There may be some increased association with relapsing pancreatitis. Patients with FHH typically have an elevated serum calcium and an iPTH that is usually within the normal range. This normal iPTH is an inappropriate response to hypercalcemia and does not allow for differentiation from PHP. A useful method of **distinguishing FHH from PHP** is the ratio of calcium clearance (Cl_{Ca}) to creatinine clearance (Cl_{Cr}). This can be calculated from the following formula:

$$Cl_{Ca}/Cl_{Cr} = (Ca_u \times Cr_s) / (Cr_u \times Ca_s)$$

where Ca_u and Cr_u represent values of creatinine and calcium from a 24-hour urine collection and Cr_s and Ca_s are spot serum values. A value of <0.01 is considered consistent with FHH and is approximately one-third that seen in those without the disease. Documenting hypercalcemia in other family members may also be a clue to the diagnosis.

There are multiple **additional laboratory abnormalities** that are less critical in the diagnostic workup of hyperparathyroid disorders. In those with PHP, the phosphate level should be low to low-normal due to renal phosphate wasting. Urine calcium excretion and levels of $1,25(OH)_2$ vitamin D may be elevated. It should be noted that the PTH–related peptide (PTHrP) produced by many malignancies is not detected by the common commercially available assays for PTH, therefore the hypercalcemia of malignancy should not masquerade as hyperparathyroidism.

It is possible to look for hyperfunctioning parathyroid tissue by either **MRI** or **technetium scanning**. A recent study suggests that in patients who remained hypercalcemic after parathyroid surgery, the sensitivity of both tests was similar and was near 85% for finding hyperfunctioning tissue. These studies may also be helpful in differentiating 4-gland hyperplasia from a functioning adenoma, which may help determine the appropriate surgical approach.

MANAGEMENT

The natural history of PHP suggests that in many cases it is a benign, nonprogressive disorder. In a case series of 52 untreated patients, there was no change in serum and urine biochemical indices in 38 individuals (73%) over the course of a decade. The natural history of PHP-related bone disease remains unclear. In this same cohort, bone densitometry remained stable for more than 10 years. However, after surgery, a 10–12% increase in density at the femoral neck and lumbar spine was found (Silverberg et al., *New Engl J Med* 1999).

Surgical Therapy

The treatment for PHP is primarily surgical. Because the disease often has such a benign course, the difficulty is in determining which patients are most appropriate for surgery. Consensus guidelines formulated in 1991 and updated in 2002 suggest that **surgery is indicated** under the following conditions:

- Age <50 years
- Serum calcium >1 mg/dL above the upper limit of normal
- Patients for whom medical follow-up is either not possible or not desirable
- Marked hypercalciuria (>400 mg daily excretion)
- Reduction in bone mineral density at any site to a T score less than –2.5
- Decrease in Cl_{Cr} to 70% of normal

By applying these guidelines, approximately 30% of those with asymptomatic disease become surgical candidates. Additional factors that may influence the decision to pursue surgical correction include neuropsychological dysfunction, menopause, GI symptoms, abnormal indices of bone turnover, or cardiovascular abnormalities.

The appropriate surgical procedure depends on the underlying cause of the disease. In a patient with an adenoma, only the diseased gland should be removed. In those with hyperplasia of all 4 glands, all tissue is removed save a small remnant left *in situ* or transplanted to the nondominant forearm. Typically, a small amount of tissue is cryopreserved should this transplant be unsuccessful. Because the half-life of iPTH is so short, intraoperative measurement of PTH is generally performed to assess for the adequacy of removal of tissue. Removal of an adenoma potentially can be done with minimally invasive surgery, whereas 4-gland hyperplasia generally requires a more extensive neck dissection. Because minimally invasive surgery can be performed with a lower risk of complications, the threshold for resection of an adenoma may be lower that that for 4-gland resection.

Common complications of parathyroid surgery include the so-called **hungry bone syndrome**, in which profound hypocalcemia develops, requiring parenteral calcium supplementation. Rates of postsurgical hypocalcemia may be higher in those with hyperplasia than in those with a single adenoma. Persistent hypoparathyroidism may also occur, mainly in those who have had surgery for parathyroid hyperplasia. Recurrent laryngeal nerve injury occurs in 1–2% of surgeries. In general, outcomes are improved with increased experience of the parathyroid surgeon.

Nonsurgical Therapy

In those patients who are not appropriate for surgical intervention, there are some guidelines for therapy. Adequate hydration should be ensured, as should a moderate calcium intake. Thiazide diuretics and other drugs that can exacerbate hypercalcemia should be avoided. Oral phosphate decreases gut uptake of calcium, inhibits bone resorption of calcium, and inhibits production of calcitriol. However, the use of phosphorus supplementation should be avoided as it may cause ectopic calcification and may increase PTH levels. It is unclear what role estrogen and bisphosphonates play. The calcium level should be followed at least semiannually, and the urinary calcium excretion and bone density should be monitored annually.

The disease course of FHH is generally benign; surgery is contraindicated. Exceptions to this include severe cases with marked elevations of serum calcium, infantile hypercalcemia, and in patients with relapsing pancreatitis. Patients with FHH should be offered genetic counseling before having children, as they are at risk for complications with pregnancy.

Management of secondary hyperparathyroidism can be problematic. The initial goal is to decrease the **calcium-phosphorus product** to <55 mg^2/dL^2. Decreasing uptake of phosphorus from the gut is the primary method of controlling phosphorus levels. In patients with CKD, the goal for daily intake of phosphorus is <800 mg/day. This is obtained primarily through limiting intake of meats and dairy products and is practically very difficult to obtain, as this represents a 60% decrease from the intake of an average American. Additionally, patients require more dietary protein intake as they reach end-stage renal disease to avoid malnutrition. Most patients eventually require therapy with **phosphorus-binding agents**. The aluminum-containing agents that had typically been used have been linked to osteomalacia and encephalopathy and are now avoided. Currently, the mainstays of therapy are calcium-based binders such as calcium carbonate and calcium acetate. Calcium acetate has the benefit of binding more phosphorus with less calcium being absorbed per milligram of elemental calcium than calcium carbonate. The dose should be titrated to maintain a PO_4 level of 4–6 mg/dL.

The next step in maintaining calcium homeostasis in secondary hyperparathyroidism is to replace vitamin D using calcitriol (Calcijex) or one of its analogues. The goals of **vitamin D therapy** are to stabilize or decrease PTH levels to an acceptable range and to normalize calcium levels. Because vitamin D increases the serum calcium-phosphate product, placing the patient at risk for calciphylaxis and hypercalcemia, the serum levels of phosphorus and calcium should be controlled before beginning vitamin D therapy.

Finally, **surgical parathyroidectomy** may become necessary in those with prolonged, uncontrolled elevations in PTH. Indications for surgical parathyroidectomy are as follows:

- Persistent hypercalcemia, especially if symptomatic
- Severe pruritus
- Serum calcium-phosphate product that persistently exceeds 70–80 mg^2/dL^2
- Progressive bone pain or pathologic fractures
- Symptomatic hypercalcemia after renal transplantation
- Calciphylaxis

KEY POINTS TO REMEMBER

- PHP and malignancy represent the two most common causes of hypercalcemia.
- Diagnosis of hyperparathyroidism is made by detecting a persistently elevated or high-normal PTH in the setting of hypercalcemia.
- PHP must be distinguished from FHH. This is done using urinary indices of calcium excretion.
- Management is primarily surgical; specific guidelines exist to determine who should be referred for surgery.

REFERENCES AND SUGGESTED READINGS

Bilezikian JP. Primary hyperparathyroidism: when to observe and when to operate. *Endocrinol Metab Clin North Am* 2000;29(3):465–478.

Bilezikian JP, et al. Summary statement from a workshop on asymptomatic primary hyperparathyroidism: a perspective for the 21st century. *J Clin Endocrinol Metab* 2002;87(12):5353–5361.

Consensus Conference on the Management of Asymptomatic Primary Hyperparathyroidism. *Ann Intern Med* 1991;114:593–597.

Marx SJ. Hyperparathyroid and hypoparathyroid disorders. *N Engl J Med* 2000;343:1863–1875.

Silverberg SJ, et al. A 10-year course with or without parathyroid surgery. *N Engl J Med* 1999;341:1249–1255.

Wermers RA, et al. Survival after the diagnosis of hyperparathyroidism: a population-based study. *Am J Med* 1998;104(2):115–122.

23

Hypocalcemia

Paul A. Kovach

INTRODUCTION

Hypocalcemia is defined as a decrease in ionized calcium and excludes pseudohypocalcemia in the hypoalbuminemic patient. It is extremely common in the inpatient setting and is estimated to occur in up to 88% of patients in an ICU and 26% of those admitted to a non-ICU ward. The prevalence of hypocalcemia in the outpatient setting is less well studied and largely depends on the prevalence of the underlying disorder.

CAUSES

Broadly stated, there are four potential causes of chronic hypocalcemia:

- Insufficient parathyroid hormone (PTH)
- Insufficient response to PTH
- Insufficient vitamin D
- Insufficient response to vitamin D

Acute hypocalcemia often occurs in response to an overwhelming metabolic insult, for example, the release of phosphate in a patient with rhabdomyolysis, and is seen in a multitude of acute medical conditions.

Hypoparathyroidism

Hypoparathyroidism is defined as an **inappropriately low secretion of PTH for a given ionized calcium**. Characteristic laboratory findings of hypoparathyroidism are hypocalcemia and hyperphosphatemia with normal renal function. 24-Hour excretion of calcium is low, as is the blood calcitriol level.

Hypoparathyroidism may have a surgical, familial, autoimmune, or idiopathic origin. **Surgical hypoparathyroidism** usually occurs on postoperative day 1–2 as a complication after surgery on the neck, though it may occur up to years after a procedure. It is caused by inadvertent injury to or removal of parathyroid tissue and may be associated more with the experience of the surgeon than with the exact procedure performed. Additionally, hypocalcemia in the postoperative setting may occur after multiple blood transfusions, as the citrate preservative in the blood chelates calcium. Postoperative hypocalcemia may also be seen in the "hungry bone syndrome" after surgery for hyperparathyroidism. It is caused by rapid precipitation of calcium-containing hydroxyapatite crystals in bone after correction of the hyperparathyroidism. Hungry bone syndrome can be distinguished from hypoparathyroidism by the phosphorous level, which is low, and a PTH level that is appropriately elevated.

Hypoparathyroidism may also be associated with type 1 polyglandular syndrome, also known as **polyglandular autoimmune syndrome**. This disorder is either idiopathic or acquired as an autosomal-recessive trait. It consists of the classic triad of hypoparathyroidism, adrenal insufficiency, and mucocutaneous candidiasis and usually presents between age 6 months and 20 years. The hypoparathyroidism often presents years after the other conditions. The disease may also be associated with pernicious anemia, type 1 diabetes mellitus, and thyroiditis.

Idiopathic hypoparathyroidism typically presents in childhood but may present any time through the eighth decade of life. It has a 2:1 female predominance and may be associated with anti-PTH antibodies. The familial form of the disorder may be transmitted in an autosomal-dominant, recessive, or x-linked pattern.

Hypoparathyroidism may also result from agenesis or dysgenesis of the parathyroid glands. This is often associated with the **DiGeorge syndrome**, in which malformation of the third and fourth branchial pouches causes absence of the thymus and parathyroid. The mnemonic used for the symptoms of DiGeorge syndrome is CATCH-22 (*c*ardiac anomalies, *a*bnormal facies, *t*hymic aplasia, *c*left palate, and *h*ypocalcemia seen with a deletion in chromosome *22*).

Pseudohypoparathyroidism

This cluster of inherited disorders is caused by **decreased end-organ responses to PTH**. The biochemical abnormalities mimic that of hypoparathyroidism (low calcium, high phosphorous); however, the PTH level is elevated. There are multiple possible defects in the PTH-receptor complex; thus, there are several phenotypic presentations of the disease that have been described.

The molecular basis of type 1 pseudohypoparathyroidism is a defect in the membrane-bound PTH-receptor/adenylate cyclase complex, which yields cyclic adenosine monophosphate (cAMP) as a secondary messenger in the cell. Patients with pseudohypoparathyroidism will not have a physiologic increase in cAMP in the urine after infusion of PTH.

Pseudohypoparathyroidism type 1A presents with the physical stigmata of **Albright's hereditary osteodystrophy** (AHO), which include short metatarsals and metacarpals, short stature, rounded facies, obesity, mental retardation, and heterotopic ossification. The disease is caused by a defect in G_s alpha and leads to deficits in the cAMP cascade. Patients may also show resistance to thyrotropin and other hormones that use cAMP as a second messenger. Inheritance of the disease is autosomal dominant and the expression of the gene is tissue specific and imprinted, with the maternal allele being expressed in the kidney. Thus, if one inherits the defective allele from the mother, hypocalcemia is present. If the allele is inherited from the father, there is the physical appearance of AHO but serum calcium homeostasis is maintained. This latter disorder is termed **pseudopseudohypoparathyroidism**.

Pseudohypoparathyroidism type 1B is characterized by a defective kidney response to PTH, with the associated biochemical sequelae. The patients do not have AHO; instead, they often have skeletal findings consistent with hyperparathyroidism.

Pseudohypoparathyroidism type 2 is associated with an appropriate increase in cAMP in the urine with PTH but a defective phosphaturic response. This disorder is quite rare, with <50 cases having been described.

Vitamin D Deficiency

Vitamin D deficiency leads to the syndromes of **rickets** and **osteomalacia**. Rickets occurs in growing bone, typically in children, and results from abnormal calcification of cartilage at the physis. The typical presentation involves bowing of the limbs and cupping of the costochondral junctions (the rachitic rosary). Osteomalacia occurs after growth plates close and has a clinical appearance that is difficult to distinguish from osteoporosis.

Vitamin D deficiency may occur with **inadequate exposure to sun, inadequate dietary supply of vitamin D**, or **intestinal malabsorption of fatty acids**. Patients with inadequate sun exposure are often hospitalized or institutionalized, very young or very old, and may live in extremes of latitude. Patients of darker skin color have less conversion of vitamin D_2 to calcidiol for a given amount of sunlight. Dietary insufficiency may occur in those who live in areas where vitamin D supplementation of dairy products is not standard practice. Additionally, an inadequate dietary intake may occur in the elderly or in breastfed infants of vegetarian mothers. Malabsorption may occur in patients with underlying biliary, pancreatic, or intestinal pathology.

There are two familial states of relative vitamin D deficiency. Patients with vitamin D–dependent rickets type 1, also known as **pseudovitamin D deficiency**, have a deficiency of 25(OH)D 1-hydroxylase. This condition is rare and is inherited in an autosomal recessive fashion. Treatment is with pharmacologic doses of both vitamin D and calcitriol. Vitamin D–dependent rickets type 2, also known as **hereditary calcitriol resistant rickets**, involves typical symptoms of rickets as well as alopecia. It is inherited as an autosomal recessive disease and is the result of a mutation in the vitamin D receptor gene. It can be treated with high doses of calcium as well as calcitriol.

Miscellaneous Causes of Acute Hypocalcemia

There are several disorders that can result in acute hypocalcemia by overwhelming the normal mechanisms of control of calcium. Hypocalcemia often coincides with hypomagnesemia in patients with poor oral intake. An acute fall in calcium is seen in patients with acute pancreatitis. The degree of hypocalcemia with pancreatitis can be a prognosticator, with lower levels predicting a worse prognosis; the mechanism may be due to release of free fatty acids into the peritoneum. Rapid release of phosphorous from injured muscle cells or dying tumor cells can rapidly complex calcium in patients with rhabdomyolysis or tumor lysis. This can be compounded by the acute renal failure often associated with these conditions. In addition, malignancy can cause hypocalcemia as a result of osteoblast activation in patients with blastic metastases from breast or prostate cancer. Endotoxins cause hypocalcemia by poorly understood mechanisms in septic patients.

PRESENTATION

History

Neuromuscular symptoms are the most pronounced and correlate with the rate and magnitude of the fall in serum calcium. The most pronounced symptom is tetany. Patients typically complain of circumoral paresthesias and carpopedal spasm—the classic example of which is the *main d'accoucheur* posture. This involves adduction of the thumb, flexion of the metacarpal joints, and flexion of the wrist. Patients may also develop potentially life-threatening laryngeal stridor due to laryngeal spasm.

CNS manifestations of hypocalcemia include seizures, irritability, confusion, and delirium. Children with chronic hypocalcemia may have mental retardation. Calcification of the basal ganglia may result in movement disorders. Patients may also complain of muscle cramping, particularly in the legs, feet, and lower back.

Physical Exam

The two classic physical exam findings include Chvostek's sign and Trousseau's sign. **Chvostek's sign** is elicited by tapping the facial nerve 2 cm in front of the earlobe and observing for ipsilateral contraction of facial muscles. The sign is neither sensitive (27%) nor specific and may be seen in 25% of patients who do not have hypocalcemia. **Trousseau's sign** is elicited by inflating a blood pressure cuff to 20 mm Hg above the systolic blood pressure for 3 minutes and observing for *main d'accoucheur* posturing of the hand. It is reported to have a sensitivity of 66% and a false-positive rate of 4%.

The primary dermatologic manifestation of hypocalcemia is impetigo herpetiformis, a form of acute pustular psoriasis associated with hypocalcemia in pregnancy. This appears as clusters of pinpoint pustules. Patients may also have less specific findings such as dry, flaky skin and brittle nails.

Laboratory Evaluation

A low total serum calcium should be interpreted in conjunction with the patient's serum albumin level, as a common cause of hypocalcemia is hypoalbuminemia. To correct the total serum calcium in the setting of hypoalbuminemia, use the equation:

$$[4 - \text{serum albumin (g/dL)}] \times 0.8 + \text{serum Ca}^{++} \text{ (mg/dL)} = \text{corrected Ca}^{++}$$

Alternatively, one can measure serum free (ionized) calcium directly. Other laboratory studies should include assessment of serum phosphorus, magnesium, creatinine, intact PTH, and, potentially, vitamin D metabolites. The classic ECG finding of hypocalcemia includes prolongation of the QT interval. This is the result of prolongation of phase 2 of the cardiac muscle cell. T-wave inversion may also occur, which does not revert with acute correction of the calcium.

TREATMENT

The real treatment for hypocalcemia is appropriate **correction of the underlying condition** causing hypocalcemia. In patients with pseudohypocalcemia secondary to decreased serum albumin, nutritional status should be optimized. The magnesium should be corrected in hypomagnesemic patients.

The indications for **acute correction of hypocalcemia** include severe symptomatic tetany, stridor, or seizures. Calcium may be replaced with either calcium gluconate or calcium chloride as an IV bolus. 10–20 mL (1–2 standard amps) of a 10% calcium gluconate solution may be given over 10 minutes; calcium chloride is equally effective. Care should be taken not to give the bolus more rapidly, as cardiac dysfunction may result. The effect of this bolus is transient, and prolonged IV therapy should probably follow.

For urgent, but not emergent, replacement of calcium, 1 mg/kg/hour of elemental calcium may be given as an IV piggyback over several hours. Each 10-mL amp of calcium gluconate contains 90 mg/2.25 mmol of elemental calcium. As such, if 6 amps of calcium gluconate are mixed in 500 mL of D_5W, a drip rate of 0.92 mL/kg/hour will provide 1 mg/kg/hour of elemental calcium. Because calcium is irritating, care should be given to ensure that the IV solution used as replacement doesn't extravasate. Additionally, bicarbonate and phosphate solutions cause calcium to precipitate. Serum calcium should be measured every 4–6 hours during IV infusion and rate adjusted to maintain a serum calcium level of 8–9 mg/dL.

The goal of **chronic calcium replacement** therapy is to keep the calcium in the low range of normal. If the calcium is kept below this, the patient remains at risk for symptoms of hypocalcemia or cataracts. A higher calcium level may predispose patients to nephrolithiasis. Approximately 1.5–3 g of elemental calcium should be given as a dietary supplement to ensure adequate intake. There are multiple different preparations of oral calcium, so care must be taken to ensure the appropriate dose of elemental calcium has been prescribed. In general, calcium carbonate is the cheapest, although absorption may be less than with other products.

Vitamin D supplementation is typically given as ergocalciferol (vitamin D_2). This preparation is the least expensive and has the longest half-life. The typical dose range for patients with hypoparathyroidism is on the order of 50,000–100,000 IU PO daily (1.25–2.5 mg/day). Serum 25(OH) vitamin D levels can be measured along with serum calcium levels to assess for adequacy of treatment. Vitamin D is extremely lipophilic and may require several weeks to reach a steady state with a new dose. Calcitriol, which has a shorter half-life, may also be given with a typical starting does of 0.25–0.5 mcg PO daily.

Because the hypoparathyroid patient is dependent on renal excretion of calcium to maintain calcium homeostasis, careful attention should be paid to renal function. Any medication causing an acute decrease in glomerular filtration rate may cause symptomatic hypercalcemia. Additionally, thiazide diuretics, by blocking calcium excretion, may lead to hypercalcemia in those taking chronic calcium or vitamin D replacement. Corticosteroids and antiepileptics may cause hypocalcemia by increasing the hepatic metabolism of vitamin D.

KEY POINTS TO REMEMBER

- Pathophysiology of chronic hypocalcemia relates to a functional deficiency of either PTH or vitamin D.

- The most worrisome symptoms of acute hypocalcemia are neurologic (i.e., seizures) or neuromuscular (i.e., tetany).
- Acute management is with IV calcium supplementation.
- Chronic management is generally with vitamin D and oral calcium supplementation.

REFERENCES AND SUGGESTED READINGS

Becker KL, ed. *Principles and practice of endocrinology and metabolism,* 2nd ed. Philadelphia: Lippincott, 1995:532–546.

Favus MJ, ed. *Primer on the metabolic bone diseases and disorders of mineral metabolism,* 4th ed. Philadelphia: Lippincott Williams & Wilkins, 1999:226–240.

Shoback D, et al. Mineral metabolism and metabolic bone disease. In: Greenspan FS, Gardner DG, eds. *Basic and clinical endocrinology.* New York: Lange Medical Books, 2001:273–333.

Simpson JA. The neurological manifestations of idiopathic hypoparathyroidism. *Brain* 1952;75:76–90.

Vanderark CR. Electrolytes and the electrocardiogram. *Cardiovasc Clin* 1973;5(3):269–294.

24

Osteoporosis

Jason S. Goldfeder

INTRODUCTION

Osteoporosis is a disorder characterized by low bone mass and microarchitectural deterioration of bone that leads to a **decrease in bone mass, enhanced bone fragility,** and a consequent **increase in the risk of fractures**. Osteoporosis is the most common metabolic bone disorder in humans and is generally an asymptomatic condition until complications develop. The prevalence, adverse outcomes, and economic cost associated with osteoporotic fractures, particularly hip fractures, are quite significant. The association of osteoporosis as an asymptomatic risk factor for fractures is similar to that of hypertension with stroke and hypercholesterolemia with coronary heart disease. Significant advances in diagnostic testing since the early 1990s have made osteoporosis relatively easy to diagnose, and several national societies have developed guidelines endorsing routine screening for osteoporosis. Several pharmaceutical agents that vary in their impact on enhancing bone density, decreasing the rates of fracture at various clinical sites, and side effects are approved for the prevention and treatment of osteoporosis. However, a significant percentage of patients with osteoporosis, including those who have already experienced fractures, are not appropriately diagnosed and treated.

Definition

Before 1994, making a diagnosis of osteoporosis required the presence of a clinical fracture. In 1994, the World Health Organization changed the definition of osteoporosis to include criteria based on bone densitometry testing. There are four diagnostic categories based on the comparison of a patient's bone mineral density (BMD) with that of a young adult reference mean (the T score; see the section Bone Mineral Density Testing).

- **Normal:** BMD within 1 standard deviation (SD) of the young adult reference mean (T $\geq$ –1.0)
- **Osteopenia:** BMD between 1 and 2.5 SDs below the young adult reference mean (–2.5 <T <–1.0)
- **Osteoporosis:** BMD >2.5 SDs below the young adult reference mean (T $\leq$ –2.5)
- **Established or severe osteoporosis:** BMD >2.5 SDs below the young adult reference mean (T $\leq$ –2.5) and the presence of one or more fragility fractures

Classification

Osteoporosis can be classified as primary or secondary osteoporosis. In primary osteoporosis, the deterioration of bone mass is related to aging or decreased gonadal function, typically in postmenopausal women or aging men. Secondary osteoporosis results from chronic conditions or medications that accelerate bone loss (see the section Risk Factors, Table 24-2).

Epidemiology

Approximately 30 million postmenopausal women in the United States have either osteopenia or osteoporosis. The majority of available data on the epidemiology of osteopenia and osteoporosis is in white women. Current estimates of the prevalence of osteoporosis come from the NHANES III epidemiologic study, which was conducted from 1988 to 1994. In this study, which used young white women as the referent for comparison, osteopenia and osteoporosis were estimated to be present in 41% and 17% of white women, 28% and 8% of black women, and 37% and 12% of Mexican-American women > age 50 years. The ratio of the age-adjusted prevalence of osteoporosis in white vs black women ranged from 1.5 to 2.8, depending on the site of measurement. The ratio in white vs Mexican-American women ranged from 0.8 to 1.2. Extrapolating the NHANES data to the current population, the National Osteoporosis Foundation currently estimates that 52% and 20% of postmenopausal white women have osteopenia and osteoporosis, respectively, and that there are currently approximately 22 million and 8 million women of all races in the United States with osteopenia and osteoporosis, respectively.

CAUSES

Pathogenesis

An adult's total bone mineral content is dependent on his/her peak bone mass achieved during early adulthood and his/her level of bone remodeling. Bone remodeling takes place throughout childhood and adulthood and is a result of the balance of concurrent bone resorption and new bone formation. Osteoporosis can result from poor bone acquisition and the failure to achieve expected peak bone or increased bone remodeling.

Peak bone mass is generally reached at approximately age 25–30 years. Peak bone mass is primarily determined by genetic factors, including race and gender. However, potentially modifiable environmental and metabolic conditions, such as nutritional status, calcium intake, physical activity level, tobacco use, hormonal deficiencies, and other medical comorbidities, can also affect the level of peak bone mass achieved. Black women and men of all races typically achieve higher levels of peak bone mass than white women, which is a key reason why the rates of osteoporosis and fractures are lower in these groups. Adults who do not achieve their predicted peak bone mass are at risk of developing osteoporosis at an earlier age.

When the rate of bone resorption exceeds that of new bone formation, the overall increased rate of bone turnover leads to a net loss of bone mass. Men and women slowly begin to lose peak bone mass at a rate of approximately 0.5–1% per year starting at approximately age 35 years. The rate of net bone loss is frequently increased after menopause in women as estrogen deficiency alters cytokine production and enhances osteoclast activity. This accelerated rate of bone loss is most prominent in areas of trabecular bone, such as the spine, and may result in a loss of bone mass of 3–5% per year for up to 10 years. The rate of bone loss in areas with more cortical bone, such as the hips, tends to be delayed and less rapid. As men achieve a higher peak bone mass initially and do not usually go through a rapid period of bone loss in the absence of secondary disorders, bone loss does not tend to reach levels that increase the risk for fractures until age 65–70 years.

Risk Factors

Several risk factors have been shown to be independently associated with low bone mass (Table 24-1). Some of these risk factors are modifiable and are important to address in a regimen to prevent or treat osteoporosis. There are also multiple chronic medical conditions and medications that are risk factors for causing secondary osteoporosis (Table 24-2). Osteoporosis typically results in fractures when adults with low bone density fall. As such, risk factors for falling that are independent of low BMD are important risk factors for experiencing osteoporotic fractures (Table 24-3).

PRESENTATION

Most patients with osteoporosis are asymptomatic until they develop fractures. As such, the history and physical exam are usually not sensitive enough to make a diagnosis of osteoporosis in the absence of diagnostic testing (see the sections Screening for Osteoporosis and Bone Mineral Density Testing). Once a patient is clinically diag-

TABLE 24-1. RISK FACTORS FOR OSTEOPOROSIS

Female sex
White race
Advanced age
Personal history of a fracture
Family history of osteoporosis/fracture in a first-degree relative
Small body habitus/low body weight (<127 lbs)
Sedentary lifestyle/lack of physical activity
Tobacco use
Excessive alcohol intake (>2 drinks/day)
Insufficient intake of calcium or vitamin D
Excessive caffeine intake
Early menopause (< age 45 yrs)
   Premature ovarian failure
   Medical or surgical menopause

TABLE 24-2. CAUSES OF SECONDARY OSTEOPOROSIS

Endocrine disorders
   Acromegaly
   Amenorrhea (primary or secondary amenorrhea of any cause)
   Anorexia
   Cushing's syndrome/hypercortisolism
   Diabetes mellitus, type 1
   Hyperparathyroidism
   Hyperprolactinemia
   Hyperthyroidism
   Hypogonadism (primary or secondary)
   Porphyria
Genetic/collagen disorders
   Ehlers-Danlos
   Glycogen storage diseases
   Homocystinuria
   Hypophosphatasia
   Osteogenesis imperfecta
GI/hepatic disorders
   Celiac sprue
   Chronic cholestatic liver disease
   Chronic malabsorptive conditions
   Cirrhosis
   Gastric bypass/gastrectomy

(continued)

TABLE 24-2. *(Continued)*

Hemochromatosis
Inflammatory bowel disease
Hematologic disorders
  Amyloidosis
  Leukemia/lymphoma
  Mastocytosis
  Multiple myeloma
Infectious diseases
  HIV/AIDS
Metabolic/nutritional disorders
  Alcoholism
  Hyperhomocystinemia
  Hypocalcemia
  Vitamin D deficiency
Pulmonary disorders
  COPD
Renal disorders
  Chronic kidney disease (of any cause)
  Renal tubular acidosis
Rheumatologic disorders
  Ankylosing spondylitis
  Rheumatoid arthritis
Medications
  Aluminum
  Cyclosporine
  Dilantin
  Glucocorticoids
  Gonadotropin agonists (e.g., Lupron)
  Heparin (prolonged use)
  Methotrexate
  Phenobarbital
  Phenothiazines
  Protease inhibitors
  Thyroxine (excessive replacement)

nosed with osteoporosis, the history should focus on assessing for modifiable risk factors (see Table 24-1), medical conditions associated with secondary osteoporosis (see Table 24-2), and risk factors for falling (see Table 24-3).

Screening for Osteoporosis

No randomized, controlled, prospective clinical trial has proven that screening for osteoporosis and subsequent intervention decreases the incidence of osteoporotic fractures or

TABLE 24-3. RISK FACTORS FOR FALLING

History of falls
Dementia
Impaired vision
Poor physical condition/frailty
Foot problems or inappropriate footwear
History of stroke or Parkinson's disease
Environmental hazards
Use of benzodiazepines, anticonvulsants, or anticholinergic medications

other complications. However, based on the prevalence of the condition, frequency of complications, accessibility of diagnostic testing, and available treatment options, several national societies have issued consensus statements supporting routine screening for osteoporosis (Table 24-4). In general, all groups agree that women who present with fragility fractures in the absence of trauma should be screened, but opinions vary on whether and under what conditions routine screening of asymptomatic adults should be conducted. Of note, even though the majority of data on the diagnosis and treatment of osteoporosis are in white women, the recommendations for screening for osteoporosis in women are irrespective of race.

Osteoporotic Fractures

Fragility Fractures
Fragility fractures are the primary cause of morbidity and mortality in adults with osteoporosis. The most common sites for osteoporotic fractures are the **hip**, the **spine**,

TABLE 24-4. SOCIETAL RECOMMENDATIONS ON ROUTINE SCREENING FOR OSTEOPOROSIS

Group	Recommendations
National Osteoporosis Foundation	Screen all women > age 65 yrs regardless of risk factors
	Screen younger postmenopausal women with ≥1 risk factor besides sex, race, and menopausal status
U.S. Preventive Services Task Force	Screen all women > age 65 yrs regardless of risk factors
	Screen women aged 60–65 yrs who are at increased risk for fractures primarily based on low body weight (<70 kg) or lack of hormone replacement therapy
NIH	Routine screening is not recommended
American College of Obstetricians and Gynecologists	Screen all women > age 65 yrs regardless of risk factors
	Screen postmenopausal women < age 65 yrs with additional risk factors
European Foundation for Osteoporosis and Bone Disease	Routine screening is not recommended

and the **distal radius** (forearm or wrist). Approximately 1.5 million osteoporotic fractures occur each year in the United States, including 700,000 vertebral fractures, 300,000 hip fractures, 200,000 wrist fractures, and 300,000 other fractures. In white women aged 65–85 years, it is estimated that 90% of all vertebral fractures, 90% of all hip fractures, 70% of all forearm fractures, and 50% of all other fractures are attributable to osteoporosis. The corresponding rates in black women are 80% for vertebral fractures, 80% for hip fractures, 60% for forearm fractures, and 40% for all other fractures. In both races, a smaller percentage of fractures can be attributed to osteoporosis in women < age 65 years, but a larger percentage can be attributed to osteoporosis in women > age 85 years. A 50-year-old white woman has an approximate 50% risk of experiencing an osteoporotic fracture during her lifetime, including a 32% risk of a having a vertebral fracture, a 16% risk of having a hip fracture, and a 15% risk of having a wrist fracture. With the anticipated aging of the population, osteoporotic fractures are predicted to increase several-fold worldwide by 2050.

Hip Fractures

Hip fractures are the most devastating cause of morbidity and mortality attributable to osteoporosis. Mortality rates are increased 5–6-fold during the first month after a hip fracture and approximately 3-fold over the first year, resulting in a 1-year mortality rate from hip fractures in women of 10–20%. 15–30% of women require nursing home placement for at least 1 year. Up to one-half of women able to walk before a hip fracture require long-term placement or help with activities of daily living after fracture. Only 30–40% of women regain their prefracture level of function. Treatment of hip fractures and their associated complications are responsible for the majority of the cost associated with treating osteoporosis, with cost estimates of $14 billion to treat hip fractures in 1995 and $17 billion in 2001.

Vertebral Fractures

Vertebral fractures are also associated with significant morbidity and mortality. Vertebral fractures tend to be more occult than hip fractures and are often present radiographically but not clinically. As opposed to hip and wrist fractures, most vertebral fractures are not related to acute trauma and can result from routine everyday activities or minor stresses on the spine such as bending or lifting. Only approximately one-third of radiographically confirmed vertebral compression fractures come to medical attention, and <10% result in hospital admissions. However, asymptomatic vertebral fractures are a major risk factor for subsequent fractures, including hip fractures. Treatment to prevent subsequent hip fractures with antiresorptive therapy is more beneficial in adults with prevalent vertebral fractures. Vertebral fractures are associated with chronic back pain, loss of height, and kyphosis. Having multiple vertebral fractures can result in the development of restrictive lung disease or GI complications such as chronic abdominal pain, constipation, and anorexia. Vertebral fractures have been shown to decrease quality of life across several domains. Most important, long-term prospective studies have shown that the presence of vertebral fractures, whether symptomatic or not, is associated with a 15–30% increased rate of overall mortality, including an increased risk of mortality secondary to all cancers, specifically lung cancer, and pulmonary disease.

MANAGEMENT

Bone Mineral Density Testing

The standard of care to diagnose and evaluate adults for osteoporosis is to assess their BMD. Several radiologic tests are available to measure BMD, including central and peripheral dual energy x-ray absorptiometry (DEXA), quantitative CT, and peripheral ultrasonography.

DEXA is the gold standard and is recommended for adults who have had osteoporotic fractures or who are undergoing general screening. DEXA imaging results in a low level of radiation exposure (approximately one-tenth that of a traditional x-ray) and has excellent precision and reproducibility. The most common sites to measure with DEXA are the spine, the hip, and the distal forearm. BMD results are calculated as the bone mineral content divided by the area of bone measured (g/cm^2). In the lumbosacral spine, measurements are generally made at the L-1, L-2, L-3, and L-4 vertebrae and then averaged together for a total spine score. At the hip, measurements are made at the femoral neck, greater trochanter, intertrochanteric area, and Ward's triangle and then averaged. Results of BMD testing are then reported in comparison to reference ranges in SDs as the T score and the Z score.

- The *T score* compares the patient's BMD in SDs with the average peak BMD of young healthy adults of the same gender.
- The *Z score* compares the patient's BMD in SDs with the average BMD of adults of the same age and gender.

The **diagnoses of osteoporosis and osteopenia are made based on the T score**. The Z score can occasionally be helpful if it is very abnormal as it suggests the possibility of a secondary cause of osteoporosis. Decreased BMD is a strong predictor of subsequent fracture. On average, the risk of fracture approximately doubles for each 1 SD decrease in the T score. Although decreased bone density at one site allows the diagnosis of osteoporosis to be made and increases the risk for fracture at all sites, the best predictor of fracture at a specific site is the bone density at that site. This is most important at the hip, which is the fracture site most associated with morbidity and mortality. For each 1-SD decrease in hip BMD, the risk of hip fractures increases by 2.6-fold, the risk of vertebral fractures increases by 1.8-fold, the risk of wrist fractures increases by 1.4-fold, and the risk of all fractures increases by 1.5-fold. The risk of a subsequent hip fracture associated with decreased BMD at other sites is somewhat lower. This is explained by the fact that different parts of the skeleton are affected differently at different periods and by different medical conditions. In the early postmenopausal period, bone loss occurs most rapidly in the spine. However, in adults > age 65 years, the bone density of the spine may be falsely elevated by osteoarthritis of the spine or vascular calcification. Adults with primary hyperparathyroidism lose bone most rapidly in the distal radius. If insurance coverage allows, bone density testing should be obtained of both the spine and the hip. However, if only one site is covered, bone density testing of the spine is often more helpful in women < age 65 years or within 15 years of menopause, as bone is more apt to be lost more rapidly in the spine, and vertebral fractures are the most common type of fracture in this age group. In women > age 65 years, bone density of the hip is often more clinically useful, as hip fractures become more of a clinical concern and the spine bone density has a greater chance of being falsely elevated.

Although results of bone density testing are an important risk factor for subsequent fracture, other factors (particularly age) also play prominent roles. The 10-year risk of experiencing osteoporotic fractures at multiple sites increases significantly with age at the same level of BMD.

Quantitative CT scanning and **central bone densitometry** have a similar ability to predict fractures. Quantitative CT scanning actually is a measure of volumetric density and reports results in g/cm^2. Quantitative CT can be obtained of the hip or spine and is less affected by superimposed osteoarthritis. However, quantitative CT scanning is more expensive, requires a larger dose of radiation, and is not frequently used clinically.

Peripheral bone density testing can be performed with either DEXA or single x-ray energy absorptiometry. Sites that can be measured include the forearm, finger, or heel. Studies using single x-ray energy absorptiometry that were performed before central DEXA was available found that abnormal results were associated with complications such as hip fractures. Peripheral ultrasonography can also be performed on the heel, tibia, or patella. The primary benefits of peripheral DEXA and ultrasonography are the portability of the equipment and the ability of the tests to be performed in a primary care office. However, there are not universally agreed on diagnostic criteria for the different machines available. In addition, the precision of the machines does not allow their use for monitoring response to therapy. Peripheral testing has not been fully endorsed for use in the diagnosis of osteoporosis, but if peripheral testing is performed, abnormal results should be followed up with a central DEXA to establish or confirm the diagnosis.

Laboratory Evaluation

Multiple laboratory tests are available to evaluate for **secondary causes of osteoporosis** (see Table 24-2). There is not a uniform consensus on how much of a workup, if any, is required in adults with a new diagnosis of osteoporosis. Secondary osteoporosis is more common in premenopausal women and men in whom the threshold for diagnostic testing might be somewhat lower. One study of patients from a tertiary referral center found that most patients would be diagnosed with the combination of a serum calcium, parathyroid hormone (PTH), 24-hour urine for calcium, and thyroid-stimulating hormone (TSH) if the patient was taking levothyroxine (Synthroid). The National Osteoporosis Foundation endorses consideration of limited biochemical testing in some patients with initial tests, possibly including a TSH, PTH, vitamin D level (25OH-VitD), serum protein electrophoresis, and 24-hour urine for calcium and cortisol. Other tests to consider if disorders are suggested by the history and physical exam include assessment of renal and liver function, testosterone screening, and luteinizing hormone (LH) and follicle-stimulating hormone (FSH) levels.

Serum and urinary markers of bone turnover are frequently increased in patients with osteoporosis. Markers of bone formation include serum alkaline phosphatase and osteocalcin. Markers of bone resorption include urinary hydroxyproline, and N- and C-terminal collagen telopeptides. Markers of bone turnover may predict the risk of fracture independent of BMD and allow assessment of the response to treatment, but at this point their role in clinical practice is unclear, and testing is generally unnecessary.

Plain film x-rays are generally unreliable markers of bone mass, as 20–50% of bone must be lost before changes are evident on x-ray. Although not routinely necessary, a baseline lumbosacral spine x-ray could be considered in an adult with newly diagnosed osteoporosis to assess for any baseline vertebral fractures, which are a prominent risk factor for subsequent clinical fractures.

Indications for Treatment

All postmenopausal women should be evaluated for risk factors for osteoporosis. Bone density testing should be performed in all adults with fractures and should be considered in postmenopausal women based on their age and risk factors. The nonpharmacologic and lifestyle recommendations should be suggested to all adults, including those who do not meet criteria for specific pharmacologic therapy for osteoporosis to prevent the development of osteoporosis. The following are indications to initiate specific therapy for osteoporosis. It is important to be aware that the prospective randomized controlled pharmacologic trials for the treatment of osteoporosis have taken place mainly in white women (85% to >95% in most treatment trials), so limited data are available on the therapeutic benefit of pharmacologic agents in minority groups.

- All adults with osteoporotic fractures of the hip or spine
- Adults with a T score ≤–2.0 SD who do not have specific risk factors for osteoporosis
- Adults with a T score of ≤–1.5 SD who have risk factors for osteoporosis

Nonpharmacologic Treatment Options

Adults with osteoporosis should be encouraged to stop smoking and avoid excessive alcohol intake. **Weight-bearing exercise** should be encouraged. Multiple small observational and randomized controlled trials have shown that regular exercise can help maximize peak bone mass in young women, decrease age-related bone loss, actually improve BMD in some circumstances, and help maintain muscle balance and strength. The goal should be to exercise for 30–60 minutes at least 3 times per week. High-impact weight-bearing activities, such as brisk walking, jogging, weight lifting, and racket sports, are beneficial forms of exercise. Non–weight-bearing activities, such as swimming, are of more questionable benefit. Exercise has never been proven to prospectively decrease the risk of fracture, but it does improve function and decrease the rate of falls. Patients should be assessed for reversible causes of falls such as overmedication, vision problems, and poor footwear. For patients at high risk of falling, hip protectors worn under their clothes have been shown to decrease the rate of hip fractures by 60%. A combined aggressive program of nonpharmacologic treatment has been shown to decrease the rate of hip fractures by up to 25%.

Pharmacologic Treatment Options

Calcium and Vitamin D

Adequate intake of calcium is essential to achieve peak bone mass in early adulthood and to maintain bone mass throughout postmenopausal life. Vitamin D increases calcium absorption in the intestine and calcium reabsorption in the kidney. Vitamin D is supplied in both the diet and conversion from skin precursors in the presence of sunlight. Elderly adults, especially those who are chronically ill or institutionalized, frequently have a high prevalence of vitamin D deficiency, as they have limited exposure to sunlight. The majority of clinical trials have found that **supplementation with calcium and vitamin D** has a modest beneficial effect on BMD. Most important, one study of elderly women in nursing homes found that supplementation with calcium and vitamin D decreased the rate of hip and other fractures. In essentially all of the randomized, placebo-controlled clinical trials with antiresorptive and bone forming agents, patients in both the placebo and treatment groups received supplemental calcium and either received supplemental vitamin D or had serum levels checked with supplementation if vitamin D levels were low.

The recommended daily allowance of calcium varies somewhat in different consensus guidelines, but in general is at least 1000–1200 mg/day (Table 24-5).

Foods rich in calcium include milk, yogurt, cheeses, sardines, and fortified juices. The average daily calcium intake in adults from nondairy foods is 250 mg/day. The estimated amount of elemental calcium in common dairy products is as follows:

- 8-oz glass of milk: 300 mg
- 8 oz of yogurt: 400 mg
- 1 oz of cheese: 200 mg
- Fortified juices: varies

Most adults do not regularly eat enough dairy products in their diets to meet recommended intakes. Essentially all of the clinical trials in adults with osteoporosis that have included dietary assessments of calcium intake have found that most adults'

TABLE 24-5. RECOMMENDED DAILY CALCIUM INTAKE

Organization	Age (yrs)	Recommended daily allowance of elemental calcium
National Osteoporosis Foundation	All ages	1200 mg/day
NIH	11–24	1200–1500 mg/day
	25–50	1000 mg/day
	50–65	Men: 1000 mg/day
		Women on HRT: 1000 mg/day
		Women not on HRT: 1500 mg/day
	>65	1500 mg/day

HRT, hormone replacement therapy.

dietary calcium intake is significantly below recommended levels. As such, most adults both with and without osteoporosis require calcium supplementation. There are a multitude of calcium supplements available, most as either calcium carbonate or calcium acetate. It is important to realize that the recommendations for calcium are for elemental calcium and that many over-the-counter calcium supplements are labeled by the amount of calcium carbonate or acetate per pill. Calcium salts are best absorbed when taken between meals. The recommended daily allowance of vitamin D is 400–800 IU PO daily, with the higher amount recommended for adults at highest risk of being vitamin D deficient. Foods rich in vitamin D include fortified milk and cereals, egg yolks, and liver. Some calcium supplements include vitamin D (Os-Cal D).

Bisphosphonates: Alendronate (Fosamax) and Risedronate (Actonel)
The bisphosphonates are the best agents currently available for treating osteoporosis. Bisphosphonates bind to mineralized bone and inhibit osteoclast activity. Bisphosphonates inhibit both bone resorption and bone formation but **inhibit bone resorption** to a greater degree. Alendronate and risedronate are the two FDA-approved bisphosphonates for osteoporosis (Table 24-6). Both agents have been shown to **improve bone density** at various sites in the skeleton and **decrease the rates of total, hip, and symptomatic and asymptomatic vertebral fractures**. Randomized controlled trials showing a benefit in reducing fractures have lasted up to 4 years. Sustained benefit in improving bone density has been shown with as long as 10 years of treatment with alendronate and 7 years of risedronate. Alendronate and risedronate are the only agents to date that have been consistently shown to decrease hip fractures in patients with osteoporosis. However, the significant decrease in hip fractures is primarily seen only in patients with established osteoporosis (T <–2.5) who have preexisting vertebral fractures. The benefit in absolute terms in reducing fractures of all types with both agents is more prominent in patients with preexisting vertebral fractures.

Bisphosphonates should be taken early in the morning with a glass of water at least **30 minutes before any food or other medications** to prevent retention of the pills in the esophagus. Absorption is limited by antacids and calcium. In the randomized, placebo-controlled trials with alendronate and risedronate, there was no significant difference in the rate of significant GI side effects between the agents and placebo. However, in clinical practice, esophageal and gastric side effects and complications have been reported, reinforcing the need for proper dosing. Once-a-week formulations of alendronate and risedronate are available for both osteoporosis prevention and treatment and may increase compliance.

Zoledronate (Zometa) and ibandronate (Boniva) are two potent bisphosphonates that have been studied in clinical trials. When given IV, including as a one-time dose, zoledronate has been shown to lead to persistent improvements in BMD and markers of bone turnover after 1 year. Ibandronate has been shown to improve BMD when given once weekly either PO or IV. Although both agents show promise for the treatment of osteoporosis, neither has been studied in large enough trials for a long enough period so far to find a reduction in clinical fractures.

Raloxifene (Evista)
Raloxifene is a selective estrogen receptor modulator that exhibits proestrogen effects on certain tissues and antiestrogen effects on other tissues. Raloxifene exhibits beneficial effects on bone by blocking the activity of cytokines that stimulate osteoclast-mediated bone resorption. Raloxifene has been shown in randomized controlled trials lasting up to 3–4 years to **improve BMD** at the spine and the hip and to **decrease the rate of new vertebral fractures** (MORE study). Raloxifene has not been found to have a significant impact on hip or total nonvertebral fractures. An ideal candidate for raloxifene is a woman who has predominantly decreased BMD at the spine with more preserved levels of bone density at the hip. Raloxifene decreases total cholesterol and low-density lipoprotein (LDL) cholesterol similarly to estrogen, but does not raise high-density lipoprotein (HDL) cholesterol and triglycerides as estrogen does. Raloxifene does not reduce hot flashes. It does increase the risk of deep venous thrombosis and pulmonary embolism in a fashion similar to estrogen. However, raloxifene does

TABLE 24-6. AVAILABLE AGENTS FOR OSTEOPOROSIS: DOSING AND SIDE EFFECTS

Agent	FDA approved for prevention	Dose for prevention	FDA approved for treatment	Dose for treatment	Side effects
Alendronate (Fosamax)	Yes	5 mg PO/day 35 mg PO once/wk	Yes	10 mg PO/day 70 mg PO once/wk	Abdominal pain, dyspepsia, nausea, esophagitis, musculoskeletal pain
Risedronate (Actonel)	Yes	5 mg PO/day 35 mg PO once/wk	Yes	5 mg PO/day 35 mg PO once/wk	Abdominal pain, dyspepsia, gastritis, esophagitis
Zoledronate (Zometa)	No	Not applicable	No	4 mg IV for 1 dose	Myalgias, arthralgias, fever
Ibandronate (Boniva)	No	Not applicable	No	20 mg PO or IV once/wk	Abdominal pain, dyspepsia, back pain, myalgias
Raloxifene (Evista)	Yes	60 mg PO/day	Yes	60 mg PO/day	Hot flashes, leg cramps, lower extremity edema, increased risk of DVT/PE
Estrogen (alone or with a progesterone); multiple combinations available	Yes	Multiple types Usually 0.625 mg PO/day conjugated estrogen	No	Not applicable	Vaginal bleeding, breast tenderness, increased risk of CHD, stroke, DVT/PE, breast cancer
Calcitonin (Miacalcin)	Yes	100 IU intranasally/day	Yes	200 IU intranasally/day	Nasal congestion, rhinorrhea
Teriparatide (Forteo)	No	Not applicable	Yes	20 mcg SC/day	Dizziness, leg cramps, headache, nausea, mild hypercalcemia

CHD, coronary heart disease; DVT, deep vein thrombosis; PE, pulmonary embolism.

not stimulate the endometrium or breast and does not increase the risk of endometrial hyperplasia or cancer or breast cancer. In fact, the largest clinical trial of raloxifene found a significant decrease in estrogen receptor–positive breast cancer as a secondary end point. With activity similar to estrogen on some tissues, but different at others, the cardiovascular impact of raloxifene is uncertain at this point. The ongoing international Raloxifene Use for the Heart (RUTH) study is currently evaluating the cardiovascular effects of raloxifene.

Estrogen/Hormone Replacement Therapy

Estrogen replacement therapy (ERT) improves bone density by inhibiting osteoclast activity. Little of the clinical data assessing the impact of estrogen has been in women with documented osteoporosis. As a result, most of the data on estrogen are more appropriate to interpret for prevention rather than treatment of osteoporosis. In addition, until the recent publication of the Women's Health Initiative (WHI), most of the fracture data with estrogen was from observational trials. Prospective randomized, controlled trials lasting up to 3 years have found that ERT, with or without concomitant progesterone, improved BMD at the spine and hip. A meta-analysis found that ERT increased BMD at the spine by 7% and the hip by 4% after 2 years. The beneficial effects on BMD are lost within a few years after stopping hormone replacement therapy (HRT). One of the largest prospective observational trials found that women on ERT for an average of 5 years experienced 34% fewer fractures. Previous users of ERT who were no longer taking it had fracture rates similar to those who had never taken it. The benefit of estrogen on decreasing fractures was only evident in patients who started it within 5 years of menopause. Until recently, the prospective clinical trial data assessing the ability of estrogen to prevent fractures was limited by the fact that many of the trials were too small, too short in duration, or studied women who were to low-risk to independently find a significant decrease in fractures. In a recent meta-analysis of prospective trials published before the WHI, ERT was found to decrease the rate of total fractures by 27%, with the benefit being more significant in women < age 60 years than in women > age 60 years.

The recent WHI answered many important questions about the use of ERT for prevention of chronic conditions. The WHI is the first large-scale prospective randomized, controlled trial that has individually found that combination estrogen/progesterone replacement therapy decreased the rate of fractures. Total fractures, vertebral fractures, hip fractures, and other osteoporotic fractures were decreased by 24%, 34%, 34%, and 23%, respectively. Although the rate of colon cancer was also decreased by 37%, overall, the rate of adverse events, including a 29% increase in coronary heart disease, a 41% increase in stroke, a 111% increase in deep venous thrombosis/pulmonary embolism, and a 26% increase in breast cancer, exceeded the benefits, including fracture reduction. Similar decreases in fracture rates were found in women on estrogen alone who had undergone a previous hysterectomy in the estrogen-only arm of the WHI study.

Little prospective data actually exist in patients with known osteoporosis; only one published small trial found a decrease in vertebral fractures with transdermal estrogen. Based on the lack of data in treating known osteoporosis and the balance of adverse events shown in the WHI, ERT has fallen out of favor for the prevention or treatment of osteoporosis. ERT is actually not FDA-approved for the treatment of osteoporosis; other forms of therapy are more potent with less toxicity to use in prevention.

Calcitonin (Miacalcin)

Calcitonin enhances BMD by **inhibiting osteoclast formation**. Calcitonin is available in both SC and intranasal forms, but the intranasal route is the one that has been most studied in osteoporosis. The beneficial effects on BMD of the spine are generally less with calcitonin than most of the other agents available to treat osteoporosis. Minimal to no impact has been seen on BMD of the hip. In the Prevent Recurrences of Osteoporotic Fracture (PROOF) study, one of the doses of intranasal calcitonin was found to decrease vertebral fractures after 5 years. There was not a dose-dependent response for vertebral fractures, and there was not a significant benefit in decreasing hip or nonvertebral fractures. Calcitonin is typically a **second- or third-line agent** for the treatment of osteoporosis and is primarily reserved for patients with either contraindications to or intolerable side effects from other agents, particularly bisphosphonates. However, intranasal calcitonin has been found to be **beneficial in treating the pain of acute vertebral compression fractures**.

Teriparatide (Forteo)

Teriparatide is a recombinant formulation of the active 34 N-terminal peptide portion of parathyroid hormone. Although continuous exposure to PTH (as in patients with primary hyperparathyroidism) leads to increased bone resorption, intermittent exposure has been shown to stimulate bone formation. Teriparatide is the first pharmacologic agent that primarily increases bone formation by **stimulating osteoblast activity**. As opposed to all of the other agents for osteoporosis that work by decreasing bone turnover more than new bone formation, teriparatide works by stimulating new bone formation more than it stimulates bone resorption. Teriparatide has been studied in high-risk women with a history of vertebral fractures for up to 2 years. The improvement in bone density was greater than that seen with any of the other available agents for osteoporosis (Table 24-7). Spinal fractures and total nonvertebral fractures decreased significantly, but the trial was too small and too short for there to be enough hip fractures to assess that end point. Because of its significant cost, teriparatide should generally be **reserved for patients with severe or established osteoporosis,** particularly those who cannot take or have had unsuccessful results with bisphosphonates. Mild hypercalcemia occasionally develops. Rats that were treated with high doses of teriparatide had an increased rate of developing osteosarcomas. Although this has not been seen in human trials, teriparatide's package insert contains a black box warning about osteosarcomas. Teriparatide is contraindicated in patients with preexisting hypercalcemia or metastatic bone disease and in those at increased risk for osteosarcoma, such as those with Paget's disease, prior radiation therapy to bone, and in children. Treatment is not recommended for >2 years.

Combination Therapy

Several different combination regimens have been studied with variable results. Studies assessing combination regimens have primarily studied the impact on BMD and have not been large enough or long enough to assess fracture risk. Adding alendronate or risedronate to patients already taking HRT has been shown to improve bone density compared to placebo. Combination therapy with alendronate and HRT was shown to improve bone density more after 3 years than either agent alone. Larger trials are needed to study whether this improvement in bone density with two agents that have a similar mechanism of action translates into better fracture results. In the absence of such data, the possible adverse effects of HRT need to be considered before initiating dual therapy. Adding teriparatide to HRT has been shown to improve BMD. The most promise was held for combining teriparatide with a bisphosphonate using the most potent agents for bone resorption and bone formation. However, a recent trial found that combination therapy with teriparatide and alendronate was less effective than teriparatide alone at improving BMD and increasing new bone formation. As a result, combination therapy with teriparatide and a bisphosphonate is contraindicated at this time. Starting a bisphosphonate after completing 2 years of teriparatide makes theoretical sense and is currently being evaluated in clinical trials.

Impact of Other Medical Therapies on Fractures

Two common forms of medical therapy that have been thought to possibly impact the risk of osteoporotic fractures are **thiazide diuretics** and **hepatic 3-methylglutaryl coenzyme A (HMG-COA) reductase inhibitors**. Thiazide diuretics are thought to be helpful because they decrease urinary calcium excretion. A large population cohort study found that adults taking thiazide diuretics experienced significantly fewer hip fractures, especially if they had been on treatment for >1 year. Initial case-control studies with HMG-COA reductase inhibitors suggested an association of the agents with less hip fractures, but more recent studies have not found a significant benefit.

TABLE 24-7. AVAILABLE AGENTS FOR OSTEOPOROSIS: IMPACT ON BONE MINERAL DENSITY (BMD) AND FRACTURES

Agent	Increase in BMD of spine	Decrease in rate of vertebral fractures	Increase in BMD of hip	Decrease in rate of hip fractures	Decrease in rate of nonvertebral fractures
Alendronate (Fosamax)	6–9%	40–50%	4–7%	50–55%	20–47%
Risedronate (Actonel)	5–6%	40–60%	2–5%	40–60%	20–40%
Zoledronate (Zometa)	4–5%	Not studied	3–4%	Not studied	Not studied
Ibandronate (Boniva)	3–4%	Not studied	2–3%	Not studied	Not studied
Raloxifene (Evista)	3%	30–50%	2%	Not significant	Not significant
Estrogen/hormone replacement therapy[a]	4–7%	34–40%	2–4%	34–36%	24–27%
Calcitonin (Miacalcin)	1–2%	33%	No change	Not significant	Not significant
Teriparatide (Forteo)	8–14%	65–70%	3–5%	Studies not powered	53%

[a]Data for estrogen/hormone replacement therapy is from studies in postmenopausal women and not in women with known osteoporosis.

Follow-Up

Follow-up of patients with osteoporosis includes **monitoring for complications, side effects, and response to treatment.** Continued assessment should take place for modifiable risk factors for fall such as gait disorders, visual problems, or sedating medications (see Table 24-3). Height should be followed on a regular basis to screen for asymptomatic vertebral fractures. In general, antiresorptive therapy needs to be continued long term, as the beneficial effect on BMD is lost over time after stopping treatment, especially with HRT. BMD should be reevaluated after 12–18 months to assess response to therapy. Repeat measurements made sooner than that can be difficult to interpret, as the expected change in bone density over a shorter period may be similar to the precision of the machine. BMD changes generally need to be at least 3% to be considered significant, as the precision of most bone densitometers is approximately 1–1.5%. Repeat measurements need to be made on the same bone density machine to allow results to be accurately compared. Patients who are being screened for osteoporosis but are not on treatment should wait at least 2 years before undergoing repeat bone density testing.

Osteoporosis in Men

Much less is known about osteoporosis in men than women. The prevalence of osteoporosis and osteoporotic fractures is less common in men than women because men achieve a higher peak bone mass, lose bone at a slower rate, and have a shorter life expectancy. Men typically have a BMD that is 8–18% greater at different sites than women. Men begin to experience complications from osteoporosis approximately 15–20 years later than women. Complications of osteoporosis are significant in men, as 50-year-old men have a 13% lifetime risk of an osteoporotic fracture. Approximately 30% of hip fractures occur in men, and men have higher mortality rates after hip fractures than women. Men have a 31% 1-year mortality after a hip fracture, 79% are in a nursing home or assisted living facility at 1 year, 60% have a permanent disability, and only 41% return to the prefracture level of function.

Estimates of the prevalence of osteoporosis in men depend on the bone density cutoff used to make a diagnosis of osteoporosis. There are differences of opinion on whether male or female bone density cutoffs should be used. 2–6% of men > age 50 years meet the diagnostic criteria for osteoporosis, with the number varying based on whether female or male cutoffs are used for comparison. BMD testing should be considered in men with nontraumatic fractures, osteopenia on x-rays, use of chronic steroids, hypogonadism, hyperparathyroidism, and other risk factors for secondary osteoporosis. There are no universal consensus guidelines for routine screening in men, although some experts recommend considering screening in men > age 70 or 75 years. Men are more likely to have secondary osteoporosis than women. A laboratory evaluation, including testosterone screening, is generally recommended in men, as 30–60% have a specific cause of their osteoporosis.

Nonpharmacologic therapy, including weight-bearing exercise, smoking cessation, decreasing alcohol intake, and decreasing fall risks, are recommended to men just as they are to women. **Calcium and vitamin D supplementation** are recommended. **Alendronate** has been shown to improve bone density and decrease the rate of vertebral fractures in men. Alendronate is FDA approved for osteoporosis, including steroid-induced osteoporosis, and risedronate is approved for steroid-induced osteoporosis. Teriparatide has been shown to improve BMD and is another option for men. Testosterone replacement with IM injections, topical patches, or topical gels should be prescribed for men with documented hypogonadism. Studies have consistently found that a small percentage of men with fragility fractures are diagnosed with and treated for osteoporosis.

KEY POINTS TO REMEMBER

- The clinical consequences of osteoporosis are primarily related to fragility fractures, which most commonly occur at the spine, hip, and wrist.
- The key part of the evaluation in patients with suspected osteoporosis is to evaluate their bone density by DEXA. Osteoporosis and osteopenia are defined as T scores >2.5 and 1–2.5 SDs below the young adult reference mean.
- All patients with osteoporotic fractures, a T score <−2.0, or a T score <−1.5 with additional risk factors should be treated for osteoporosis.
- It is vital to ensure that all patients with osteoporosis have an adequate intake of calcium and vitamin D, which usually requires supplementation.
- Bisphosphonates (alendronate, risedronate) are generally the first-line agents in the treatment of osteoporosis as they are the only treatment options that have been proven to decrease the development of vertebral and hip fractures.
- ERT and HRT can prevent the development of osteoporotic fractures, but this benefit must be weighed against the increased risk of several adverse outcomes.

SUGGESTED READING

National Osteoporosis Foundation. *Physician's guide to the prevention and treatment of osteoporosis*. National Osteoporosis Foundation: Washington, DC, 2003.

NIH Consensus Development Panel on Osteoporosis Prevention, Diagnosis, and Therapy. Osteoporosis prevention, diagnosis, and therapy. *JAMA* 2001;285:785–795.

U.S. Preventive Services Task Force. Screening for osteoporosis in postmenopausal women: recommendations and rationale. *Ann Intern Med* 2002;137:526–528.

Writing group for the Women's Health Initiative Investigators. Risks and benefits of estrogen plus progestin in healthy postmenopausal women. Principal results from the Women's Health Initiative randomized controlled trial. *JAMA* 2002; 288:321–333.

REFERENCES

Black DM, Cummings SR, Karpf DB, et al. Randomised trial of effect of alendronate on risk of fracture in women with existing vertebral fractures. *Lancet* 1996;348:1535–1541.

Black DM, Greenspan SL, Ensrud KE, et al. The effects of parathyroid hormone and alendronate alone or in combination in postmenopausal osteoporosis. *N Engl J Med* 2003;349:1207–1215.

Blake GM, Fogelman I. Applications of bone densitometry for osteoporosis. *Endocrinol Metab Clin North Am* 1998;27:267–288.

Brunader R, Shelton DK. Radiologic bone assessment in the evaluation of osteoporosis. *Am Fam Physician* 2002;65:1357–1364.

Cauley JA, Seeley DG, Ensrud K, et al. Estrogen replacement therapy and fractures in older women. *Ann Intern Med* 1995;122:9–16.

Chapuy MC, Arlot ME, Duboeuf F, et al. Vitamin D3 and calcium to prevent hip fractures in elderly women. *N Engl J Med* 1992;327:1637–1642.

Chestnut CH, Silverman S, Andriano K, et al. A randomized trial of nasal spray salmon calcitonin in postmenopausal women with established osteoporosis: the prevent recurrence of osteoporotic fractures study. *Am J Med* 2000;109:267–276.

Cummings SR, Black DM, Nevitt MC, et al. Bone density at various sites for prediction of hip fractures. *Lancet* 1993;341:72–75.

Cummings SR, Black DM, Thompson DE. Effect of alendronate on risk of fractures in women with low bone density but without vertebral fractures. *JAMA* 1998;280:2077–2082.

Delmas PD, Bjarnason NH, Mitlak BH, et al. Effects of raloxifene on bone mineral density, serum cholesterol concentrations and uterine endometrium in postmenopausal women. *N Engl J Med* 1997;337:1641–1647.

Eastell R. Treatment of postmenopausal osteoporosis. *N Engl J Med* 1998;338:736–745.

Ettinger B, Black DM, Mitlak BH, et al. Reduction of vertebral fracture risk in postmenopausal women with osteoporosis treated with raloxifene. *JAMA* 1999;282:637–645.

Ettinger MP. Aging bone and osteoporosis: strategies for preventing fractures. *Arch Intern Med* 2003;163:2237–2246.

Greenspan SL, Resnick NM, Parker RA. Combination therapy with hormone replacement and alendronate for prevention of bone loss in elderly women. *JAMA* 2003;289:2525–2533.

Harris ST, Watts NB, Genant HK, et al. Effects of risedronate treatment on vertebral and nonvertebral fractures in women with postmenopausal osteoporosis. *JAMA* 1999;282:1344–1352.

Hulley S, Furberg C, Barrett-Connor E, et al. Noncardiovascular disease outcomes during 6.8 years of hormone therapy: heart and estrogen/progestin replacement study follow-up (HERS II). *JAMA* 2002;288:58–66.

Kado DM, Browner WS, Palermo L. Vertebral fractures and mortality in older women. *Arch Intern Med* 1999;159:1215–1220.

Kannus P, Parkkari J, Niemi S. Prevention of hip fracture in elderly people with the use of a hip protector. *N Engl J Med* 2000;343:1506–1513.

Looker AC, Orwoll ES, Johnston CC, et al. Prevalence of low femoral bone density in older U.S. adults from NHANES III. *J Bone Miner Res* 1997;12:1761–1768.

Lufkin EG, Wahner HW, O'Fallon WM, et al. Treatment of postmenopausal osteoporosis with transdermal estrogen. *Ann Intern Med* 1992;117:1–9.

Marshall D, Johnell O, Wedel H. Meta-analysis of how well measures of bone mineral density predict occurrence of osteoporotic fractures. *BMJ* 1996;312:1254–1259.

McClung MR, Geusens P, Miller PD, et al. Effect of risedronate on the risk of hip fracture in elderly women. *N Engl J Med* 2001;334:333–340.

Melton LJ, Thamer M, Ray NF, et al. Fractures attributable to osteoporosis: Report from the National Osteoporosis Foundation. *J Bone Miner Res* 1997;12:16–23.

Neer RM, Arnaud CD, Zanchetta JR, et al. Effect of parathyroid hormone (I-34) on fractures and bone mineral density in postmenopausal women with osteoporosis. *N Engl J Med* 2001;344:1434–1441.

Nelson HD, Helfand M, Woolf SH, et al. Screening for postmenopausal osteoporosis: a review of the evidence for the U.S. Preventive Services Task Force. *Ann Intern Med* 2002;137:529–541.

NIH Consensus Development Panel on Optimal Calcium Intake. Optimal calcium intake. *JAMA* 1994;272:1942–1948.

Orwoll E, Ettinger M, Weiss S, et al. Alendronate for the treatment of osteoporosis in men. *N Engl J Med* 2000;343:604–610.

Reid IR, Brown JP, Burckhardt P, et al. Intravenous zoledronic acid in postmenopausal women with low bone mineral density. *N Engl J Med* 2002;346:653–661.

Schoofs MW, van der Klift M, Hofman A, et al. Thiazide diuretics and the risk for hip fracture. *Ann Intern Med* 2003;169:476–482.

Todd JA, Robinson RJ. Osteoporosis and exercise. *Postgrad Med* 2003;79:320–323.

Torgerson DJ, Bell-Syer SEM. Hormone replacement therapy and prevention of nonvertebral fractures—a meta-analysis of randomized trials. *JAMA* 2001;285:2891–2897.

World Health Organization. WHO technical report series 843. Assessment of fracture risk and its application to screening for postmenopausal osteoporosis. Geneva: World Health Organization, 1994.

Writing group for the PEPI trial. Effects of hormone replacement on bone mineral density. Results from the postmenopausal estrogen/progestin interventions (PEPI) trial. *JAMA* 1996;276:1389–1396.

Paget's Disease

Jason S. Goldfeder

INTRODUCTION

Paget's disease is a disorder of focal abnormal bone turnover characterized by **increased skeletal remodeling, hypertrophy, and abnormal bone structure** that lead to mechanically weaker bone. Paget's disease can be localized to one skeletal area (monostotic Paget's disease) or can simultaneously affect multiple parts of the skeleton (polyostotic Paget's disease). It was first described in 1877 by Sir James Paget and is also referred to as **osteitis deformans**. Pain is the most common symptom of Paget's disease, and multiple complications can occur, but the majority of patients are asymptomatic and are diagnosed incidentally after abnormalities are found on laboratory tests or x-rays done for other reasons. Treatment decisions in patients with Paget's disease are based on symptoms, the areas of the skeleton that are involved, and the degree of bone turnover.

Epidemiology

Paget's disease is the second most common metabolic bone disorder in older adults after osteoporosis. It has a distinctive geographic distribution throughout the world. Paget's disease occurs most commonly in western Europe, especially Great Britain, North America, Australia, and New Zealand. It is quite uncommon in Asia, Africa, and the Middle East. Paget's disease is a disorder of the elderly and is extremely uncommon in adults < age 40 years. The prevalence increases significantly with each decade after age 50 years. Population studies using x-rays and autopsies have found prevalence rates of 1–3% in adults > age 50 years in the United States. The prevalence of symptomatic Paget's disease is several-fold lower. Prevalence and incidence rates are higher in men than women. The prevalence of Paget's disease is similar in both white and African American populations. Since the 1980s, the prevalence of Paget's disease has declined in several countries, including the United States, Great Britain, and Australia.

Etiology

The exact etiology of Paget's disease has been debated for several decades and remains somewhat unclear. A **viral infection of osteoclasts** has been postulated since the 1970s. Viruses that have been proposed as possible causative agents include members of the paramyxovirus family, such as respiratory syncytial virus and the measles virus, and canine distemper virus. Indirect evidence supporting a viral etiology has included the description of viral-like inclusion bodies in osteoclasts on electron microscopy and viral-like antigens on immunohistochemical studies. However, no viral pathogen has ever been cultured from bone or detected in PCR testing.

Genetic factors also appear to play a role in Paget's disease. Up to 15–30% of patients with Paget's disease (40% in one isolated Spanish study) have a positive family history. The mode of transmission appears to be autosomal dominant. The relative risk of developing Paget's disease is increased 7-fold in first-degree relatives of those with Paget's disease. Familial cases typically are diagnosed at a younger age and have a more aggressive disease course. Possible susceptibility genes have been located on chromosomes 6 and 18. Additionally, a homozygous gene deletion on chromosome 8 has recently been discovered that leads to osteoprotegerin deficiency, which can result in juvenile Paget's disease. The leading hypothesis for the development of Paget's disease is that a viral infection of osteoclasts in genetically susceptible hosts acts to trigger the increased osteoclast activity that initiates the enhanced bone turnover.

CAUSES

Normal bone remodeling depends on the coupled metabolic response of bone-forming osteoblasts and bone-resorbing osteoclasts. The primary abnormality in Paget's disease is enhanced osteoclast activity. The osteoclasts in patients with Paget's disease are multinucleated and are markedly increased in number and size. Pagetic osteoclasts have up to 100 nuclei compared to the normal 5–10 nuclei. The increased osteoclastic activity results in three distinct phases of the disease. Different parts of the skeleton may simultaneously go through different stages.

- The **initial osteolytic phase** is characterized by intense bone resorption by the abnormally large osteoclasts, usually in the long bones or the skull.
- In the **mixed osteolytic/osteoblastic phase**, active bone resorption by osteoclasts is coupled with increased bone formation by reactive osteoblasts.
- The **late sclerotic phase** is characterized primarily by continued new bone formation, resulting in the overproduction of thickened disorganized bone of poor quality.

PRESENTATION

The majority of patients with Paget's disease are **asymptomatic**, and the disease is diagnosed incidentally on x-rays done for other reasons or in the follow-up of an elevated alkaline phosphatase. Recent studies have found that only 5–30% of patients with Paget's disease are symptomatic. Paget's disease predominates in the axial skeleton and long bones. There is only one skeletal area involved (monostotic Paget's disease) in 10–30% of patients, whereas the remainder have multiple foci of disease (polyostotic Paget's disease) that may be at different stages of disease. Once the initial sites of disease have been detected, it is uncommon for new foci of disease to develop. The rates of skeletal involvement by location are shown in Table 25-1.

Common Symptoms

The two most common symptoms in adults with Paget's disease are **bone pain** and **joint pain**. Bone pain typically is constant and deep seated and may be worse at night. Pain frequently increases with weight bearing. The severity of pain does not always

TABLE 25-1. FREQUENCY OF SKELETAL SITES INVOLVED IN PAGET'S DISEASE (%)

Pelvis	72
Lumbosacral spine (esp. L3-4)	58
Femur	55
Thoracic spine	45
Sacrum	43
Skull	42
Tibia	35
Humerus	31
Scapula	23
Cervical spine	14

correlate with x-ray findings and tends to be more prominent in advanced lytic lesions. Secondary osteoarthritis and corresponding pain frequently develop, particularly in weight-bearing joints such as the hip and the knee. Several mechanisms contribute to the development of osteoarthritis, including uneven bony expansion resulting in an uneven base for articular cartilage, limited joint space due to bony overgrowth, and altered joint mechanics secondary to bony deformities. Bony deformities include bowing of the limbs, kyphosis or scoliosis of the spine, and enlargement of the skull (osteoporosis circumscripta). Local skin warmth may also occur secondary to increased bony vascularity.

Complications

Multiple complications can occur in patients with Paget's disease (Table 25-2), although most are infrequent. **Fractures** are one of the most common complications and occur in 6–7% of patients. Fractures occur most commonly in the femur, tibia, and humerus and are often associated with poor healing and nonunion. Multiple possible **neurologic complications** can occur because of either direct nerve root compression by expanding bone or diversion of blood flow to bone. Spinal stenosis is the most common of the neurologic complications. Deafness occurs in 10–30% of patients with disease affecting the skull. Most of the cardiovascular complications are much less common than previously thought, particularly high-output heart failure. As Paget's disease is a focal process, bone marrow involvement and the development of anemia or thrombocytopenia do not occur.

TABLE 25-2. POSSIBLE COMPLICATIONS IN PAGET'S DISEASE

Organ system	Possible complications
Long bones	Fractures
Neurologic	Spinal stenosis
	Chronic headaches
	Cranial neuropathies (especially II, V, VII, VIII)
	Noncommunicative hydrocephalus
	Dementia
	Seizure disorder
Dental	Loss of teeth/malocclusion
ENT	Deafness
	Tinnitus
	Vertigo
Rheumatologic	Hyperuricemia/gout
	Increased susceptibility to seronegative spondyloarthropathies, psoriatic arthritis
Cardiovascular	Increased vascular disease
	High-output heart failure
	Valvular heart disease (aortic > mitral)
Metabolic	Hypercalcemia (usually with immobility)
	Primary hyperparathyroidism
Tumors	Benign giant cell tumors
	Malignant sarcoma

Malignant Sarcomatous Degeneration

Malignant sarcomatous degeneration is an uncommon but severe and usually life-threatening complication of Paget's disease. It occurs in <1% of patients and occurs most commonly in those with severe polyostotic disease. Sarcomas occur more commonly in men than women and usually occur in older adults. The majority of tumors are osteosarcomas, whereas much smaller percentages are malignant fibrous histiocytomas, fibrosarcomas, and chondrosarcomas. The most common bones involved in descending order are the femur, humerus, pelvis, skull, and facial bones. Malignant transformation may be heralded by a sudden or severe increase in pain, a palpable mass, an increase in the alkaline phosphatase, or a pathologic fracture. The prognosis is poor, with a 50% mortality rate at 6 months and a 5-year survival rate of only 5–15%. A small percentage of patients with limb bone sarcomas without evidence of metastatic disease can be treated with wide surgical excision/amputation and aggressive chemotherapy and/or radiation therapy.

MANAGEMENT

Diagnostic Evaluation

The evaluation of patients with Paget's disease includes plain films, a bone scan, and laboratory assessment of markers of bone turnover. A **bone scan** is the best test for extent of disease and should be performed in all patients with Paget's disease. The bone scan is more sensitive, but less specific than traditional x-rays. It can pick up 15–30% of lesions that are not detected by plain films. The order in which the tests are obtained typically depends on whether the patient is diagnosed based on symptoms or incidentally.

Symptomatic patients usually are diagnosed after x-rays are obtained to evaluate the cause of pain. Characteristic features on plain films include localized bony enlargement, cortical thickening, sclerotic changes, and osteolytic areas. A bone scan should subsequently be obtained to assess what additional parts of the skeleton are involved. Subsequent plain film x-rays can be obtained of painful areas or high-risk areas that are abnormal on the bone scan (spine, skull, joints) to assess for the degree of abnormalities. Markers of bone turnover should also be obtained (see later).

The most frequent way Paget's disease presents clinically is in asymptomatic patients who are found to have an **elevated alkaline phosphatase**. Sources of an elevated alkaline phosphatase include the liver and bone. If there are no other evident abnormalities on routine liver function tests (AST, ALT, bilirubin), a serum gamma-glutamyltransferase should be obtained to further rule out occult hepatic disease. If the gamma-glutamyltransferase is normal, a bone scan should be obtained to assess for lesions consistent with Paget's disease. X-rays should be obtained of abnormal areas to confirm the diagnosis of Paget's disease.

Several laboratory tests are available to assess the degree of bone formation and bone resorption. There is not uniform agreement about which tests are necessary, particularly with regard to bone resorption. The alkaline phosphatase is the most useful clinical marker of bone formation to assess the degree of osteoblast activity. The alkaline phosphatase level correlates well with the extent of disease on bone scan. Bone-specific alkaline phosphatase is more specific than the total alkaline phosphatase, but is more difficult to obtain. It can be considered in patients with monostotic Paget's disease who may have a normal total alkaline phosphatase. Serum osteocalcin and procollagen type I C-terminal peptide are additional markers of bone formation that have been studied, but are less reliable and should not be routinely obtained.

Laboratory markers of bone resorption assess the degree of osteoclastic activity. The majority of available tests are urinary measurements that are obtained from the second voided morning urine after an overnight fast. Several different tests have been evaluated. Two of the most clinically useful are urinary type I collagen **pyridoline crosslinks** and **N-telopeptide**, which have supplanted urine hydroxyproline as the tests of choice for bone resorption. These tests of bone resorption often have to be sent to a referral laboratory.

At the time of initial diagnosis, markers of both bone formation and bone resorption should be obtained. The alkaline phosphatase is sufficient to serve as the sole marker for **monitoring disease activity** in many patients, particularly those with primarily increased osteoblastic activity. However, patients with a normal alkaline phosphatase or high levels of osteoclastic activity should have markers of bone resorption followed. The effectiveness of treatment is typically judged by the degree of decline in markers of bone turnover, percentage of decline, and the time required until markers normalize.

Additional radiographic testing is generally unnecessary except to evaluate for complications. A CT or MRI is most commonly used to evaluate for neurologic complications, such as spinal stenosis. A bone biopsy is usually not required to make a diagnosis of Paget's disease and is primarily obtained when concern arises for malignant sarcomatous degeneration.

Treatment

The primary goals of treatment are to decrease pain and decrease the rate of bone turnover to prevent progression of disease and the development of complications.

Pharmacologic Therapy

Therapeutic options have significantly improved since the early 1990s with the development of more potent bisphosphonates. **Bone pain** is the one indication for which there is proven benefit of treatment from randomized controlled clinical trials. Most experts recommend treating asymptomatic patients who are at risk for developing complications based on the skeletal sites involved and the degree of bone turnover. However, there are not prospective clinical trial data to support this approach. Asymptomatic disease in areas that are at low risk of developing complications, such as the ribs, scapula, distal bones, or the sacrum, generally does not require treatment. The following are generally accepted **indications to initiate treatment** in Paget's disease.

* Symptomatic disease: bone pain, deformities, or neurologic symptoms
* Asymptomatic patients with evidence of increased bone turnover at risk for complications based on the areas involved
  - Lytic lesions in long bones with fractures
  - Disease in proximity of joints with risk of developing osteoarthritis
  - Disease in the spine because of the risk of spinal stenosis
  - Disease in the skull because of the risk of deafness and cranial nerve dysfunction
* Patients preparing for elective orthopedic surgery on involved joints should receive treatment for at least 6 weeks to decrease bony vascularity

A **second-generation bisphosphonate** is recommended for treatment in patients requiring therapy. When used to treat Paget's disease, bisphosphonates are given as pulse courses of therapy at higher doses than are traditionally used to treat osteoporosis. Alendronate (Fosamax), risedronate (Actonel), and pamidronate (Aredia) are recommended as first-line agents (Table 25-3). These agents typically decrease bone turnover, as measured by the decline in serum alkaline phosphatase by 60–80%. Bone markers are normalized in approximately 50–70% of patients. Etidronate (Didronel) and tiludronate (Skelid) are older bisphosphonates that are less effective on improving symptoms and markers of bone turnover. **Supplemental calcium and vitamin D** are recommended to prevent defective bone mineralization, although this is much less common with the newer bisphosphonates. The oral bisphosphonates should be taken with water only. The patient should remain upright, and food and other medications should be avoided for at least 30 minutes to decrease the likelihood of developing esophageal complications. Calcitonin (Miacalcin) is another second-line agent that can be considered in patients who are unable to tolerate bisphosphonates. Calcitonin is more effective in Paget's disease when given IM than when given via inhalation. The rates of bone turnover are decreased by approximately 50% and normalized in approximately 25% of patients. Symptoms and bone turnover usually recur soon after stopping therapy. More potent bisphosphonates that are given as a one-time IV dose are being evaluated (see Table 25-3). Plicamycin (Mithracin) and gallium nitrate (Ganite)

TABLE 25-3. TREATMENT OPTIONS IN PATIENTS WITH PAGET'S DISEASE

Agent	Dose
First-line agents	
Alendronate (Fosamax)	40 mg PO qd for 6 mos
Risedronate (Actonel)	30 mg PO qd for 2 mos
Pamidronate (Aredia)	30–60 mg IV qd for 3 days or
	30 mg IV q wk for 6 wks or
	30 mg IV q mo for 6 mos
Second-line agents	
Tiludronate (Skelid)	400 mg PO qd for 3 mos
Etidronate (Didronel)	400 mg PO qd for 6 mos
Calcitonin (Miacalcin)	50–100 IU/IM qd SC for 6–12 mos
	200–400 IU qd intranasally for 6–12 mos
Agents currently being investigated	
Zoledronate (Zometa)	400 mcg IV × 1 dose
Ibandronate (Boniva)	2 mg IV × 1 dose

are experimental agents with potential serious adverse effects that can be considered in patients with severe disease that does not respond to bisphosphonates, but only after referral to an expert in bone metabolism.

Surgery
Surgical therapy is **indicated for complications** of Paget's disease. The most common indication for surgery is a joint replacement, usually of the hip or the knee, for secondary osteoarthritis. Other reasons to consider surgical intervention are for a complicated or nonhealing fracture, bowing deformities of long bones, spinal stenosis, and focal nerve root compression syndromes. Bisphosphonate therapy is typically prescribed for at least 6 weeks before elective surgery to decrease bone vascularity and the risk of intraoperative bleeding.

Follow-Up
Follow-up of patients with Paget's disease includes **monitoring their symptoms** and **markers of bone turnover**, occasionally supplemented with plain film x-rays. Symptoms should initially be monitored every 3 months in those on therapy and every 6–12 months in those not on treatment. The markers of bone resorption typically improve quickly within days, whereas the markers of bone formation take longer to improve, often up to 1 month. The goal of therapy is to normalize the markers of bone turnover. The **alkaline phosphatase** is the easiest of the markers of bone turnover to follow and is usually the only one needed in follow-up. The alkaline phosphatase should be checked every 3–4 months while on therapy until it normalizes. The urine type I collagen pyridoline crosslinks or N-telopeptide should be followed in those with highly active lytic disease, especially if the alkaline phosphatase is relatively normal. The alkaline phosphatase should be followed annually in those not on treatment. Repeat x-rays should be obtained after 1 year of treatment in those with high-risk lytic lesions. Other indications for subsequent x-rays are new symptoms or worsening of stable symptoms, trauma, a concern for a fracture, and concern for sarcomatous degeneration.

Patients whose alkaline phosphatase normalizes on therapy should have it serially followed. Retreatment with another course of a bisphosphonate should be considered if the alkaline phosphatase increases by >20–25% above the posttreatment nadir.

KEY POINTS TO REMEMBER

- Paget's disease is a disorder of enhanced osteoclast activity that leads to increased bone remodeling, bony hypertrophy, and abnormal bony architecture.
- The primary risk factors for developing Paget's disease are advanced age, a positive family history, and male gender.
- Paget's disease predominates in the axial skeleton, long bones, and skull.
- Most patients with Paget's disease are asymptomatic and are diagnosed after finding an isolated elevated alkaline phosphatase.
- The most common symptoms of Paget's disease are bony pain and joint pain related to secondary osteoarthritis.
- Multiple complications can develop in patients with Paget's disease, but most are uncommon except for fractures, spinal stenosis, and hearing loss.
- The initial diagnostic evaluation should include a bone scan, x-rays of high-risk areas, and measurement of the serum alkaline phosphatase and urinary markers of bone resorption.
- Symptomatic patients and those who are asymptomatic but have evidence of disease in high-risk areas, such as long bones, near joints, the spine, and the skull, should be treated, but asymptomatic patients who do not have disease in high-risk areas can be followed without treatment.
- Standard therapy for Paget's disease is a several-month course of high doses of a bisphosphonate.
- The goal of treatment is to normalize markers of bone turnover, particularly the alkaline phosphatase. Retreatment should be considered in patients whose markers of bone turnover increase by >25% over their posttreatment nadir.

REFERENCES AND SUGGESTED READINGS

Altman RD, Bloch DA, Hochberg MC, et al. Prevalence of pelvic Paget's disease of bone in the United States. *J Bone Miner Res* 2000;15:461–465.

Ankrom MA, Shapiro JR. Paget's disease of bone (osteitis deformans). *J Am Geriatr Soc* 1998;46:1025–1033.

Delmas PD. Biochemical markers of bone turnover in Paget's disease of bone. *J Bone Miner Res* 1999;14(Suppl 2):66–69.

Delmas PD, Meunier PJ. The management of Paget's disease of bone. *N Engl J Med* 1997;336:558–566.

Drake WM, Kendler DL, Brown JP. Consensus statement on the modern therapy of Paget's disease of bone from a western osteoporosis alliance symposium. *Clin Therapeut* 2001;23:620–626.

Fraser WD. Paget's disease of bone. *Curr Opin Rheumatol* 1997;9:347–354.

Hadjipavlou AG, Gaitanis IN, Kontakis GM. Paget's disease of bone and its management. *J Bone Joint Surg* 2002;84:160–169.

Hamdy RC. Clinical features and pharmacologic treatment of Paget's disease. *Endocrinol Metab Clin North Am* 1995;24:421–435.

Harrington KD. Surgical management of neoplastic complications of Paget's disease. *J Bone Miner Res* 1999;14(Suppl 2):45–48.

Hosking DJ. Prediction and assessment of the response of Paget's disease to bisphosphonate treatment. *Bone* 1999;24(Suppl 5):69S–71S.

Kaplan FS. Surgical management of Paget's disease. *J Bone Miner Res* 1999;14(Suppl 2):34–38.

Klein RM, Norman A. Diagnostic procedures for Paget's disease. Radiologic, pathologic, and laboratory testing. *Endocrinol Metab Clin North Am* 1995;24:437–450.

Leach RJ, Singer FR, Roodman GD. Genetics of endocrine disease. The genetics of Paget's disease of the bone. *J Clin Endocrinol Metab* 2001;86:24–28.

Lombardi A. Treatment of Paget's disease of bone with alendronate. *Bone* 1999;24 (Suppl 5):59S–61S.

Lyles KW, Siris ES, Singer FR, et al. A clinical approach to diagnosis and management of Paget's disease of bone. *J Bone Miner Res* 2001;16:1379–1387.

Ooi CG, Fraser WD. Paget's disease of bone. *Postgrad Med J* 1997;73:69–74.

Poncelet A. The neurologic complications of Paget's disease. *J Bone Miner Res* 1999;14 (Suppl 2):88–91.

Reddy SV, Menaa C, Singer FR, et al. Cell biology of Paget's disease. *J Bone Miner Res* 1999;14(Suppl 2):3–7.

Roux C, Dougados M. Treatment of patients with Paget's disease of bone. *Drugs* 1999; 58:823–830.

Russell RGG, Rogers MJ, Frith JC, et al. The pharmacology of bisphosphonates and new insights into their mechanisms of action. *J Bone Miner Res* 1999;14(Suppl 2):53–65.

Selby PL, Davie MWJ, Ralston SH, Stone MD. Guidelines on the management of Paget's disease of bone. *Bone* 2002;31:366–373.

Singer FR. Update on the viral etiology of Paget's disease of bone. *J Bone Miner Res* 1999;14(Suppl 2):29–33.

Siris ES. Goals of treatment for Paget's disease of bone. *J Bone Miner Res* 1999;14 (Suppl 2):49–52.

Staa TPV, Selby P, Leufkens HGM, et al. Incidence and natural history of Paget's disease of bone in England and Wales. *J Bone Miner Res* 2002;17:465–471.

Tiegs RD. Paget's disease of bone: indications for treatment and goals of therapy. *Clin Therapeutics* 1997;19:1309–1329.

Tiegs RD, Lohse CM, Wollan PC, et al. Long-term trends in the incidence of Paget's disease of bone. *Bone* 2000;27:423–427.

Whyte MP, Obrecht SE, Finergan PM, et al. Osteoprotegerin deficiency and juvenile Paget's disease. *N Engl J Med* 2002;347(3):175–184.

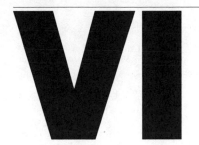

VI

Disorders of Fuel Metabolism

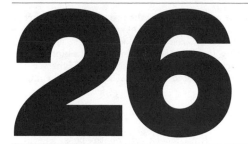

Standards of Care for Diabetes Mellitus

Michael A. DeRosa

INTRODUCTION

Diabetes mellitus (DM) requires proper health screening, patient education, and medical care to prevent acute and chronic complications. In addition to the traditional components of the standard medical history, physical exam, and laboratory evaluation, a few aspects of the care of patients with diabetes deserve further exploration. The standards of care summarized below are based primarily on those established by the American Diabetes Association (ADA). These "Clinical Practice Recommendations" are published each year in the supplement to the January *Diabetes Care* issue and are available online at http://www.diabetes.org.

GLYCEMIC CONTROL

Optimal glycemic control has many benefits, including

- Decreased incidence of acute complications, such as diabetic ketoacidosis and non-ketotic hyperosmolar coma
- Prevention/slowing of the progression of chronic microvascular complications (nephropathy, retinopathy and neuropathy)
- Reduction of diabetes-related deaths and all-cause mortality

Two primary ways to monitor glycemic control are **self-monitored blood glucose (SMBG)** and **hemoglobin (Hgb) Hb A1C**. SMBG is generally checked before meals and at bedtime. The frequency of SMBG ranges from 1–4 or more readings/day. The A1C reflects blood glucose levels over the previous 2–3 months. The A1C should be monitored every 3 months until a patient reaches goal, and then every 6 months if the patient is stable. The goals for glycemic control should be set for the individual patient based on risks of hypoglycemia, age, comorbidities, life expectancy, and complications. Normalization of A1C may be appropriate for some patients. General guidelines for glycemic control established by the American Diabetes Association are as follows:

- A1C: <7.0%
- Preprandial plasma glucose: 90–130 mg/dL
- Peak postprandial plasma glucose: <180 mg/dL

Note that capillary blood glucose levels are 10–15% lower. Newer blood glucose meters are calibrated to report plasma glucose values, so each patient should be informed whether his or her meter reports blood or plasma glucose values. If there is a discrepancy between SMBG values reported by the patient and the A1C, it may be useful to measure SMBG 1–2 hours after a meal. To achieve these goals for glycemic control, many modalities are used in combination. Some of these tools are dietary modifications, regular exercise, and SMBG. If these fail, oral glucose–lowering agents and/or a physiologically based insulin regimen should be added.

HYPERTENSION

Management of hypertension is important in all people but is especially important in diabetic patients, because blood pressure control reduces the frequency of diabetes-related deaths and cerebrovascular disease, as well as slows the progression of nephropathy and retinopathy. **Blood pressure should be checked at every visit.** Lifestyle modifications and medical treatment should be considered if the blood pressure is >130/80 mm Hg. Preferred initial medical therapy is with ACE inhibitors, beta-blockers, or diuretics, because these agents are beneficial in reducing cardiac events. Hypertensive patients with diabetic nephropathy should be treated with an ACE inhibitor or angiotensin receptor blocker (ARB).

RETINOPATHY

Patients with diabetes are at risk for retinopathy. Diabetic retinopathy poses a serious threat to vision and is the leading cause of blindness in middle-aged Americans. To monitor for this complication, patients with diabetes require **yearly dilated ophthalmologic evaluations.** People with type 1 diabetes require a regular exam within 3–5 years after onset of their disease. Because people with type 2 diabetes may have evidence of retinopathy at the time they are diagnosed, they should undergo yearly eye exams from the time of diagnosis.

NEPHROPATHY

Diabetic nephropathy is the leading cause of end-stage renal disease in the United States and the leading cause of diabetes-related morbidity and mortality. The earliest sign of diabetic nephropathy is microalbuminuria. The most common screening test for microalbuminuria is measurement of microalbumin:creatinine ratio in a spot urine collection. **Microalbuminuria** is defined as a microalbumin:creatine ratio of 30–300 mcg/mg. This screening test should be performed in patients with type 1 DM within 5 years of initial diagnosis and in patients with type 2 DM at the time of diagnosis. This test should be repeated annually. For accurate diagnosis, microalbuminuria should be confirmed in 2 of 3 tests within 3–6 months to eliminate positive tests due to transient conditions such as exercise, urinary tract infections, and hyperglycemia. Once microalbuminuria is diagnosed, treatment should begin with either an **ACE inhibitor or ARB** (even if normotensive), hypertension should be corrected, and glycemia should be normalized. These treatments can slow the progression of diabetic nephropathy. If the patient develops clinical macroalbuminuria (>300 mcg/mg or 300 mg/24 hours) a dietary protein restriction can be instituted to help slow progression of this renal complication. Early referral to a nephrologist is encouraged.

NEUROPATHY

Neuropathy is a common long-term complication of diabetes. There are several specific types of neuropathy that can occur. These include distal symmetric sensorimotor polyneuropathy, autonomic neuropathy (involving GI, genitourinary, and cardiovascular systems, as well as contributing to hypoglycemic unawareness), and focal neuropathy. To evaluate for neuropathy, the patient should be asked about symptoms such as pain, numbness, paresthesias, or early satiety. A **neurologic exam should be performed at each visit** and should evaluate sensation (pain/temperature, vibration, light touch, and joint position sense) and deep tendon reflexes. Strict control of glycemia decreases the incidence and slows the progression of neuropathy. After identification, medical treatment may be necessary or the person may require referral to specialty services.

LOWER EXTREMITY COMPLICATIONS

Patients with diabetes develop foot problems due to a combination of vascular and neurologic compromise and poor wound healing. DM is the leading cause of nontraumatic lower extremity amputation in the United States. **Annual foot exams** should include evaluation of touch and vibration sense (Semmes-Weinstein 10-g monofilament and tuning fork), deep tendon reflexes, and pedal pulses. At every visit, the feet should be visually inspected for skin breakdown, callus, discoloration, or other signs of vascular or neurologic disease.

Patients should be educated in the importance of well-fitting shoes and frequent self-inspection of their feet. High-risk patients should be referred to specialists in foot care.

HYPERLIPIDEMIA

Diabetic patients should have a **fasting lipid profile** [low-density lipoprotein (LDL) cholesterol, total cholesterol, high-density lipoprotein (HDL) cholesterol, and triglycerides] **checked yearly.** Goals for patients with diabetes are as follows (see Chap. 30, Diagnosis, Standards of Care, and Treatment of Hyperlipidemia, for a more detailed discussion of lipid profile goals):

- LDL cholesterol: <100 mg/dL [<70 mg/dL in patients with known coronary heart disease (CHD)]
- Triglycerides: <150 mg/dL
- HDL cholesterol (males): >40 mg/dL
- HDL cholesterol (females): >50 mg/dL

Therapy is first directed to meeting the LDL cholesterol goal. A secondary goal is to raise HDL cholesterol above the gender-specific target. For those with triglycerides ≥200 mg/dL, current National Cholesterol Education Program/Adult Treatment Panel III guidelines establish a non-HDL cholesterol (total – HDL cholesterol) <130 mg/dL as the secondary goal. If the triglyceride level is >500 mg/dL, therapy should first be directed at lowering triglycerides to prevent pancreatitis. For specific recommendations on treatment of hyperlipidemia, please refer to Chap. 30, Diagnosis, Standards of Care, and Treatment of Hyperlipidemia.

CARDIOVASCULAR DISEASE

Cardiovascular disease is the leading cause of death among patients with diabetes. Cardiovascular disease risk factor reduction is as important in the management of diabetes as glycemic control. These risk factors include hypertension, dyslipidemia, positive family history of premature CHD, presence of urinary microalbumin, smoking, and sedentary lifestyle. Antiplatelet therapy with 75–162 mg of **enteric-coated aspirin daily** reduces cardiovascular events in individuals with diabetes who have CHD. Primary prevention with aspirin should be considered in adults > age 40 years with diabetes or one or more of the following risk factors:

- A family history of CHD
- Smoking history
- Hypertension
- Albuminuria
- Hyperlipidemia

Screening Recommendations

The American Diabetes Association recommends that people with a history of CHD as well as selected people without a prior history or symptoms of CHD undergo **testing for CHD.** The American Diabetes Association 2004 Clinical Practice Recommendations suggest screening exercise stress testing in patients with any of the following:

- Typical or atypical cardiac symptoms
- Abnormal resting ECG
- Peripheral or carotid occlusive arterial disease
- Age >35 years with sedentary lifestyle planning to begin a vigorous exercise program
- ≥2 cardiac risk factors in addition to diabetes

A consultation with a cardiologist is recommended regarding further workup of patients with an abnormal exercise ECG.

Additional Recommendations

- Individualized nutritional recommendations, preferably by a registered dietitian.

- Individualized exercise recommendations based on cardiac status and the presence of retinopathy or neuropathy.
- Patient education consistent with the National Standards for Diabetes Self-Management Education Programs.
- Women of childbearing age should be informed of the importance of optimal blood glucose control before conception and throughout pregnancy.
- Influenza vaccine should be administered annually to patients with diabetes, beginning each October. The pneumococcal vaccine should be administered once the diagnosis of diabetes is established.
- Smoking cessation should be recommended for all diabetic patients who smoke.

Optimum care of people with diabetes prevents the acute complications and reduces the risk of development of long-term complications of this disease. This can be accomplished through patient education, regular health screening, medical care, laboratory evaluation, and timely referral to specialists.

KEY POINTS TO REMEMBER

- Tight glycemic control reduces the microvascular complications of diabetes.
- Establish goals for glycemic control based on the individual patient.
- The most important facet of diabetes care may be to identify and reduce cardiac risk factors (treat hypertension and hyperlipidemia, prescribe aspirin, advise smoking cessation).
- Screen for albuminuria and treat it with ACE inhibitors or ARBs.
- Provide/refer patients for annual dilated retinal exams.
- Inspect the feet at each visit and provide a yearly comprehensive exam.
- Use other specialists, including diabetes nurse educators, dietitians, ophthalmologists, cardiologists, podiatrists, and orthopedists.

REFERENCES AND SUGGESTED READINGS

American Diabetes Association. Standards of medical care for patients with diabetes mellitus (position statement). *Diabetes Care* 2004;27:S1–S137.

Bild DE, Shelby JV, Sinnock P, et al. Lower-extremity amputation in people with diabetes. Epidemiology and prevention. *Diabetes Care* 1989;12:24–31.

Chobanian AV, et al. The seventh report of the Joint National Committee on prevention, detection, evaluation, and treatment of high blood pressure (the JNC 7 report). *JAMA* 2003;289:2560–2572.

The Diabetes Control and Complications Trial Research Group. The effect of intensive treatment of diabetes on the development and progression of long-term complications in insulin-dependent diabetes mellitus. *N Engl J Med* 1993;329:977–986.

Executive summary of the third report of the National Cholesterol Education Program (NCEP) expert panel on detection, evaluation, and treatment of high blood cholesterol in adults (Adult Treatment Panel III). *JAMA* 2001;285:2486–2497.

Klein R, Klein BE. Vision disorders in diabetes. In: Harris MI, et al., eds. Diabetes in America, DHHS publication number 85-1468. Washington, DC: United States Government Printing Office, 1985.

Harris MI, Klein R, Welborn TA, et al. Onset of NIDDM occurs at least 4–7 years before clinical diagnosis. *Diabetes Care* 1992;15:815–819.

Perneger TV, Brancati FL, Whelton PK, et al. End-stage renal disease attributable to diabetes mellitus. *Ann Intern Med* 1994;121:912–918.

UK Prospective Diabetes Study Group. Intensive blood-glucose control with sulphonylureas or insulin compared with conventional treatment and risk of complications in patients with type 2 diabetes (UKPDS 33). *Lancet* 1998;352:837–853.

UK Prospective Diabetes Study Group. Tight blood pressure control and risk of macrovascular and microvascular complications in type 2 diabetes: UKPDS 38. *BMJ* 1998;317:703–713.

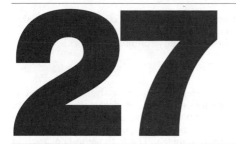

Diabetes Mellitus Type 1

Janet B. McGill and
Michael A. DeRosa

INTRODUCTION

Type 1 diabetes mellitus (T1DM) is an illness in which autoimmune destruction of pancreatic beta cells causes **insulin deficiency** and **hyperglycemia**. The overall prevalence of the disease is 0.25–0.5% of the population, or 1/400 children, and 1/200 adults in the United States. The incidence of T1DM is increasing in developed countries, and it is appearing at younger ages. The peak onset occurs at age 10–12 years; however, it can be diagnosed from a few months of age into the ninth decade of life. Males and females are equally affected. T1DM accounts for 5–10% of all cases of diabetes and needs to be accurately diagnosed so that insulin therapy is not delayed or withheld inappropriately. Insulin deficiency can lead to acute metabolic decompensation known as **diabetic ketoacidosis (DKA)**, as well as chronic hyperglycemia that leads to microvascular complications. The treatment goal of T1DM is normalization of blood glucose (BG) by physiologically based insulin replacement therapy.

CAUSE

Etiology and Pathogenesis

The autoimmune process that **selectively destroys pancreatic beta cells** is T-cell mediated with an unknown antigenic stimulus. Environmental factors, including coxsackie and rubella viruses, and dietary factors, such as early exposure to cow's milk, have been implicated. Insulitis (lymphocytic infiltration of pancreatic islets) is an early finding, followed by apoptosis of beta cells, which leads to their virtual absence later in the disease course. Antibodies to beta-cell antigens can be found in the majority of patients before diagnosis and for some time after the onset of clinical diabetes. These disease markers are antibodies to glutamic acid decarboxylase (GAD65), to tyrosine phosphatases IA-2 and IA-2 beta, and to insulin (IAA). Of these markers, GAD65 is positive in 80% of children and adults near the time of diagnosis, whereas IA-2 and IAA are positive in approximately 50% of children and are less likely to be present in adults. The presence of two antibodies has high sensitivity and specificity for rapid progression to insulin dependency and may help clarify the diagnosis in some patients. In cases of T1DM in which no evidence of autoimmunity can be detected, the classification used is idiopathic T1DM.

Several organ-specific **autoimmune diseases occur with increased frequency in patients with T1DM**, including autoimmune thyroiditis (Hashimoto's and Graves' diseases), Addison's disease, pernicious anemia, celiac sprue, vitiligo, alopecia, and chronic active hepatitis. In a study of 265 adults with T1DM, the risk of thyroid disease was 32% for the proband, 25% for siblings, and 42% for parents, with females more commonly affected than males. The risk of developing autoimmune thyroid disease increases with age, so periodic screening should continue throughout adulthood in patients with T1DM and their family members.

The **genetic susceptibility** to T1DM is manifested by linkage with several gene loci and association with HLA-DR and DQ. The IDDM1 gene located in the HLA region of chromosome 6p21.3, and the IDDM2 gene in the region 5' upstream of the insulin gene on chromosome 11p15.5 contribute 42% and 10%, respectively, to the observed familial clustering. In the family of a patient with T1DM, there is a 30% risk of diabetes developing in an identical twin, 6% in an offspring, and 5% in siblings. The striking familial discordance supports the importance of environmental factors.

Pathogenesis of Complications

Patients with both T1DM and T2DM are susceptible to organ dysfunction that is caused by long-term exposure to hyperglycemia and leads to devastating morbidity and mortality. The **microvascular complications** of retinopathy, nephropathy, and neuropathy share some pathogenic features but may not appear at the same time or with the same severity in all individuals with diabetes. The pathogenesis of each of these complications includes increased oxidative stress or the generation of reactive oxygen species with inadequate scavenger activity. **Advanced glycation end-products** are formed by processes of glycation and/or oxidation of proteins, nucleotides, and lipids, and have intrinsic cellular toxicity. High glucose and reactive oxygen species levels have been shown to increase diacylglycerol and stimulate protein kinase C activity, causing alterations in intracellular signal transduction and production of cytokines and growth factors. Glucose enters peripheral nerves by mass action, is converted first to sorbitol by aldose reductase, then to fructose by sorbitol dehydrogenase. These saccharides produce osmotic stress, increase glycation, and cause alterations in the NADH/NAD ratio, which collectively contribute to nerve fiber damage and loss. Diabetic retinopathy is associated with the adverse effects of hyperglycemia on the vascular endothelium and cytokines such as vascular endothelial growth factor. In renal mesangial cells, hyperglycemia induces transforming growth factor-beta, which stimulates matrix synthesis and inhibits matrix degradation. Investigational agents that target these processes are currently in clinical development.

PRESENTATION

History

T1DM develops most commonly in childhood but can present at any age. Because 80% of cases occur without a positive family history, symptoms may be overlooked until hyperglycemia reaches critical levels. The **prodromal symptoms are related to hyperglycemia** and include weight loss, polyuria, polydipsia, polyphagia, and blurred vision. If ketoacidosis is present, the patient might complain of abdominal pain, nausea, vomiting, myalgias, and shortness of breath and exhibit changes in mental and hemodynamic status.

In previously diagnosed patients, the **history of present illness** should document the duration of the illness, frequency of hyper- and hypoglycemia, results of self-monitored BG testing (SMBG), dietary habits, and the status of any microvascular or macrovascular complications. The history of present illness or medication history should **record the insulin regimen in detail** and should provide an assessment of adequacy or problems with the regimen. In adolescent and adult women, menstrual, sexual, and gestational histories should be elicited, and the method of birth control should be documented. Smoking behavior, alcohol and drug use, and socioeconomic status and social support are all important factors in the care of a patient with T1DM.

Physical Exam

If the patient presents in **DKA**, signs of dehydration and acidosis, such as tachycardia, orthostatic hypotension, and dry mucous membranes, might be evident. Fruity odor to the breath reflects the presence of ketones. Routine follow-up physical exams should document height, weight, and Tanner staging in children to determine that growth and development are advancing normally. Blood pressure and heart rate are important measures for all patients with T1DM. At least annually, the physical exam should include skin, funduscopic, oral, thyroid, and cardiovascular exams, as well as sensory testing and foot screening. Dilated eye exam by an ophthalmologist is recommended at 3–5 years of T1DM duration, with scheduling of repeat exams based on clinical findings.

Diagnostic and Laboratory Evaluation

The diagnosis of T1DM is typically made when a **random plasma glucose** ≥**200 mg/dL** is accompanied by signs and symptoms of diabetes (e.g., DKA). If the diagnosis of T1DM versus T2DM is unclear and the patient has not had DKA, testing for antibodies to GAD65, IA-2B (also known as *ICA*), or IAA or C-peptide level can be useful. C-peptide levels are typically low or undetectable in patients with T1DM. **Hgb A1C** should be measured 2–4 times per year, and a lipid profile, serum creatinine and electrolytes, and urine microalbumin:creatinine ratio should be checked at least annually in adolescents and adults. Screening for thyroid antibodies is recommended, and thyroid-stimulating hormone (TSH) should be checked annually if the patient is antibody positive or has a goiter.

Treatment Goals

The goal of diabetes treatment is to **maintain the BG as close to normal as possible** and to **avoid hypoglycemia.** All patients with T1DM require insulin therapy, and early achievement of a near-normal A1C has been shown to preserve residual beta-cell function and to reduce long-term complications. The Diabetes Control and Complications Trial (DCCT) and its follow-up study have shown that every 1% reduction in A1C reduces retinopathy by 33%, microalbuminuria by 22%, and neuropathy by 38%. Tight control for the first 5–10 years of diabetes confers long-term risk reduction, supporting the hypothesis that hyperglycemia induces organ toxicity that can be self-perpetuating (glycemic memory). In children, the therapeutic goals include ensuring normal growth and development and the scrupulous avoidance of severe hypoglycemia at young ages. In the postpubertal adolescent and adult patient, maintenance of normal blood pressure, achieving target lipid levels, smoking cessation, aspirin use in patients > age 40, and preconception counseling are important treatment parameters. Please refer to Chap. 26, Standards of Care for Diabetes Mellitus, for detailed recommendations.

MANAGEMENT

Glucose Monitoring

Patients with T1DM should be encouraged to do **SMBG** at least 4 times daily so that appropriate insulin adjustments can be made based on ambient glucose levels. These recommendations may be modified for children with school considerations. Increased monitoring is required during acute illnesses, for intense exercise, and before and during pregnancy. Alternate site testing, rapid readings, and meters with averaging, graphing, and download functions have helped patients with the challenging task of SMBG. Periodic monitoring during the nighttime is recommended for all patients to check for nocturnal hypoglycemia.

Dietary Therapy

Dietary therapy involves **individualized assessment and instruction** and is most effectively provided by a registered dietitian. The caloric requirement for people with moderate physical activity is approximately 35 kcal/kg/day, with significant variation. The usual diet for patients with diabetes provides 50% of calories derived from carbohydrates and fiber. Protein should make up 10–20% of calories and <30% should come from fat, keeping saturated fat to a minimum. Individualized instruction should consider the patient's caloric needs, ethnicity, habits, constraints, and the prescribed insulin regimen. Most patients are instructed in either an exchange system or carbohydrate-counting techniques and use meal planning as an integral part of their diabetes treatment. Review of dietary principles is a cost-effective way to help the patient achieve treatment targets.

Insulin Therapy

Insulin therapy must be individualized, and numerous regimens have been used. The DCCT and other studies have clearly demonstrated that patients are more likely to

TABLE 27-1. INSULIN TYPES AND PHARMACOKINETICS[a]

Insulin	Onset	Peak	Duration
Rapid acting[b]			
Insulin aspart (Novolog)	10–20 mins	1–3 hrs	3–5 hrs
Insulin lispro (Humalog)	10–15 mins	1–2 hrs	3–4 hrs
Insulin glulisine (Apidra)	10–20 mins	1 hrs	3–4 hrs
Short acting			
Regular ("R")	0.5–1.0 hr	2–4 hrs	6–8 hrs
Intermediate acting			
NPH ("N")[c]	1.5–3 hrs	4–10 hrs	12–22 hrs
Lente ("L")[c]	2–4 hrs	7–12 hrs	16–22 hrs
Long acting			
Ultralente ("UL")[c]	4–8 hrs	Variable	18–30 hrs
Insulin glargine (Lantus)[d]	1–2 hrs	None	24 hrs

[a]Insulin pharmacokinetics show significant inter- and intrasubject variation. The onset, peak, and duration may be influenced by the dose administered, the injection site, skin temperature, and other less well-defined factors.
[b]Rapid-acting insulin should be administered immediately before or after meals. Also suitable for insulin pump use.
[c]Cloudy, suspended formulations require resuspension by rolling and tipping (but not shaking) the vial before administration. Resuspension is a potential source of erratic pharmacokinetics.
[d]Do not mix with any other type of insulin in the same syringe due to incompatible pH. Clear preparation, no resuspension needed.

achieve glycemic targets using **intensified insulin therapy with basal and bolus components** than with conventional therapy with one or two injections. Intensive insulin therapy is provided by either multiple daily injections (MDIs) or continuous subcutaneous insulin infusion (CSII) using an insulin pump. Insulin pharmacokinetic properties are highlighted in Table 27-1.

Decisions about the appropriate insulin regimen should be made with the patient's abilities and scheduling constraints in mind. In general, patients need an **intermediate- or long-acting insulin to cover basal needs** and a **rapid- or short-acting insulin to provide meal coverage**. When initiating or changing an insulin regimen, an estimation of **total daily insulin dose (TDD)** should be made. Individual requirements vary, but usually range from 0.5 to 1 U/kg/day, with the majority of patients requiring approximately 0.6 U/kg/day.

Historically, the most widely prescribed regimen was "split-mixed," which used NPH or Lente as the basal insulin and a short or rapid-acting analog before breakfast and dinner as follows:

Time	Dose	Regimen
Before breakfast	0.4 × TDD	NPH or Lente
	0.2 × TDD	Humalog, NovoLog, or Regular
Before dinner	0.2 × TDD	Humalog, NovoLog or Regular
	0.2 × TDD	NPH or Lente (this dose is sometimes given at bedtime)

Use of this regimen presumed that the patient would eat lunch at a standard time, because the morning NPH or Lente is likely to peak at about midday. Patient scheduling problems and the erratic pharmacokinetics of NPH and Lente have made this regimen less popular.

The most commonly prescribed regimens for patients with T1DM by endocrinologists are MDI or CSII. These regimens use the concepts of basal and bolus (pre-meal) dosing. The **basal dose** is generally 45–55% of the TDD, or approximately 0.3 U/kg/day, and is often given in 1 injection of insulin glargine at bedtime. If NPH or Lente are used, the dose will be about 0.15 U/kg twice a day. The basal insulin dose is adjusted so that the fasting BG is routinely within the target of 80–120 mg/dL, and there is <30 mg/dL variation between evening and morning values. Changes in weight, exercise, persistent hyperglycemia, or frequent hypoglycemia should prompt reconsideration of the basal insulin dose.

Bolus doses are administered to cover caloric intake and to correct high BG readings. Pre-meal bolus doses are determined by one or more of the following methods:

- Fixed amount before each meal, approximately 0.1 U/kg or one-sixth of the TDD
- Fixed dose before each meal as above plus a sliding scale "correction factor" (see below) based on the pre-meal SMBG
- Carbohydrate counting plus "correction factor" uses variable amounts depending on anticipated carbohydrate intake and the pre-meal SMBG

Both the patient and the physician need to learn important concepts to succeed in the use of MDI regimens. If fixed amounts of pre-meal insulin are to be used, the patient should have a clear idea of the prescribed meal plan and be able to follow it precisely. Alternatively, the patient can adjust the pre-meal dose based on the anticipated carbohydrate content, which allows greater flexibility. To do this, the physician or diabetes educator must determine the **"insulin to carbohydrate" ratio**, which can be calculated by dividing 500 by the TDD. A patient who takes 50 U of insulin daily needs 1 U of insulin for every 10 g of carbohydrate intake. The patient needs to learn which foods contain carbohydrate, how to estimate the grams of carbohydrate in the serving provided, and how to calculate the pre-meal dose. Additional adjustments are sometimes made for high-fat meals or for meals that have high fiber content. Occasional postprandial SMBG is needed to test whether the "insulin to carbohydrate" ratio is correct or whether the patient has been able to estimate the carbohydrate content of the meal appropriately.

In addition to covering calories, the patient must be able to compensate for high or low BG readings. An individualized sliding scale, known as the **correction factor** is determined, which provides the number of units to be added (or subtracted) to each pre-meal dose. The correction factor is estimated by dividing 1800 by the TDD.

Sample Calculations

Example 1: An overweight patient takes 60 U of insulin daily. His current BG is 178 mg/dL, and he is about to eat a meal with 90 g of carbohydrate. His physician has told him that his target SMBG is 120 mg/dL. What dose of rapid-acting insulin should he take?

Insulin to carbohydrate ratio = 500/60 = 1 U insulin/8.33 g

Correction factor = 1800/60 = 30 (predicts that 1 U insulin drops the BG 30 mg/dL)

90 g carbohydrates/8.33 g/U insulin = approximately 10 U insulin to cover carbohydrates.

SMBG – target BG = 178 mg/dL – 120 = 58 mg/dL. He will take 2 U insulin as correction.

Thus, the patient should take 12 U of rapid-acting insulin.

Example 2: A thin, insulin-sensitive patient takes 30 U of insulin per day. If this patient has a current BG of 178 and is about to eat the same meal as the patient in Example 1, how much insulin should she use?

Insulin to carbohydrate ratio = 500/30 = 1 U insulin/16.66 g

Correction factor = 1800/30 = 60 (predicts that 1 U insulin will drop the BG 60 mg/dL)

90 g carbohydrates/16.66 g/U insulin = approximately 5 U insulin to cover carbohydrates.

SMBG – target BG = 178 – 120 = 58 mg/dL. She will take 1 U insulin as correction.

Thus, this patient should take 6 U of rapid-acting insulin.

Continuous Subcutaneous Insulin Infusion

Insulin pump therapy has become an accepted alternative to MDI and has both advantages and disadvantages. Technologic advances have contributed to smaller pumps with features such as multiple basal rates, dose calculators, and alternate dosing modalities. CSII offers the patient with T1DM the greatest flexibility, and is more socially acceptable than needles and syringes for frequent dosing. Insulin pumps are the size of a pager and contain 180–300 U of insulin in a specialized syringe that is connected to a subcutaneous (SC) catheter by thin tubing. The SC catheter should be changed and repositioned every 3 days. The pump is pre-programmed to infuse the basal rate of insulin, but the patient must activate the pump to deliver bolus doses at the time of the meal or when a correction is needed. Only rapid-acting insulin is used. Diabetes education from an educator experienced in CSII is necessary to teach the patient how to use the pump, which requires several hours of instruction.

Insulin dose prescribing is conceptually similar to MDI; however, the TDD is reduced 10–20%, and the basal rate (equal to one-half of the new TDD) is divided by 24 and programmed as an hourly rate. For example, a patient taking 48 U/day with MDI will need approximately 20 U for basal requirements, or approximately 0.8 U/hour to start. The basal rate can be adjusted to accommodate nighttime low BG, morning rise, and increased or decreased activity during the day. The basal rate can be temporarily reduced for exercise or the pump can be put in suspended mode for hypoglycemia. Bolus dosing is handled similarly to MDI, with a key exception. Today's insulin pumps can administer doses in very small quantities, so the correction factor can be prescribed as a fraction. The opportunity to give smaller doses is helpful for children and insulin-sensitive patients.

The **major disadvantage** of CSII is the high cost of an insulin pump and supplies. Because only rapid-acting insulin is used, if there is a pump or catheter failure, the BG can rise quickly and DKA can ensue within 12 hours of the interruption of insulin delivery. Another potential disadvantage is the risk for catheter site infection, which is minimized by instruction in semi-sterile techniques.

Adjusting Insulin Doses

Insulin dose adjustments are made after evaluating SMBG values and looking for patterns. The efficacy of a specific rapid-acting insulin dose is monitored by the SMBG that follows the dose in question (e.g., postprandial or noon SMBG reflects the breakfast dose of rapid-acting insulin). Intermediate and long-acting insulin doses are evaluated by scrutinizing the SMBG after the injection (e.g., morning SMBG to determine adequacy of evening dose), and review of overall frequency of hyper- and hypoglycemia. Diabetes educators are often skilled at insulin dose adjustments and provide a valuable resource for patients who are experiencing problems keeping their glucose values near the target range. Diabetes education is cost-effective and necessary to achieve tight glycemic control while avoiding hypoglycemic episodes.

DIABETIC KETOACIDOSIS

DKA is the direct result of insulin deficiency; however, dehydration and excess counterregulatory hormones (glucagon, epinephrine, and cortisol) are accelerating factors. Typically, an **exacerbating factor** can be identified: new diagnosis of diabetes, omission of insulin doses, infections, pregnancy, trauma, emotional stress, excessive alcohol ingestion, myocardial infarction, stroke, intercurrent illness, hyperthyroidism, Cushing's disease, or, rarely, pheochromocytoma. The major clinical features of DKA are hyperglycemia, dehydration, acidosis, abdominal pain, nausea, vomiting, change in hemodynamic status, and altered mental status.

Pathophysiology

The pathophysiology of DKA begins with insulin levels that are insufficient to support peripheral glucose uptake and to suppress hepatic gluconeogenesis. Hyperglycemia is

TABLE 27-2. DIFFERENTIAL DIAGNOSIS OF ANION-GAP ACIDOSIS (THE MUDPILES MNEMONIC)

Condition	Clinical associations
M: methanol ingestion	Visual impairment/blindness; osmol gap between the calculated and measured osmolality (seen with any alcohol ingestion)
U: uremia	History of renal failure; increased serum urea and creatinine
D: diabetic ketoacidosis	History of diabetes, hyperglycemia
P: paraldehyde	Formaldehyde-like breath odor; increased paraldehyde level
I: iron; isoniazid	Increased serum iron level; patient may have elevated hepatic transaminases with isoniazid toxicity
L: lactic acidosis	May be due to hypovolemia/sepsis, infarction, metformin, cyanide, hydrogen sulfide, CO, methemoglobin; lactate levels are elevated
E: EtOH; ethylene glycol	Osmol gap between the calculated and measured osmolality (seen with any alcohol ingestion); increased EtOH level seen with EtOH intoxication; calcium oxalate crystals seen in the urine with ethylene glycol
S: salicylates	Tinnitus, increased salicylate level, may have a concurrent respiratory alkalosis

EtOH, ethanol.

further driven by increases in the counterregulatory hormones glucagon, catecholamines, cortisol, and growth hormone. Activation of catabolic pathways in muscle and fat produce amino acids and free fatty acids, which fuel hepatic gluconeogenesis and ketone production. The osmotic diuresis imposed by hyperglycemia causes marked fluid and electrolyte losses, further stimulating catecholamine release. Catecholamines are antagonistic to insulin action and contribute to increased lipolysis, which pumps free fatty acids into the circulation that then undergo fatty acid oxidation to ketone bodies. Volume depletion decreases renal blood flow, which contributes to reduced excretion of glucose and ketones and increased serum levels of creatinine and potassium. Acidosis ensues when the levels of acetone, acetoacetate, and beta-hydroxybutyrate exceed the buffering capacity of bicarbonate and the respiratory response. Low $PaCO_2$ reflects the respiratory effort and the severity of the metabolic acidosis. The presence of an anion gap and low bicarbonate in the setting of high BG and an ill-appearing patient should prompt immediate treatment for DKA while confirmatory laboratory evaluation is under way. The differential diagnosis for anion-gap acidosis is outlined in Table 27-2.

Symptoms

The symptoms of DKA are nonspecific and include anorexia, nausea, vomiting (coffee ground emesis in 25%), abdominal pain, and myalgias or weakness. Polyuria and polydipsia are characteristic of high BG, but may become blunted due to vomiting, reduced renal clearance, and altered mental status as the severity of DKA worsens. Hyperpnea is noted with mild acidosis, and the patient may complain of shortness of breath. Kussmaul breathing is a sign of a critically ill patient. The physical exam reveals tachycardia, hypotension or orthostatic hypotension, dry mucous membranes, poor skin turgor, abdominal tenderness, and other signs of clinical events that may have prompted the DKA episode. Mental status can be normal or severely compromised. Signs of a concurrent illness or event that precipitated the DKA may be present.

Laboratory Findings

Laboratory findings of DKA include the following: glucose >250 mg/dL, glycosuria, an elevated anion gap, and the presence of serum or urine ketones. The anion gap should exceed 12 and is calculated as follows: [Anion gap = $Na^+ - (Cl + HCO_3)$]. The serum bicarbonate is typically <15 mEq/L, the P_{CO_2} <40 mm Hg, and the arterial pH <7.3. Creatinine and K^+ are generally increased above baseline. If hypokalemia is present at the time of diagnosis, the patient has severe K^+ depletion and requires careful monitoring. The initial ECG should be checked for signs of hyperkalemia, which include peaked T waves, shortened QT intervals, widened QRS complexes, and flattened or absent P waves. Later in the course of treatment, if hypokalemia occurs, a repeat ECG might show ST segment depression, flattened or inverted T waves, a prolonged QT interval, and appearance of U waves. Hyponatremia may be present, but the measured serum sodium should be corrected for the high glucose (add 1.6 to the reported sodium for every 100 mg/dL that the glucose is >100 mg/dL), and may be further depressed by high triglycerides. Amylase and lipase may be elevated via unclear mechanisms, do not necessarily indicate pancreatitis, and resolve with treatment of the DKA.

Treatment

Clinical Evaluation and Triage

Intensive care admission is required for patients with hemodynamic instability or mental status changes, pediatric patients, or if frequent monitoring is not possible on a medical ward. Hemodynamic monitoring may be required for patients in shock, with possible sepsis, with DKA complicated by myocardial infarction, or in patients with end-stage renal disease or chronic heart failure. Nasogastric tube placement may be needed for patients with hematemesis or comatose patients.

Fluids and Electrolytes

Fluid resuscitation in adults should begin with normal saline at 1 L/hour unless there is a contraindication (chronic heart failure, end-stage renal disease). The typical total body water deficit is 4–6 L, sodium deficit is 7–10 mEq/kg, K^+ deficit is 3–5 mEq/kg, and PO_4 deficit is 5–7 mmol/kg. If the corrected sodium is normal or high on repeat testing, change the IV fluids to 0.45% NaCl; continue 0.9% saline if it is low. When the K^+ drops to <5.0 mEq/L and the patient has adequate urine output, add 20–30 mEq K^+ to each liter of IV fluid. Plan to correct the water and salt deficits over 24 hours, slower in children. The starting fluid administration rate for children should be 10–20 mL/kg/hour and should not exceed 50 mL/kg over the first 4 hours of therapy.

Patients presenting with DKA have a total body PO_4 depletion due to osmotic diuresis, although this may not be apparent on presentation because insulin deficiency and acidosis cause PO_4 to shift out of cells. Serum PO_4 levels decrease with insulin therapy. Except in very severe cases of hypophosphatemia (serum PO_4 <1.0 mg/dL) or concomitant cardiorespiratory compromise, routine administration of PO_4 has not been shown to be beneficial and may, in fact, be harmful because excess replacement can cause hypocalcemia.

Bicarbonate should not be routinely administered to patients in DKA unless the serum pH is <7.0 or the patient has life-threatening hyperkalemia.

Insulin and Glucose

Initial IV loading bolus 0.1 – 0.15 U/kg of regular (R) insulin followed by continuous infusion 0.1 U/kg/hour (100 units R insulin/100 cc normal saline solution). Children should not receive IV bolus doses of insulin; begin with the infusion.

Monitor serum glucose every hour and expect the BG to decline by 50–75 mg/dL/ hour. A slower response could indicate insulin resistance, inadequate fluid resuscitation, or improper insulin delivery. As the acidosis clears, the glucose is likely to fall more rapidly. When the serum glucose is <250 mg/dL, add 5% dextrose to the IV fluids, and decrease the insulin infusion rate by up to one-half. If the glucose infusion rate is kept stable, the insulin infusion requirements will be more predictable. Continue intensive insulin therapy and monitoring until the patient is tolerating oral intake and the anion-gap acidosis has resolved. As the acidosis resolves, the anion gap closes, arterial and venous pH rise, and serum bicarbonate rises. The American Diabetes Association position paper regarding the treatment of DKA states that criteria for the resolution of DKA include a glucose <200 mg/dL, a serum bicarbonate ≥18 mEq/L, and a venous pH >7.3. Patients recovering from DKA may develop a transient non–anion gap hyperchloremic metabolic acidosis that occurs due to urinary loss of "potential bicarbonate" in the form of ketoanions and their replacement by chloride ions from IV fluids. This non–anion-gap acidosis is transient and has not been shown to be clinically significant except in renal failure.

Common error: The hyperglycemia will respond to treatment faster than the acidosis will resolve. **Do not decrease or discontinue the insulin infusion when glucose levels approach the normal range.** This can lead to worsening of the ketoacidosis. Instead, continue the IV insulin infusion, but adjust the dose and/or add 5% dextrose. If 5% dextrose is infused at excessively rapid rates, the BG will increase, and the transition to SC insulin will be delayed.

Monitoring

- Fingerstick BG every hour during insulin infusion.
- Electrolytes, BUN, and creatinine every 2–4 hours until the K^+ has stabilized and the anion gap acidosis is resolved.
- Serum ketones or beta-hydroxybutyrate level by fingerstick on admission only. Use of the fingerstick beta-hydroxybutyrate test to follow DKA treatment is under review.
- Intake and output, weight.

Transition to SC Insulin

Continue the IV insulin infusion and IV fluids until the acidosis has cleared, the glucose is <250 mg/dL, and the patient is able to eat. **Note:** It is possible for the patient to attempt a small or clear liquid meal while on an insulin drip, but the drip rate may need to be increased for the meal hour then returned to the usual rate. Make the transition to SC insulin before a meal or at bedtime, but not during the middle of the night or between meals. If the patient has been previously diagnosed, give the usual pre-meal insulin dose plus any correction factor, and cover basal needs with intermediate- or long-acting insulin. For example, if the drip can be stopped at noon, give a pre-meal dose of short-acting insulin according to the patient's usual schedule and add a partial dose of NPH to cover until dinner or bedtime. Start basal insulin (NPH, Lente, or Lantus) and short-acting insulin 1–2 hours before stopping the insulin drip. Reduce the rate of IV dextrose to ≤ 100 cc/hour or discontinue it if the patient is unable to eat. Note that IV fluids may need to be continued until the serum creatinine has returned to baseline.

Problem Solving

Recurring DKA should prompt additional history to search for precipitating causes. Insulin pump malfunction, noncompliance with insulin doses, social distress, medication problems, or concomitant illness should warrant attention of an experienced diabetes care provider. Newly diagnosed patients require additional time in the hospital for the institution of an insulin regimen and diabetes education.

CHRONIC COMPLICATIONS

Care of the patient with T1DM includes screening for microvascular and macrovascular complications, and the application of proven therapies to reduce morbidity and mortality. The best-studied intervention in T1DM is the use of ACE inhibitors (ACEIs) to prevent progression of microalbuminuria to macroalbuminuria and slow the progression of diabetic nephropathy. ACEIs may also slow the progression of retinopathy. ACEIs should be started if blood pressure increases above the normal range for the patient's age or when microalbuminuria is identified. ACEIs should be avoided in premenopausal women who are not using effective birth control, are planning a pregnancy, or who are pregnant, due to the risk of birth defects. Blood pressure control, lipid parameters, and other prevention measures are covered in Chap. 26, Standards of Care for Diabetes Mellitus, and Chap. 28, Diabetes Mellitus Type 2.

KEY POINTS TO REMEMBER

- Several organ-specific autoimmune diseases occur with increased frequency in patients with T1DM, including autoimmune thyroiditis (Hashimoto's and Graves' diseases), Addison's disease, pernicious anemia, celiac sprue, vitiligo, alopecia, and chronic active hepatitis.
- Dietary therapy is a crucial component of therapy for patients with T1DM.
- Insulin therapy for T1DM is commonly given as either MDI or CSII, both of which use the concepts of basal/bolus dosing with pre-meal dose adjustments.
- In DKA, remember that even though initial serum levels of K^+ may be elevated, patients are actually total body K^+ depleted. Add K^+ to IV fluids when serum K^+ is <5 and the patient has adequate urine output.
- During treatment of DKA, hyperglycemia will respond faster than acidosis to treatment with insulin and IV fluids. Make sure the anion gap acidosis has resolved before transitioning to subcutaneous insulin.
- Once DKA has resolved, start basal SC insulin and short-acting SC insulin 1–2 hours before turning off the insulin drip.

SUGGESTED READING

The Diabetes Control and Complications Trial Research Group. The effect of intensive treatment of diabetes on the development and progression of long-term complications in insulin-dependent diabetes mellitus. *N Engl J Med* 1993;329:977–986.

Kitabchi AE, et al. for the American Diabetes Association. Hyperglycemic crises in diabetes. *Diabetes Care* 2004;27(Suppl 1):S94–S102.

Lewis EJ, Hunsicker LG, Bain RP, et al. For the Collaborative Study Group. The effect of angiotensin-converting enzyme inhibition on diabetic nephropathy. *N Engl J Med* 1993;329:1456–1462.

The Writing Team for the Diabetes Control and Complications Trial/Epidemiology of Diabetes Interventions and Complications Research Group. Sustained effect of intensive treatment of type 1 diabetes mellitus on development and progression of diabetic nephropathy. The epidemiology of diabetes interventions and complications (EDIC) study. *JAMA* 2003;290(16):2159–2166.

REFERENCES

American Diabetes Association. Standards of medical care in diabetes. *Diabetes Care* 2004;27:S15–S46.

Atkinson MA. Maclaren NK: The pathogenesis of insulin-dependent diabetes mellitus. *N Engl J Med* 1994;331:1428–1436.

Bode BW, ed. *Medical management of type 1 diabetes*, 4th ed. Alexandria, VA: American Diabetes Association, 2004.

Brownlee M. Biochemistry and molecular cell biology of diabetic complications. *Nature* 2001;414(6865):813–820.

Chen Q, Kukreja A, Maclaren NK. Classification of the autoimmune polyglandular syndromes. In: Gill RG, Harmon JT, Maclaren NK, eds. *Immunologically mediated endocrine diseases*. Philadelphia: Lippincott Williams & Wilkins, 2002:167–187.

Cook A. Etiology/pathogenesis of type 1 diabetes. In: Gill RG, Harmon JT, Maclaren NK, eds. *Immunologically mediated endocrine diseases*. Philadelphia: Lippincott Williams & Wilkins, 2002:287–301.

Imagawa A, et al. for the Osaka IDDM Study Group. A novel subtype of type 1 diabetes mellitus characterized by a rapid onset and an absence of diabetes-related antibodies. *N Engl J Med* 2000;342(5):301–307.

Kitabchi AE, et al. Management of hyperglycemic crises in patients with diabetes. *Diabetes Care* 2001;24(1):131–153.

Laffel LMB, McGill JB, Gans DJ, for the North American Microalbuminuria Study Group. The beneficial effect of angiotensin-converting enzyme inhibition with captopril on diabetic nephropathy in normotensive IDDM patients with microalbuminuria. *Am J Med* 1995;99:497–504.

Ratner RE, Hirsch IB, Neifing JL, et al. Less hypoglycemia with insulin glargine in intensive insulin therapy for type 1 diabetes. U.S. study group of insulin glargine in type 1 diabetes. *Diabetes Care* 2000;23:639–643.

28

Diabetes Mellitus Type 2

Janet B. McGill and
Dawn D. Smiley

INTRODUCTION

Type 2 Diabetes Mellitus (T2DM), formerly known as non–insulin-dependent diabetes, is a metabolic syndrome with carbohydrate intolerance as the cardinal feature. T2DM accounts for >90% of all cases of diabetes in the United States and Canada and is a growing public health concern, with an estimated total prevalence of 18 million among people ≥ age 20 years, or 8.7% of the adult population. Diabetes is the sixth leading cause of death in the United States and a leading cause of morbidity and mortality in other countries. The disease is the leading cause of end-stage renal disease and of blindness in individuals age 20–74 years, and of nontraumatic limb amputation. The major cause of mortality in diabetes is cardiovascular, and the diagnosis of diabetes confers a 2- to 4-fold increase in cardiovascular risk.

CAUSES

Etiology and Pathophysiology

The etiology of T2DM is multifactorial. **Insulin resistance** can be identified in >90% of persons with T2DM and may be present for many years before diabetes is diagnosed. Hyperglycemia becomes apparent when the insulin secretory response is inadequate to meet the metabolic demand. Both insulin resistance and insulin deficiency can progress over time, prompting the need for additional therapy to manage worsening hyperglycemia. **Genetic factors** are implicated in insulin resistance, but probably account for only 50% of the disordered metabolism. Obesity, in particular visceral adiposity, increasing age, and physical inactivity contribute significantly to insulin resistance and, in epidemiologic studies, are the factors associated with increasing incidence of T2DM. Insulin resistance can be induced or aggravated by pregnancy, endocrine disorders such as Cushing's disease, exogenous steroids, protease inhibitors, serious medical or surgical illness, and a number of commonly used drugs. The definitive tests for insulin resistance are only available in research settings, and they measure insulin-mediated glucose uptake or hepatic glucose output. In the clinical setting, insulin resistance is inferred when features of the metabolic syndrome are present, with or without a diagnosis of diabetes. There are no definitive histopathologic findings of insulin resistance; however, studies have demonstrated a correlation between increased fat in the liver and level of insulin resistance. Increased muscle triglyceride is also seen in this syndrome.

Before the onset of diabetes, persons with insulin resistance often have elevated insulin and C-peptide levels, and this relative hyperinsulinemia can persist through the stage of pre-diabetes. Insulin deficiency relative to the demand required to accommodate insulin resistance leads to hyperglycemia and an ultimate diagnosis of T2DM. The initial defects in insulin secretion are loss of first-phase insulin release and loss of the oscillatory secretion pattern. The clinical correlate of this early defect is postprandial hyperglycemia. Further decline in insulin secretion leads to inadequate suppression of hepatic glucose output and presents clinically as both fasting and postprandial hyperglycemia. Insulin secretory insufficiency can worsen as the blood glucose (BG) increases, a phenomenon known as **glucose toxicity**. Chronic elevation of free fatty acids, another characteristic of T2DM, may contribute to reduced insulin secretion and islet cell apoptosis. Structural changes in the islets of Langerhans' cells that are seen in long-standing T2DM include amyloid accumulation and a reduction in the number of insulin-producing beta cells. Early in the course of diabetes, improvement in insulin secretion can be achieved by reducing insulin resistance and improving hyperglycemia, thus reducing the functional deficits imposed by hyperglycemia and elevated free fatty acids. Whether insulin secretory capacity can be preserved over time by therapeutic interventions that reduce insulin resistance or by maintenance of near normal glycemia is not known. Longitudinal data from the UK Prospective Diabetes Study (UKPDS) suggest that loss of insulin secretory capacity over time is common in T2DM.

The American Diabetes Association (ADA) classifies a heterogeneous group of disorders that cause or are strongly associated with diabetes as "**Other specific types**." The most common problems in this group of disorders are the drug- or chemical-induced forms of diabetes. Typical offending agents include glucocorticoids, nicotinic acid, thiazides, beta-adrenergic agonists, the newer atypical antipsychotic agents, and some antiretroviral agents. Hyperglycemia can be relatively mild or quite severe with the institution of these therapies. Screening for new-onset diabetes or for deterioration in glycemic control if the patient has been previously diagnosed with diabetes is warranted. Diseases of the exocrine pancreas can result in partial or complete insulin deficiency. Patients with hemochromatosis or advanced cystic fibrosis may present with nonketotic hyperglycemia. Pancreatitis, pancreatectomy, pancreatic neoplasia, or fibrocalculous pancreatopathy may cause insulin deficiency, and insulin therapy may be needed early in the course of the illness. Diabetes can occur with other endocrine diseases such as Cushing's syndrome, acromegaly, and others. Resolution of the diabetes often occurs when the hormonal excess is corrected.

Diabetes is a feature of a number of **genetic disorders**. Patients with Down syndrome, Prader-Willi syndrome, and others may develop diabetes as a consequence of obesity. Mild to moderate hyperglycemia that presents in young adults with a family history that suggests a dominantly inherited trait may represent maturity-onset diabetes in the young (MODY), of which there are six types. Obesity and insulin resistance are not characteristic features of MODY. Most of the T2DM that is diagnosed in children and teenagers is not MODY, but is rather early-onset classic T2DM. Other rare forms of diabetes that present in adulthood include mitochondrial gene defects and defects of the insulin molecule or of the insulin receptor (type A insulin resistance).

A common clinical problem is the patient who does not have features of insulin resistance and who may not respond to oral hypoglycemic agents as expected. These patients should be tested for autoimmune markers such as anti-GAD65 and ICA antibodies (see Chap. 27, Diabetes Mellitus Type 1). **Latent autoimmune diabetes in adults (LADA)** is an insulin-deficient form of diabetes that develops more slowly than classic type 1 diabetes and is associated with other autoimmune diseases. The majority of patients with LADA require exogenous insulin within 5 years of diagnosis. Later in the course of the illness, patients with LADA may become C-peptide negative and are at risk for ketoacidosis. The prevalence of autoimmune beta cell destruction in a population of T2DM is unknown, but will likely vary by ethnicity. Approximately 10% of the UKPDS study cohort was positive for beta-cell antibodies, and that subgroup had a rapid progression to insulin therapy for control of hyperglycemia.

PRESENTATION

Individuals at high risk for the development of T2DM can often be identified before the onset of clinical diabetes. **Risk factors** for the development of T2DM include older age, obesity [body mass index (BMI) ≥ 27 kg/m^2], sedentary lifestyle, history of glucose intolerance (i.e., gestational DM, impaired glucose tolerance, stress hyperglycemia), history of intrauterine growth retardation, family history, and ethnicity. T2DM is 2–6 times more prevalent in African Americans, Asians, Hispanic Americans, Native Americans, and Pima Indians than in non-Hispanic whites.

TABLE 28-1. DIAGNOSIS OF DIABETES

Stage	FPG	Oral glucose tolerance test	Random blood glucose
Normal	FPG <100 mg/dL	2-hr PG <140 mg/dL	—
Pre-diabetes			
Impaired fasting glucose	FPG ≥100 and <126 mg/dL	—	—
Impaired glucose tolerance	—	2-hr PG ≥140 mg/dL and <200 mg/dL	—
Diabetes	FPG ≥126 mg/dL, confirmed	2-hr PG ≥200 mg/dL	≥200 mg/dL with symptoms

FPG, fasting plasma glucose; PG, plasma glucose.

The **metabolic syndrome,** defined as ≥3 of the following characteristics, may precede the diagnosis of T2DM and may confer increased risk of cardiovascular disease.

- Abdominal obesity (waist circumference)
  Men: >102 cm (>40 in.)
  Women: >88 cm (>35 in.)
- Triglycerides ≥150 mg/dL
- High-density lipoprotein (HDL) cholesterol
  Men: <40 mg/dL
  Women: <50 mg/dL
- Blood pressure ≥130/85 mm Hg
- Fasting glucose ≥110 mg/dL

The **diagnosis of T2DM** is made when the fasting plasma glucose (FPG) is ≥126 mg/dL, confirmed on a second sample; or when a random BG of ≥200 mg/dL is accompanied by symptoms; or by finding that the 2-hour BG on a 75-g oral glucose tolerance test is ≥200 mg/dL. Patients with impaired fasting glucose or impaired glucose tolerance are at higher risk for the development of T2DM and may be at higher risk for cardiovascular events even in the absence of T2DM. The diagnostic criteria for diabetes and pre-diabetic conditions are listed in Table 28-1.

Because mild hyperglycemia is asymptomatic, patients presenting with symptoms of polyuria, nocturia, polydipsia, polyphagia, fatigue, weight changes, or blurred vision are likely to have significant BG elevation and may have been undiagnosed for some time. Patients who present with complaints of extremity pain, sexual dysfunction, or visual changes from diabetic retinopathy are likely to have been hyperglycemic for years before the actual diagnosis of diabetes.

The **medical history** of a patient with diabetes should include documentation of the onset and progression of diabetes, with information about episodes of diabetic ketoacidosis (DKA), prior response to medications, and level of glycemic control. Health behaviors, such as frequency of self-monitoring of BG, use of medical nutrition therapy, and exercise frequency and intensity, should be recorded. Usual BG values and problems with both hyperglycemia and hypoglycemia require assessment to plan changes in therapy. Symptoms of hyperglycemia and hypoglycemia should be elicited to augment the careful exam of glucose records or meter readings.

The past medical history (PMH) should include a review of cardiovascular risk factors, including duration (e.g., hypertension since 1994 and hyperlipidemia with elevated LDL first identified in 2001) and cardiovascular event history. Notation should be made of the level of retinopathy, including eye procedures, evidence of nephropathy, history of neuropathy, and history of foot ulceration or joint problems. The most recent eye exam and vaccine status should be recorded. Menstrual history, pregnancy history, and use of contraception need to be addressed in the PMH of adolescent and adult women.

Review of systems for a patient with diabetes should target pertinent positive and negative cardiovascular, visual, and neuropathic complaints.

The **physical exam** may be completely normal or may include hypertension, obesity, or acanthosis nigricans. Funduscopic exam may be normal or abnormal (dot hemorrhages, exudates, neovascularization, or laser scars). The cardiovascular exam is crucial for patients with diabetes and should include carotid and peripheral pulses. Exam of the feet, including skin, nails, joints, and sensation with a 10-g Semmes-Weinstein monofilament, should be done at regular intervals. The diagnosis of neuropathy is based on a combination of symptoms and physical findings, with documented decrease in >1 sensory modality (e.g., absent reflexes plus loss of vibratory sensation).

Laboratory Evaluation

Suspected diabetes can be diagnosed via three different studies: FPG, random plasma glucose + symptoms, or the oral glucose tolerance test. Positive studies include either an FPG ≥126 mg/dL, a random plasma glucose ≥200 + symptoms of hyperglycemia, or a 2-hour plasma glucose ≥200 after a 75-g glucose challenge (see Table 28-1). A positive FPG must be confirmed with a second sample. A patient can also be diagnosed with new-onset diabetes if he or she presents with DKA. Determination of whether the diabetes diagnosis is type 1 or type 2 is accomplished by

- Thorough review of PMH, medication history, and family history.
- Physical exam looking for findings that are consistent with hyperinsulinemia (i.e., obesity, acanthosis nigricans).
- Laboratory findings consistent with the metabolic syndrome.
- Immunologic markers such as anti-GAD 65 or islet cell antibodies.
- Measurement of C-peptide.

Routine laboratory testing of a patient with T2DM should include a fasting lipid profile, Hgb A1C, renal profile, urine microalbumin, and a baseline ECG. Hgb A1C should be done at least semiannually, and most physicians agree that quarterly is appropriate if it is out of the desired range or treatment is changed. Liver function testing is required for monitoring of statin and thiazolidinedione (TZD) therapies, and should be considered for all patients with insulin resistance due to the increased risk of nonalcoholic fatty liver disease (NAFLD). Patients with T2DM and proteinuria or renal insufficiency require increased surveillance of renal parameters.

MANAGEMENT

T2DM is best managed with a multidisciplinary team, including doctors, diabetes educators, pharmacists, dietitians, and support groups. Diabetes therapy should be individually designed to achieve glycemic, blood pressure, lipid, and prevention targets while accommodating the patient's age and socioeconomic and cultural status. The glycemic target is an A1C value of <7%; however, the ADA recommendations state that there is no lower limit, even into the normal range of <6%, on most assays. Treatment options include (see Tables 28-2, 28-3, and 28-4)

- Diet and exercise alone
- Oral hypoglycemic agents
- Oral agents + nightly or basal insulin
- Pre-mixed insulin with or without oral agents
- Complex insulin regimens using intermediate- or long-acting insulin plus a rapid- or short-acting insulin for pre-meal doses
- Continuous subcutaneous (SC) insulin infusion (via SC insulin pump)

Instructions for self-monitoring of BG are tailored to the type of therapy and risk of hypoglycemia and may vary from once to four or more times daily.

TABLE 28-2. ORAL ANTIDIABETIC DRUGS

Drug	Dose	Mode of action	Efficacy	Advantages	Disadvantages
Biguanide: Metformin	500–2000 mg daily, divided doses	Reduces hepatic glucose output	↓ A1C by 1–2%	No weight gain, ↓ triglycerides	GI side effects (nausea, diarrhea); risk of lactic acidosis. Avoid if creatinine is >1.4 in women; >1.5 in men; chronic heart failure, age >80 yrs, liver impairment.
Sulfonylureas: glyburide (DiaBeta), glipizide (Glucotrol), glimepiride (Amaryl)	2.5–20 mg; 2.5–40 mg; 2–8 mg	Stimulate insulin release	↓ A1C by 1–2%	Well tolerated, inexpensive	Hypoglycemia, weight gain, allergy. Use with caution in the elderly or liver or renal insufficiency.
Meglitinides: repaglinide (Prandin), nateglinide (Starlix)	Dose tid before meals: 0.5–2 mg; 60–120 mg	Short-acting insulin secretagogue	↓ A1C by 1–1.5%	Well tolerated, may have less risk of hypoglycemia compared to sulfonylureas	Hypoglycemia, tid dosing, more expensive than sulfonylureas.
Thiazolidinediones: pioglitazone (Actos), rosiglitazone (Avandia)	15, 30, 45 mg qd; 2, 4, 8 mg qd or 2–4 mg bid	Insulin sensitizer; reduces insulin resistance peripherally	↓ A1C by 0.8–1.8%	Possible favorable endothelial effects and favorable lipid profile effects	Weight gain, fluid retention, risk of congestive heart failure, anemia; variable lipid effects, expensive. Rare liver toxicity.
Alpha-glucosidase inhibitors: acarbose (Precose), miglitol (Glyset)	Both agents: 50–100 mg tid before meals, start with lower doses	Inhibit gut enzymes that break down carbohydrates	↓ A1C by 0.7–1.5%	No weight gain	GI side effects, including flatulence, diarrhea, and cramping. Rare liver toxicity.

↓, decreased.

TABLE 28-3. ORAL COMBINATION PILLS

Trade name	Medications
Glucovance	Glyburide/metformin: 1.25 mg/250 mg; 2.5 mg/500 mg; 5 mg/500 mg
Metaglip	Glipizide/metformin: 2.5 mg/250 mg; 2.5 mg/500 mg; 5 mg/500 mg
Avandamet	Avandia/metformin: 1 mg/500 mg; 2 mg/500 mg; 4 mg/500 mg, 2 mg/ 1000 mg, 4 mg/1000 mg

Diet and Exercise

Lifestyle modification, incorporating both diet and exercise, is the first-line therapy for the prevention of diabetes and treatment of new-onset T2DM. Lifestyle modification that includes modest weight loss and adherence to 150 minutes (2.5 hours) of exercise per week is effective in reducing the progression from prediabetes to diabetes. Use of the Dietary Approaches to Stop Hypertension (DASH) diet that is enriched in fruits and vegetables and low in fat and salt has been shown to reduce some indicators of insulin resistance. Individualized medical nutrition therapy is recommended for all patients with diabetes and generally requires several encounters with a registered dietitian or group education program. The UKPDS study showed that only 3% of patients treated with dietary therapy alone were able to achieve and maintain glycemic control over a 6-year period. Institution of insulin therapy should prompt additional dietary counseling to help the patient maintain consistent caloric intake or to instruct the patient in carbohydrate-counting techniques.

Pharmacologic Treatment

Oral Hypoglycemic Agents

Oral hypoglycemic agents (see Tables 28-2 and 28-3) fall into 4 major groups: biguanide sensitizers, insulin secretagogues, TZDs, and glucosidase inhibitors. Additional classes of oral and injectable antidiabetic drugs are in clinical development.

Insulin

Insulin may be required to achieve glycemic targets in patients with T2DM. Worsening hyperglycemia over time is likely due to both increasing insulin resistance and loss of insulin secretory capacity. In most cases, the oral antidiabetic agents should be continued and a basal insulin dose started at bedtime. If the response to ≥1 oral agents has been poor, or a contraindication develops, a more complex insulin regimen might be required to achieve glucose targets. **Diabetes education** is highly recommended when insulin is started or when the regimen is changed. The regimen should be tailored to the patient's needs and abilities and advanced quickly to avoid prolonged hyperglycemia. Instruction in signs and symptoms of hypoglycemia and in methods of treatment is required. Instruction in the use of a **glucagon pen** should be provided to the patient's household members. The long-acting insulin glargine (Lantus) has been shown to cause less nighttime hypoglycemia when used with oral agents in an evening dosing regimen. Multiple daily dosing regimens have been used to achieve tight glucose control and reduce the risk of hypoglycemia by carefully adjusting the pre-meal doses according to ambient BG, anticipated carbohydrate intake, and activity level. **Insulin requirements** vary with changes in weight, diet, activity, concomitant medication use, acute illnesses, and infections. Use of oral antidiabetic drugs in combination with insulin may help to reduce the insulin requirement and the complexity of the regimen; however, TZD doses should be submaximal [up to 30 mg pioglitazone (Actos) and 4 mg rosiglitazone (Avandia)] to minimize the risk of edema and congestive heart failure (see Table 28-4). Please refer to Table 27-1 in Chap. 27, Diabetes Mellitus Type 1, for an overview of insulin types and pharmacokinetics.

Concentrated insulin, as U500 (500 U/mL) is available only as regular, and is an option for patients who require exceptionally large doses of insulin. An endocrinology consultation should be sought if U500 insulin use is contemplated.

TABLE 28-4. INSULIN REGIMENS FOR DIABETES MELLITUS TYPE 2

Regimen	Oral agents	Insulin types	Glucose monitoring	Starting doses
Oral agents + basal insulin—*Usual starting regimen*	Continue all types of oral agents. Use sub-maximal doses of TZDs.	Intermediate (NPH or Lente) or long-acting (Glargine).	Fasting and as needed during the day	0.1–0.2 U/kg given at bedtime; increase until fasting plasma glucose is at target.
bid regimens, pre-mixed insulin—*OK for patients with regular meal schedules*	Continue insulin sensitizers. TZDs: use up to 30 mg pioglitazone, 4 mg rosiglitazone.	70/30 NPH/regular; Humalog mix 75/25; NovoLog mix 70/30.	2–4× daily and as needed to avoid hypoglycemia	0.1 U/kg A.M. and P.M.; increase doses equally until blood glucose near the target range; evaluate with qid self-monitored blood glucose.
MDI regimens—*Helpful for patients with irregular meal schedules; may be necessary to achieve tight control*	Continue sensitizers at doses above if the patient is insulin resistant and there are no contraindications.	Basal insulin: insulin glargine given at bedtime or NPH/Lente given qd or bid; Pre-meal insulin: lispro (Humalog), aspart (NovoLog) or regular.	4× daily is required: before meals and at bedtime	In general, a total dose of 0.5–2 U/kg will be required. Give 50% as basal; divide the remaining 50% into pre-meal doses. Use adjustable scales ± carbohydrate counting for pre-meal dosing.
Continuous SC insulin infusion—*Many attractive features for patients*	Sensitizers may still be useful for insulin-resistant patients.	Aspart (NovoLog) and glulisine (Apidra) are approved for insulin pump use, Lispro (Humalog) is also commonly used.	4× daily and as needed	Conceptually similar to MDI regimens. Intensive diabetes education is needed.

MDI, multiple daily injection; TZD, thiazolidinedione.

Nonketotic Hyperosmolar Coma

Nonketotic hyperosmolar coma (NKHC) evolves over a period of time but presents emergently when **neurologic deterioration** occurs in the setting of **high glucose levels** and dehydration. Elderly or disabled patients with significant hyperglycemia who are unable to compensate for the free water loss with oral intake are predisposed to develop this syndrome. Patients with NKHC present with a plasma glucose that is generally >600 mg/dL, increased BUN and creatinine, increased serum osmolality, and a free water deficit of 2–6 L. Typically, the anion gap is normal or only slightly elevated, and the bicarbonate is >15 mEq/L. The effective serum osmolality is >320 mOsm/kg, calculated ($[2 \times$ measured Na (mEq/L)] + [glucose (mg/dL)/18]) +[BUN(mg/dL)/3]).

The initial goal of therapy is to **replace volume** and **correct the free water** deficit with the infusion of appropriate IV fluids. The nature of the fluids (isotonic vs hypotonic) administered and the rate of infusion are determined by the clinical circumstances. In general, most patients benefit from IV infusion of 1 L normal saline over the first hour. Subsequent fluid management is determined by the patient's hemodynamic status, corrected serum sodium (measured Na + 1.6 mEq/L for every 100 mg/dL over 100 mg/dL glucose), and free water deficit. Careful monitoring of volume status and electrolytes is required to avoid fluid overload or overly rapid correction of hypernatremia. As in DKA, patients in NKHC present with total body K^+ deficit, so K^+ should be added to IV fluids as soon as adequate urine output is restored and serum K^+ is <5 mEq/L.

IV insulin can be given as repeated IV bolus doses (0.1 U/kg/1–2 hours) or via insulin drip (see Chap. 27, Diabetes Mellitus Type 1, for further details). The glucose may decline more rapidly in NKHC than in DKA, so hourly monitoring of glucose is required. Electrolytes and the clinical status of the patient should be checked every 2–4 hours and IV fluids adjusted accordingly. SC insulin should be instituted after the patient's hydration status is normalized, the patient is able to eat, and the BG is ≤250 mg/dL. The mainstay of treatment is fluid resuscitation; however, care must be exercised in the process of treating elderly patients with tenuous cardiac and renal status. Neurologic changes should be evaluated to rule out stroke or other CNS conditions.

Goals of Therapy

The goal of therapy for control of hyperglycemia is essentially to **normalize BG values**. The ADA recommends that every patient achieve an A1C of <7%, but adds that there is no lower limit at which benefit is not observed. Other groups recommend that the A1C target be set at ≤6.5%. The overriding message is that treatment should target near normal BG values, with appropriate measures taken to avoid hypoglycemia. These measures might include diabetes education, more frequent BG monitoring, occasional nighttime glucose checks, and use of more complex insulin regimens that more closely mimic normal physiology. The BG levels that are needed to achieve these glycemic targets are fasting and pre-meal glucoses, 90–130 mg/dL; postprandial, ≤180 mg/dL; and bedtime, 100–140 mg/dL.

Blood pressure control is important for prevention of nephropathy and retinopathy and for the preservation of renal function. The blood pressure goal for all patients is <130/80 mm Hg, and lower pressures may be helpful for patients with proteinuria. ACE inhibitors (ACEIs) are considered first-line therapy for patients with prediabetes and diabetes. Both ACEIs and angiotensin receptor blockers have been shown to delay progression of deterioration of renal function in patients with nephropathy. Patients with persistent proteinuria may benefit from the use of ACEI and angiotensin receptor blocker drugs in combination.

Management of **hyperlipidemia** is considered critical to reduce the risk of cardiovascular morbidity and mortality. The 3-hydroxy-3-methylglutaryl coenzyme A reductase inhibitors (statins) have been shown to reduce cardiovascular morbidity and mortality, and LDL targets of <100 mg/dL can generally be achieved with appropriate doses. Cholesterol-sequestering agents (resins) or the cholesterol absorption inhibitor ezetimibe (Zetia) can be used in combination with statins, or alone in the patient who cannot tolerate statins. Many patients with the metabolic syndrome, prediabetes, and T2DM have elevated triglycerides and low HDL. Diet and exercise, fibrates, niacin, and fish oil are effective for this form of dyslipidemia (see Chap. 30, Diagnosis, Standards of Care, and Treatment for Hyperlipidemia, for further details about treatment goals and modalities). Low-dose aspirin (81–162 mg daily) is recommended for patients > age 40 years and can be initiated at younger ages. Smoking cessation should be recommended for all patients.

Screening and treatment for **retinopathy** is handled by ophthalmology colleagues, but the physician treating the patient for diabetes is expected to ascertain that the patient is receiving appropriate care. **Neuropathy** is arguably the most difficult complication to manage. Pain control is often an ongoing problem, and patients may require polypharmacy interventions for relief. Tricyclics, selective serotonin reuptake inhibitors (SSRIs), and other antidepressants (venlafaxine) may be useful. Often, if the patient is able to sleep through the night and uses appropriate footwear during the day with rest periods, neuropathic symptoms can be tolerated. Antiseizure medications, such as phenytoin (Dilantin) and gabapentin (Neurotonin), are used for treatment of unremitting pain. Narcotics and other addicting agents should be avoided. **Foot care** should include treatment of onychomycosis, reduction of corns and calluses, use of rubber-soled shoes with arch support, and daily inspection by the patient. Foot infections need to be evaluated immediately and treated by experienced clinicians, with referral for complex lesions.

Although **cardiovascular disease** is the leading cause of morbidity and mortality in patients with diabetes, recommendations for screening with provocative testing have not been elucidated for this high-risk group. In general, any complaints of angina or possible anginal equivalents warrant evaluation. Screening of asymptomatic diabetic patients with exercise stress testing may be considered in those with multiple cardiac risk factors, an abnormal resting ECG, known vascular disease, or plans to initiate an exercise program, but whether such screening improves outcomes is not known. Causes of unexpected weight gain or peripheral edema should be investigated. **Confounding conditions** that are more common in the overweight diabetic patient are sleep apnea, non-ischemic heart failure, anemia, and TZD-related peripheral edema. Also, depression and anxiety are more common and more persistent in patients with diabetes, and warrant evaluation and treatment. Chronic infections, such as asymptomatic bacteriuria, periodontal disease, and fungal skin and nail infections, should be managed proactively.

The incidence and prevalence of T2DM is increasing rapidly, and will severely tax future medical resources. Clinicians in every specialty will be called on to participate in the care of these patients to reduce the morbidity and mortality now observed. Increased awareness and communication will be key to effective management of this multi-faceted illness.

KEY POINTS TO REMEMBER

- At the time of presentation, screen for signs and symptoms of end-organ damage such as retinopathy, nephropathy, and neuropathy.
- When evaluating patients with hyperglycemia, consider secondary causes of diabetes such as medications, genetic disorders, and other endocrinopathies.
- Dietary modification and exercise are crucial components of every treatment regimen.
- Meeting glycemic control targets reduces the rate of diabetic complications.
- Physicians and patients should modify treatment and lifestyle regimens aggressively to achieve glycemic targets unless limited by patient safety (hypoglycemia, comorbid conditions) or circumstances.
- Treatment of hyperlipidemia, hypertension, and tobacco dependence is essential to address the leading cause of mortality in diabetic patients.
- Treatment plans must be tailored to the individual patient's needs and capabilities.

SUGGESTED READING

American Diabetes Association. Standards of medical care in diabetes. *Diabetes Care* 2004;27(Suppl 1):S5–S102. http://care.diabetesjournals.org/content/vol27/suppl_1/.

The Diabetes Control and Complications Trial Research Group. The effect of intensive treatment of diabetes on the development and progression of long-term complications in insulin-dependent diabetes mellitus. *N Engl J Med* 1993;329:977.

Kitabchi AE, Umpierrez GE, Murphy MB, et al. Hyperglycemic crises in patient with diabetes mellitus. *Diabetes Care* 2003;26(Suppl 1):S109–S117.

UKPDS publications. http://www.dtu.ox.ac.uk/index.html?maindoc=/ukpds.

REFERENCES

Beckman JA, Creager MA, Libby P. Diabetes and atherosclerosis: epidemiology, pathophysiology and management. *JAMA* 2002;287:2570–2581.

Diabetes Prevention Program Research Group. Reduction in the incidence of type 2 diabetes with lifestyle intervention or metformin. *N Engl J Med* 2002;346(6): 393–403.

Ennis ED, Stahl EJVB, Kreisberg RA. The hyperosmolar hyperglycemic syndrome. *Diabetes Rev* 1994;2:115–126.

Executive Summary of the Third Report of the National Cholesterol Education Program (NCEP) expert panel on detection, evaluation, and treatment of high blood cholesterol in adults (adult treatment panel III). *JAMA* 2001;285:2486–2497.

Hunter SJ, Garvey WT. Insulin action and insulin resistance: diseases involving defects in insulin receptor signal transduction, and the glucose transport effector system. *Am J Med* 1998;105:331–345.

Park Y, Zhu S, Palaniappan L, et al. The metabolic syndrome: prevalence and associated risk factor findings in the US population from the third national health and nutrition exam survey, 1988–1994. *Arch Intern Med* 2003;163:427–436.

Turner R et al. UKPDS 25: autoantibodies to islet-cell cytoplasm and glutamic acid decarboxylase for prediction of insulin requirement in type 2 diabetes. *Lancet* 1997;350:1288–1293.

U.S. 2000 Census Data. http://www.cdc.gov/diabetes.

Weyer C, Bogardus C, Mott DM, et al. The natural history of insulin secretory dysfunction and insulin resistance in the pathogenesis of type 2 diabetes mellitus. *J Clin Invest* 1999;104:787–794.

Zimmerman BR, ed. *Medical management of type 2 diabetes*, 4th ed. Alexandria, VA: American Diabetes Association, 1998.

Zimmet P, et al. Global and societal implications of the diabetes epidemic. *Nature* 2001;414(6865):782–787.

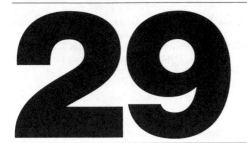

Hypoglycemia

Bharathi Raju

INTRODUCTION

Healthy individuals maintain their plasma glucose within a narrow range. In the postprandial state, insulin secretion by the beta cell rises and glucose use and energy storage by target tissues increases. In the postabsorptive (fasting) state, plasma glucose is maintained between approximately 72 and 108 mg/dL, although it can fall further without causing symptoms in some individuals, especially in young women. Hypoglycemia occurs when **plasma glucose falls <50 mg/dL**. The first defense against hypoglycemia is reduced insulin secretion. As glucose levels fall further, increased secretion of counterregulatory hormones (glucagon and epinephrine) further reduces glucose use by tissues, increases release of glucose from liver stores (glycogenolysis), and increases glucose production and release by the liver (gluconeogenesis). With prolonged fasting, other counterregulatory hormones (cortisol, growth hormone, and thyroid hormone) alter the sensitivity of the liver and kidney to insulin, glucagon, and epinephrine. These counterregulatory mechanisms are essential for survival because glucose is the sole metabolic fuel for the brain. (After a period of prolonged fasting, the brain adapts to use ketone bodies and other substrates as fuel.) Hypoglycemia may occur when there is excess insulin, decreased counterregulatory hormones, impaired responsiveness of target tissues to counterregulatory hormones, or a combination of these factors.

Hypoglycemia is classified as **reactive** or **fasting**, depending on whether it occurs primarily in the postprandial or fasting state, respectively.

CAUSES

Fasting Hypoglycemia

The most common cause of hypoglycemia is **drugs**. Insulin, sulfonylureas, and alcohol account for 70% of cases. Risk factors for insulin-induced hypoglycemia include prescription errors, skipped/delayed meals, exercise, and concomitant medications. Ingestion of alcohol during prolonged fasting may lead to hypoglycemia by inhibition of gluconeogenesis.

In severe infection and **sepsis**, glucose use may exceed production, thereby causing hypoglycemia.

Counterregulatory hormone deficiencies (**adrenal insufficiency, growth hormone deficiency**) rarely cause hypoglycemia unless there is more than one hormone deficiency. Non-islet cell **malignancies**, including lymphomas, leukemias, and teratomas, may cause hypoglycemia by secretion of IGF-2, which can increase glucose use and suppress production.

When hypoglycemia is diagnosed, the endocrinologist is often consulted to investigate whether the patient has an **insulinoma**, a life-threatening condition characterized by dysregulated insulin secretion by a pancreatic beta-cell tumor. The incidence of insulinoma is 1–2 cases per million patient years. In younger patients, insulinoma is frequently associated with multiple endocrine neoplasia 1 (MEN1). Malignant insulinomas are more common in older patients.

Factitious hypoglycemia is most frequently seen in patients who have access to insulin or oral hypoglycemics, such as health care workers or in individuals with a family history of diabetes mellitus. Medication errors may be responsible.

Reactive (Postprandial) Hypoglycemia

Reactive hypoglycemia occurs after meals. Most typically it occurs in patients with a history of **gastric surgery**. Rapid gastric emptying and glucose absorption leads to a mismatch between insulin and glucose levels. A common referral to endocrinologists is patients without a history of gastric surgery who experience symptoms of tremulousness, fatigue, anxiety, lightheadedness, decreased cognitive function, and excessive hunger within a few hours of a meal. Usually, hypoglycemia is not documented. This **idiopathic** reactive "hypoglycemia" is often inappropriately diagnosed on the basis of low blood sugars during an oral glucose tolerance test (OGTT). However, during OGTTs, healthy volunteers can have plasma glucose levels as low as 30 mg/dL without symptoms. Therefore, the **OGTT is not useful in making the diagnosis of reactive hypoglycemia.**

Other Causes of Hypoglycemia

A rare cause of hypoglycemia is the presence of **autoantibodies** against insulin or the insulin receptor. Other causes of hypoglycemia include systemic illness (renal or liver failure, heart disease, malnutrition), pregnancy, and exercise.

PRESENTATION

The diagnosis of hypoglycemia is confirmed by **Whipple's triad**:

- Symptoms of hypoglycemia
- Low plasma glucose concentration
- Relief of symptoms on raising the glucose levels

The neurogenic symptoms of hypoglycemia result from activation of the sympathetic nervous system, and the neuroglycopenic symptoms result from inadequate delivery of glucose to the brain (Table 29-1).

TABLE 29-1. SYMPTOMS OF HYPOGLYCEMIA

Neurogenic (autonomic)
    Palpitations
    Tremor
    Anxiety
    Sweating
    Hunger
    Paresthesia
Neuroglycopenic (brain glucose deprivation)
    Confusion
    Fatigue
    Seizure
    Loss of consciousness
    Focal neurologic deficit

Neurogenic and neuroglycopenic symptoms begin to occur at a glycemic threshold of approximately 50–55 mg/dL. Plasma glucose levels of approximately 40 mg/dL are associated with gross behavioral changes, and levels approximately 30 mg/dL and lower may produce coma, convulsions, and death. In individuals who experience recurrent hypoglycemia from whatever etiology, these glycemic thresholds shift to lower plasma glucose concentrations. Conversely, glucose counterregulation and symptoms of hypoglycemia occur at higher glucose concentrations in patients with poorly controlled diabetes mellitus.

Insulinomas are most frequently diagnosed between the ages of 30 and 70 years. The symptoms of insulinoma are secondary to hypoglycemia. 80% of insulinomas are benign adenomas. Insulinomas associated with MEN may be multifocal or malignant and may secrete other hormones such as gastrin or ACTH. Diagnosis can be delayed by many years. Because of frequent hypoglycemic episodes, these patients are prone to develop hypoglycemia unawareness. 50% of patients eat frequently to avoid symptoms and, therefore, gain weight. Although fasting hypoglycemia is most characteristic of insulinoma, hypoglycemia in the postprandial setting may occur.

MANAGEMENT

Management of hypoglycemia centers on the question of whether the patient has an insulinoma, which is a life-threatening but surgically curable condition. First, one must determine whether the patient really had a hypoglycemic episode with a **documented plasma glucose <50 mg/dL**. If the patient's hypoglycemia was asymptomatic, it is important to consider artifacts due to improper collection, storage, or error in analytic methods. Measured plasma glucose can drop 10–20 mg/dL/hour irrespective of initial values, so it is important for samples to be processed quickly. Also, large numbers of blood cells, such as in patients with leukemia, can consume plasma glucose, thereby artifactually lowering the measured value, even in the presence of glycolytic inhibitors.

A **detailed history** is essential and should include the following aspects: the circumstances of the episode and its temporal relationship to meals or exercise, associated symptoms, weight changes, recurrence of the episode, drug/alcohol history, medication history, history of gastric surgery, personal or family history of diabetes or of MEN1 or MEN-associated conditions, comorbid conditions, and symptoms of other hormone deficiencies.

There are no specific physical findings associated with insulinoma. Other causes of hypoglycemia may be revealed by a complete **physical exam**, including signs of chronic alcohol use, other hormone deficiencies, or of MEN1. Laboratory evaluation should focus on documentation of insulin and C-peptide levels during an episode of symptomatic hypoglycemia (plasma glucose <50 mg/dL). If the C-peptide is low in the presence of high insulin, exogenous insulin should be suspected as the etiology. With high insulin and high C-peptide, screening for sulfonylurea and other new insulin secretagogues [e.g., repaglinide (Prandin) and nateglinide (Starlix)] should be performed to rule out surreptitious or inadvertent drug use.

To elicit an episode of hypoglycemia for **biochemical evaluation**, the patient may be instructed to initiate a supervised fast. It may be necessary to admit the patient to the hospital for a supervised 72-hour fast. In normal individuals, even after 72 hours of fasting, the plasma glucose remains >50 mg/dL. However, the blood sugar of some normal women may fall below this level without symptoms. The patient may be asked to engage in moderate exercise to precipitate an episode of hypoglycemia. The fast is ended and the patient treated for hypoglycemia with IV dextrose once symptomatic hypoglycemia is documented and samples for plasma glucose, insulin, C-peptide, and screens for insulin secretagogues are obtained. In patients with insulinoma, the ratio of proinsulin to total insulin increases relative to that of healthy individuals and may be helpful in some cases. The **diagnosis of insulinoma** is suggested by documentation of hypoglycemia (plasma glucose <50 mg/dL) in a symptomatic patient with an inappropriately elevated insulin level (>5 mU/mL), inappropriately high C-peptide level (to rule out surreptitious insulin use), and a negative screen for insulin secretagogues.

Immediate treatment of severe hypoglycemia uses IV dextrose (initial bolus of 1 amp D50 followed by infusion of D_5W to maintain BG >100 mg/dL) or 1 mg IM or subcuta-

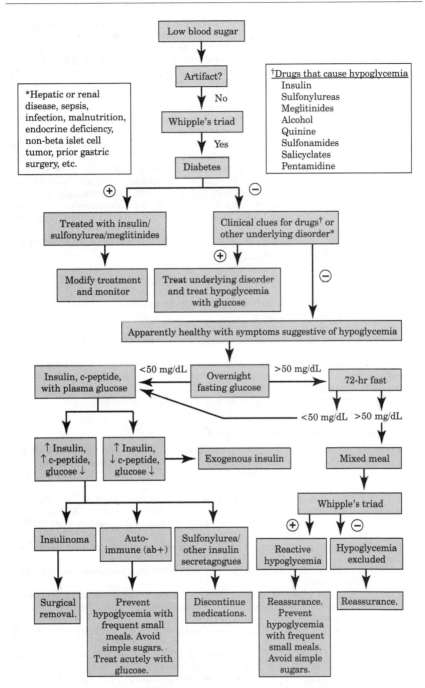

FIG. 29-1. Algorithm for the differential diagnosis and management of hypoglycemia. Adapted from Cryer PE. Glucose homeostasis and hypoglycemia. In: Larsen, PR et al., *Williams textbook of endocrinology*, 10th ed. Philadelphia: WB Saunders, 2003.

neous (SC) glucagon (in patients without ready IV access). Conscious patients may also be given readily absorbable carbohydrates (fruit juices, glucose tablets). However, to prevent recurrence, the underlying etiology must be corrected. Once a diagnosis of insulinoma is made biochemically, tumor localization is usually performed by intraoperative palpation and ultrasound. The treatment of choice is surgical resection of the insulinoma. For solitary adenomas, surgery is curative. Insulinomas associated with MEN1 may recur in another site. Medical therapy with the hyperglycemic agent diazoxide (Proglycem) is reserved for patients who are not surgical candidates, who have recurrent disease and refuse reoperation, or who have inoperable disease. Frequent, carbohydrate-rich meals may help prevent hypoglycemia.

An important role of the endocrinologist in the management of reactive hypoglycemia is reassurance of the patient and of the referring physician that the condition does not represent a life-threatening insulinoma. Treatment consists of frequent small feedings and avoidance of simple sugars. Beta-blockers, anticholinergics, and intestinal alpha glucosidase inhibitors may also have a role. Patients should be educated about the symptoms of hypoglycemia and the appropriate corrective measures (including when to seek medical attention), and diabetic patients should be given a medical alert bracelet.

One approach for the differential diagnosis and management of hypoglycemia is provided in Fig. 29-1.

KEY POINTS TO REMEMBER

- Rule out artifact from collection, storage, or error in analytic methods.
- Confirm Whipple's triad for diagnosis.
- Normal patients can have low plasma glucose.
- The most common cause of hypoglycemia is drugs (especially insulin, sulfonylureas, and alcohol).
- Draw diagnostic labs during the episode of hypoglycemia, then immediately initiate treatment.
- The treatment of choice for insulinoma is surgical resection.
- OGTTs are not appropriate for diagnosis of reactive hypoglycemia.

REFERENCES AND SUGGESTED READINGS

Consoli A, Kennedy F, Miles J, et al. Determination of Krebs cycle metabolic carbon exchange in vivo and its use to estimate the individual contributions of gluconeogenesis and glycogenolysis to overall hepatic glucose output in man. *J Clin Invest* 1987;80:1303–1310.

Cryer PE. Glucose homeostasis and hypoglycemia. In: Larsen PR, et al., eds. *Williams textbook of endocrinology*, 10th ed. Philadelphia: WB Saunders, 2003:1604

Cryer PE, Davis SN, Shamoon H. Hypoglycemia in diabetes. *Diabetes Care* 2003;26 (6):1902–1912.

Daughday W. The pathophysiology of IGF-II hypersecretion in non-islet cell tumor hypoglycemia. *Diabetes Rev* 1995;3:62–72.

Field J, Williams H. Artifactual hypoglycemia associated with leukemia. *N Engl J Med* 1961;265:946–948.

Lecavalier L, Bolli G, Cryer P, et al. Contributions of gluconeogenesis and glycogenolysis during glucose counterregulation in normal humans. *Am J Physiol* 1989;256 (6 Pt 1):E844–E851.

Luyckx A, Lefebvre P. Plasma insulin in reactive hypoglycemia. *Diabetes* 1971;20:435–42.

Mitrakou A, Fanelli C, Veneman T, et al. Reversibility of unawareness of hypoglycemia in patients with insulinoma. *N Engl J Med* 1993;329:834–839.

Owen O, Morgan A, Kemp H, et al. Brain metabolism during fasting. *J Clin Invest* 1967;46:1589–1595.

Seltzer H. Drug-induced hypoglycemia: a review of 1418 cases. *Endocrinol Metab Clin North Am* 1989;18:163–183.

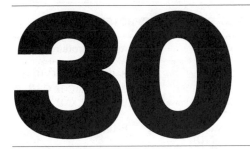

Diagnosis, Standards of Care, and Treatment for Hyperlipidemia

Michael Jakoby,
Kellie L. Flood, and
Katherine E. Henderson

INTRODUCTION

Lipids are sparingly soluble molecules that include cholesterol, fatty acids, and their derivatives. Plasma lipids are transported by lipoprotein particles composed of proteins called **apolipoproteins, phospholipids, cholesterol esters**, and **triglycerides**. Human plasma lipoproteins are separated into **5 major classes** based on hydration density: chylomicrons (least dense), very-low-density lipoproteins (VLDLs), intermediate-density lipoproteins (IDLs), low-density lipoproteins (LDLs), and high-density lipoproteins (HDLs). A sixth class, lipoprotein(a) [Lp(a)], resembles LDL in lipid composition and has a hydrated density that overlaps LDL and HDL. Physical properties of plasma lipoproteins are summarized in Table 30-1.

LIPOPROTEIN METABOLISM

Exogenous Pathway

Dietary long-chain fatty acids and cholesterol are esterified and assembled into chylomicrons as triglycerides and cholesterol-esters, respectively. Apo B-48 is the predominant chylomicron apolipoprotein, but apo C-II and apo E mediate particle clearance. After entering the venous circulation from the thoracic duct, triglycerides are hydrolyzed to non-esterified fatty acids by the activity of lipoprotein lipase (LPL), with apo C-II serving as an enzyme cofactor. Triglyceride-depleted particles are called **chylomicron remnants** and are cleared by the hepatic chylomicron remnant receptor in an interaction mediated by apo E.

Endogenous Pathway

Hepatic triglycerides and cholesterol-esters are assembled into VLDL particles and secreted into the circulation. Apo B-100 is the main VLDL apolipoprotein and is a high-affinity ligand for the apo B/E (LDL) receptor. Triglycerides are hydrolyzed through the activity of LPL and apo C-II to create a triglyceride-depleted IDL particle. IDL may be cleared from the circulation by either the LDL receptor or the remnant receptor. It also may be further depleted of triglyceride by hepatic lipase to create a cholesterol-rich LDL particle. Circulating LDL enters the liver and extra-hepatic tissues through interactions with the LDL receptor.

High-Density Lipoprotein Metabolism

Nascent HDL is secreted from the liver and small intestine as small apo A-I–containing discs. The discs acquire free cholesterol from peripheral tissues through the activity of the cholesterol efflux regulatory protein ABC1. The cholesterol is then esterified by the enzyme lecithin:cholesterol acyltransferase, with apo A-I serving as an enzyme cofactor. At this time, the particles are termed HDL_3. A larger HDL_2 particle is formed by acquisition of apolipoproteins and lipids released from delipidated chylomicrons and VLDL particles. HDL_2 is converted back to HDL_3 after removal of triglycerides by hepatic lipase or transfer of cholesterol esters to VLDL, IDL, or LDL particles. HDL

TABLE 30-1. PHYSICAL PROPERTIES OF PLASMA LIPOPROTEINS

Lipoprotein	Lipid composition[a]	Origin	Apolipoproteins
Chylomicrons	TG, 90%; chol, 3%	Intestine	B-48;C-I, C-II, C-III; E
VLDL	TG, 55%; chol, 20%	Liver	B-100; C-I, C-II, C-III; E
IDL	TG, 30%; chol, 35%	Metabolic product of VLDL	B-100; C-I, C-II, C-III; E
LDL	TG, 10%; chol, 50%	Metabolic product of IDL	B-100
HDL	TG, 5%; chol, 20%	Liver, intestine	A-I, A-II, A-IV; C-I, C-II, C-III; E
Lp(a)	TG, 10%; chol, 50%	Liver	B-100; Apo (a)

chol, cholesterol; HDL, high-density lipoprotein; IDL, intermediate-density lipoprotein; LDL, low-density lipoprotein; Lp(a), lipoprotein(a); TG, triglyceride; VLDL, very-low-density lipoprotein.
[a]Balance of particle composition: protein and phospholipid.

transports cholesterol from peripheral tissues to the liver (reverse cholesterol transport) through transfer to apo B-100–containing lipoproteins or through clearance by the putative HDL catabolic receptor.

ATHEROSCLEROSIS AND LIPOPROTEINS

Nearly 90% of patients with coronary heart disease (CHD) have some form of dyslipidemia. Increased levels of LDL, remnant lipoproteins, and Lp(a) as well as decreased levels of HDL have all been associated with an increased risk of premature vascular disease. Oxidized LDL in the subendothelium induces formation of atherosclerotic plaques by recruitment of macrophages and internalization by macrophages through activity of the CD-36 or "scavenger" receptor, leading to formation of "foam cells." Oxidized LDL also impairs normal vasomotor function. IDL appears to promote atherosclerosis through similar mechanisms. Lp(a) may promote vascular disease through internalization by macrophages and interference with normal fibrinolysis. Reverse cholesterol transport mediated by HDL appears to be anti-atherogenic by removal of cholesterol from atherosclerotic plaque and favorable effects on endothelial function, thrombosis, and red cell deformability.

CLINICAL DYSLIPOPROTEINEMIAS

Dyslipidemias may be classified according to their Fredrickson phenotype (Table 30-2). Most dyslipidemias are multifactorial in etiology and reflect the effects of uncharacterized genetic influences coupled with diet, activity, smoking, alcohol use, and comorbid conditions such as obesity and diabetes mellitus. Differential diagnosis of the major lipid abnormalities is summarized in Table 30-3. The major genetic dyslipoproteinemias are reviewed in the following sections.

Familial Hypercholesterolemia

Familial hypercholesterolemia (FH) is characterized by **increased total and LDL cholesterol** due to mutations of the LDL receptor that lead to defective uptake and degradation of LDL. FH is an autosomal-dominant disorder with a gene frequency of approximately 1:500. Plasma total cholesterol is typically >300 mg/dL, and LDL cholesterol is usually >250 mg/dL. Premature heart disease is common, with average age of onset of 45 years in men and 55 years in women. Most affected patients have **tendon xanthomas**. Other manifestations include xanthelasmata and premature arcus corneae. Homozygous FH is rare (approximately 1 per 1,000,000 of the

TABLE 30-2. FREDRICKSON CLASSIFICATION OF DYSLIPIDEMIAS

Phenotype	Lipoprotein abnormality	Lipid abnormality
I	Chylomicrons	Hypertriglyceridemia
IIa	LDL	Hypercholesterolemia
IIb	VLDL and LDL	Combined hyperlipidemia[a]
III	Chylomicron and VLDL remnants	Combined hyperlipidemia
IV	VLDL	Hypertriglyceridemia
V	Chylomicrons and VLDL	Hypertriglyceridemia

LDL, low-density lipoprotein; VLDL, very-low-density lipoprotein.
[a]Both hypercholesterolemia and hypertriglyceridemia.
Adapted from Fredrickson DS. *Ann Intern Med* 1971;75:471.

general population) and leads to severe hypercholesterolemia (total cholesterol >600 mg/dL; LDL cholesterol >550 mg/dL) and early coronary artery disease. Homozygous FH patients develop planar xanthomas at areas of skin trauma, such as elbows and knees.

Familial Combined Hyperlipidemia

Familial combined hyperlipidemia (FCH) is an autosomal dominant disorder of fairly high prevalence (0.5–2% of the general population). However, the genetic and metabolic defects of FCH remain to be established. Fredrickson type IIa, IIb, and IV lipoprotein patterns (see Table 30-2) may be observed, and the predominant lipoprotein abnormality may vary in a single person over time and among different members of an affected kindred. Patients do not develop tendon xanthomas. The major clinical manifestation is **premature vascular disease** similar in onset and severity to heterozygous FH. Lipoprotein abnormalities that characterize FCH include an abnormal cholesterol to apo B-100 ratio (>1.3) and an LDL apo B-100 level >130 mg/dL.

TABLE 30-3. DIFFERENTIAL DIAGNOSIS OF MAJOR LIPID ABNORMALITIES

Lipid abnormality	Primary disorders	Secondary disorders
Hypercholesterolemia	Polygenic, familial hypercholesterolemia, familial defective apo B-100	Hypothyroidism, nephrotic syndrome
Hypertriglyceridemia	Lipoprotein lipase deficiency, apo C-II deficiency, familial hypertriglyceridemia	Diabetes mellitus, obesity, metabolic syndrome, alcohol use, oral estrogen
Combined hyperlipidemia	Familial combined hyperlipidemia, type III hyperlipoproteinemia	Diabetes mellitus, obesity, metabolic syndrome, hypothyroidism, nephrotic syndrome
Low HDL	Familial alpha lipoproteinemia, Tangier disease, familial HDL deficiency, lecithin:cholesterol acyltransferase deficiency	Diabetes mellitus, metabolic syndrome, hypertriglyceridemia, smoking

HDL, high-density lipoprotein.

Familial Defective Apolipoprotein B-100

Familial defective apo B-100 is phenotypically similar to FH. It is caused by a mutation in apo B-100 and leads to decreased binding of mutant LDL to the LDL receptor and delayed LDL clearance. A glutamine for arginine mutation at amino acid 3500 of apo B-100 accounts for almost all cases and facilitates genetic testing to confirm the diagnosis. Gene frequency in caucasians with hypercholesterolemia is approximately 1:500–1:750.

Type III Hyperlipoproteinemia (Familial Dysbetalipoproteinemia)

Type III hyperlipoproteinemia typically occurs as an autosomal-recessive disorder in patients who are homozygous for the apo E2 isoform. Hyperlipidemia develops in adulthood and is characterized by **symmetric elevations of cholesterol and triglycerides** (300–500 mg/dL). Many apo E2 homozygotes are normolipidemic, and the emergence of hyperlipidemia often requires a secondary metabolic factor such as diabetes mellitus, hypothyroidism, or obesity. Impaired clearance leads to accumulation of cholesterol-rich remnants of chylomicrons, VLDL, and IDL. The remnant particles are called beta-VLDL and produce a characteristic peak on gel electrophoresis. Another diagnostic feature is an **elevated VLDL cholesterol to plasma triglyceride ratio** (>0.3). Premature vascular disease is common in affected individuals. Patients may develop tuberous or tuberoeruptive xanthomas. **Planar xanthomas of the palmar creases** are essentially pathognomonic for type III hyperlipoproteinemia.

Chylomicronemia Syndrome

Massive accumulation of triglyceride-rich plasma lipoproteins (chylomicrons and VLDL) is called chylomicronemia syndrome. Clinical manifestations occur when plasma triglycerides exceed 1500 mg/dL and include eruptive xanthomas, lipemia retinalis, pancreatitis, and hepatosplenomegaly. Age of onset suggests the genetic defect responsible for **hypertriglyceridemia**. Onset before puberty indicates type I hyperlipoproteinemia due to deficiency of lipoprotein lipase or apo C-II, both autosomal-recessive disorders. Severe hypertriglyceridemia developing in the fourth or fifth decades generally indicates type V hyperlipoproteinemia. These patients have no detectable abnormalities of lipoprotein lipase or apo C-II, and the causative genetic defect remains undetermined.

Most patients with hypertriglyceridemia have a milder type IV hyperlipoproteinemia phenotype, with plasma triglycerides in the range of 150–500 mg/dL. Familial hypertriglyceridemia is an autosomal-dominant disorder caused by hepatic overproduction of VLDL triglycerides that manifests as adult-onset hypertriglyceridemia. It can be diagnosed only if half of a patient's first-degree relatives are hypertriglyceridemic, and the condition may be difficult to distinguish from FCH. Familial hypertriglyceridemia and FCH patients may develop chylomicronemia syndrome in the presence of secondary factors such as obesity, alcohol use, or diabetes mellitus.

Familial Hypoalphalipoproteinemia

Familial hypoalphalipoproteinemia is an autosomal-dominant disorder that occurs with a gene frequency of approximately 1:400. The risk of premature cardiovascular disease is significantly increased, and family history is usually notable for early heart disease. There are no characteristic findings on physical exam. The diagnosis is suggested by **HDL cholesterol levels below the 10th percentile** (<30 mg/dL for men, <40 mg/dL for premenopausal women). The causative genetic defect is unknown but has been linked to a locus on chromosome 11 that contains the genes for apo A-I, apo C-II, and apo A-IV in a tandem array.

STANDARDS OF CARE FOR HYPERLIPIDEMIA

Animal models, epidemiologic studies, and genetic causes of hypercholesterolemia establish a strong causal relationship between increasing total and LDL cholesterol

TABLE 30-4. MAJOR RISK FACTORS [EXCLUSIVE OF LOW-DENSITY LIPOPROTEIN (LDL) CHOLESTEROL] THAT MODIFY LDL GOALS[a]

Cigarette smoking

Hypertension (blood pressure ≥140/90 mm Hg or on antihypertensive medication)

Low high-density lipoprotein (HDL) cholesterol (<40 mg/dL)[b]

Family history of premature coronary heart disease (CHD) (CHD in male first-degree relative < age 55 yrs; CHD in female first-degree relative < age 65 yrs);

Age (men ≥ 45 yrs; women ≥ 55 yrs)

---

[a]In Adult Treatment Panel III, diabetes is regarded as a CHD risk equivalent.
[b]HDL cholesterol ≥ 60 mg/dL counts as a "negative" risk factor; its presence removes one risk factor from the total count.
From Executive summary of the third report of the National Cholesterol Education Program (NCEP) expert panel on detection, evaluation, and treatment of high blood cholesterol in adults (Adult Treatment Panel III). *JAMA* 2001;285;2486, with permission.

levels and risk of CHD. LDL cholesterol–lowering therapy, particularly with hydroxymethylglutaryl-coenzyme A (HMG-CoA) reductase inhibitors, lowers the risk of CHD-related death, morbidity, and revascularization procedures in hypercholesterolemic patients with (secondary prevention) or without (primary prevention) known CHD. Therefore, identification and management of high LDL cholesterol is the primary goal of the National Cholesterol Education Program's third expert report on cholesterol management in adults, or Adult Treatment Program III (ATP III). The ATP III executive summary and full report can be viewed online at http://www.nhlbi.nih.gov/guidelines/cholesterol/.

Screening

Screening for hypercholesterolemia should begin **in all adults age 20 years or older**. Screening is best performed with a lipid profile (total cholesterol, LDL cholesterol, HDL cholesterol, and triglycerides) obtained after a 12-hour fast. If a fasting lipid panel cannot be obtained, total and HDL cholesterol should be measured. Measurement of fasting lipids is indicated if the total cholesterol is ≥200 mg/dL or HDL cholesterol is ≤ 40 mg/dL. If lipids are unremarkable and the patient has no major risk factors for CHD (Table 30-4), then screening can be performed every 5 years. Patients hospitalized for an acute coronary syndrome or coronary revascularization should have a lipid panel obtained within 24 hours of admission if lipid levels are unknown. Individuals with hyperlipidemia should be evaluated for potential **secondary causes**, including hypothyroidism, diabetes mellitus, obstructive liver disease, chronic renal insufficiency or nephrotic syndrome, or medications such as estrogens, progestins, anabolic steroids, and corticosteroids.

Risk Assessment

A major innovation of ATP III is a formal method of CHD risk assessment. ATP III now recognizes **five categories of CHD risk**—very high, high, moderately high, moderate, and lower risk. These CHD risk categories are defined in Table 30-5. Diabetes, noncoronary atherosclerosis (symptomatic cerebrovascular disease, peripheral artery disease, abdominal aortic aneurysm), or multiple risk factors conferring a 10-year CHD risk of more than 20% are considered CHD risk equivalents in ATP III. Risk assessment for patients without known CHD or CHD risk equivalents begins with consideration of five risk factors summarized in Table 30-4. A Framingham point score should be determined for any individual with two or more non-LDL cholesterol risk factors. (Framingham point score algorithms for men and women are summarized in Table 30-6.) Patients with multiple non-LDL cholesterol CHD risk factors are then divided into those with a 10-year CHD risk >20%, 10–20%, or <10%. Presently, emerging risk fac-

TABLE 30-5. ADULT TREATMENT PROGRAM III (ATP III) CATEGORIES OF CORONARY HEART DISEASE (CHD) RISK

Category	Definition
Very high risk	CHD and:
	Multiple risk factors (especially diabetes)
	Severe and poorly controlled risk factors (especially continued cigarette smoking)
	Multiple risk factors of the metabolic syndrome
	Acute coronary syndromes
High risk	CHD or CHD risk equivalent
Moderately high risk	2+ risk factors and 10-yr CHD risk 10–20%
Moderate risk	2+ risk factors and 10-yr CHD risk <10%
Lower risk	0–1 risk factors

Adapted from Grundy SM, Cleeman C, Merz NB, et al. Implications of recent clinical trials for the National Cholesterol Education Program Adult Treatment Panel III Guidelines. *Circulation* 2004;110:227.

tors (obesity; sedentary lifestyle; homocysteine, prothrombotic, and proinflammatory factors; and impaired fasting glucose) do not impact risk assessment, although they may influence clinical judgment when determining therapeutic options.

Therapy for Hypercholesterolemia

ATP III thresholds for initiating cholesterol-lowering therapy with **therapeutic lifestyle change** (TLC; diet and exercise) and **hypolipidemic drugs** are summarized in Table 30-7. All patients requiring cholesterol treatment should implement a diet restricted in total and saturated fat intake in accordance with ATP III recommendations (Table 30-8). Moderate exercise and weight reduction is also recommended. A registered dietitian may be helpful to plan and start a fat-restricted and weight loss promoting diet.

The ATP III LDL cholesterol treatment target for all high-risk patients is <100 mg/dL. For CHD patients in the **very-high-risk category**, an LDL cholesterol <70 mg/dL is a therapeutic option as confirmed by the Pravastatin or Atorvastatin Evaluation and Infection–Thrombolysis in Myocardial Infarction 22 (PROVE-IT) trial. An LDL cholesterol of ≥ 100 mg/dL is now identified as the threshold for simultaneous treatment with TLC and lipid-lowering agents. Based on outcomes in the Heart Protection Study (HPS), lipid-lowering drug therapy is also an option for patients with CHD and baseline LDL cholesterol <100 mg/dL. If a high-risk patient has hypertriglyceridemia or low HDL cholesterol, a fibrate or nicotinic acid (niacin) may be added to cholesterol-lowering therapy.

Patients with two or more non-LDL cholesterol risk factors and a Framingham point score predicting a 10-year CHD risk of 10–20% are considered at **moderately high risk** of CHD. Pharmacotherapy should be initiated if LDL cholesterol is ≥ 130 mg/dL. Results of the Anglo-Scandinavian Cardiac Outcomes Trial–Lipid-Lowering Arm (ASCOT-LLA) demonstrated primary CHD prevention for patients in this category treated with atorvastatin to an LDL cholesterol <100 mg/dL. ATP III identifies an LDL cholesterol target <100 mg/dL as optional for this group, with drug therapy to be considered for patients with baseline LDL cholesterol 100–129 mg/dL. Patients with two or more risk factors and a 10-year risk <10% are candidates for drug therapy when LDL cholesterol remains ≥ 160 mg/dL despite TLC.

For **low-risk patients** (0–1 risk factors), cholesterol-lowering therapy should be considered if the LDL cholesterol is ≥190 mg/dL, especially for patients who have undergone a 3-month trial of TLC. Patients with very high LDL concentrations (≥190 mg/dL) often have a hereditary dyslipidemia and require treatment with multiple lipid-lowering agents. These patients should be referred to a lipid special-

TABLE 30-6. ESTIMATE OF 10-YR RISK (FRAMINGHAM POINT SCORES) FOR MEN AND WOMEN

Estimate of 10-yr risk for men	
Age (yrs)	Points
20–34	–9
35–39	–4
40–44	0
45–49	3
50–54	6
55–59	8
60–64	10
65–69	11
70–74	12
75–79	13

Total cholesterol	Points				
	Age 20–39	Age 40–49	Age 50–59	Age 60–69	Age 70–79
<160	0	0	0	0	0
160–199	4	3	2	1	0
200–239	7	5	3	1	0
240–279	9	6	4	2	1
≥280	11	8	5	3	1

	Points				
	Age 20–39	Age 40–49	Age 50–59	Age 60–69	Age 70–79
Nonsmoker	0	0	0	0	0
Smoker	8	5	3	1	1

HDL (mg/dL)	Points	Systolic BP (mm Hg)	If untreated	If treated
≥ 60	–1	<120	0	0
50–59	0	120–129	0	1
40–49	1	130–139	1	2
<40	2	140–159	1	2
		≥160	2	3

Point total	10-yr risk (%)	Point total	10-yr risk (%)
<0	<1	9	5
0	1	10	6
1	1	11	8
2	1	12	10
3	1	13	12
4	1	14	16
5	2	15	20
6	2	16	25
7	3	≥17	≥30
8	4		

(continued)

TABLE 30-6. (*continued*)

Estimate of 10-yr risk in women	
Age (yrs)	Points
20–34	–7
35–39	–3
40–44	0
45–49	3
50–54	6
55–59	8
60–64	10
65–69	12
70–74	14
75–79	16

Total cholesterol	Points				
	Age 20–39	Age 40–49	Age 50–59	Age 60–69	Age 70–79
<160	0	0	0	0	0
160–199	4	3	2	1	1
200–239	8	6	4	2	1
240–279	11	8	5	3	2
≥280	13	10	7	4	2

	Points				
	Age 20–39	Age 40–49	Age 50–59	Age 60–69	Age 70–79
Nonsmoker	0	0	0	0	0
Smoker	9	7	4	2	1

HDL (mg/dL)	Points	Systolic BP (mm Hg)	If untreated	If treated
≥60	–1	<120	0	0
50–59	0	120–129	1	3
40–49	1	130–139	2	4
<40	2	140–159	3	5
		≥160	4	6

Point total	10-yr risk (%)	Point total	10-yr risk (%)
<9	<1	17	5
9	1	18	6
10	1	19	8
11	1	20	11
12	1	21	14
13	2	22	17
		23	22
14	2	24	27
15	3	≥25	≥30
16	4		

BP, blood pressure; HDL, high-density lipoprotein.
From Executive summary of the third report of the National Cholesterol Education Program (NCEP) expert panel on detection, evaluation, and treatment of high blood cholesterol in adults (Adult Treatment Panel III). *JAMA* 2001;285:2486, with permission.

TABLE 30-7. ADULT TREATMENT PROGRAM III (ATP III) LOW-DENSITY LIPOPROTEIN CHOLESTEROL (LDL-C) GOALS AND THRESHOLDS FOR THERAPEUTIC LIFESTYLE CHANGES (TLC) AND DRUG THERAPY

Category	LDL-C goal	Start TLC	Start drug therapy
Very high risk	<70 mg/dL	Any LDL-C	LDL-C ≥70 mg/dL
High risk	<100 mg/dL	≥100 mg/dL	≥100 mg/dL (consider if baseline LDL-C <100 mg/dL)
Moderately high risk	<130 mg/dL (<100 mg/dL optional)	≥130 mg/dL	≥130 mg/dL (optional if baseline LDL-C 100–129 mg/dL)
Moderate risk	<130 mg/dL	≥130 mg/dL	≥160 mg/dL
Lower risk	<160 mg/dL	≥160 mg/dL	≥190 mg/dL (optional if baseline LDL-C 160–189 mg/dL)

Adapted from Grundy SM, Cleeman C, Merz NB, et al. Implications of recent clinical trials for the National Cholesterol Education Program Adult Treatment Panel III Guidelines. *Circulation* 2004;110:227.

ist, and family members should be screened with a fasting lipid battery. When LDL cholesterol is 160–189 mg/dL, drug therapy should be considered if the patient has a significant risk factor for cardiovascular disease, such as heavy tobacco use, poorly controlled hypertension, strong family history of early CHD, or low HDL cholesterol.

Response to therapy should be assessed after 6 weeks and the dose of medication titrated if the LDL cholesterol treatment target is not achieved. The initial dose of a cholesterol-lowering drug should be sufficient to achieve a 30–40% reduction in LDL

TABLE 30-8. NUTRIENT COMPOSITION OF THE THERAPEUTIC LIFESTYLE CHANGE (TLC) DIET

Nutrient	Recommended intake
Saturated fat[a]	<7% of total calories
Polyunsaturated fat	Up to 10% of total calories
Monounsaturated fat	Up to 20% of total calories
Total fat	25–35% of total calories
Carbohydrate[b]	50–60% of total calories
Fiber	20–30 g/day
Protein	Approximately 15% of total calories
Cholesterol	<200 mg/day
Total calories (energy)[c]	Balance energy intake and expenditure to maintain desirable body weight/prevent weight gain

[a]Trans fatty acids are another low-density lipoprotein (LDL)–raising fat that should be kept at a low intake.
[b]Carbohydrate should be derived predominantly from foods rich in complex carbohydrates, including grains (especially whole grains), fruits, and vegetables.
[c]Daily energy expenditure should include at least moderate physical activity (contributing approximately 200 Kcal/day).
From Executive summary of the third report of the National Cholesterol Education Program (NCEP) expert panel on detection, evaluation, and treatment of high blood cholesterol in adults (Adult Treatment Panel III). *JAMA* 2001;285:2486, with permission.

cholesterol. If target LDL cholesterol has not been reached after 12 weeks, current therapy should be intensified by further dose titration, adding another lipid-lowering agent, or referral to a lipid specialist. Patients at goal should be monitored every 4–6 months.

Metabolic Syndrome

The constellation of abdominal obesity, hypertension, glucose intolerance, and an atherogenic lipid profile (hypertriglyceridemia; low HDL cholesterol; and small, dense LDL cholesterol) characterizes a condition called the **metabolic syndrome**. ATP III and World Health Organization diagnostic criteria for the metabolic syndrome are summarized in Table 30-9. Approximately 22% of Americans qualify for a diagnosis of the metabolic syndrome by ATP III criteria. Prevalence is increased in older individuals, women, Hispanic Americans, and African Americans. Two large epidemiologic studies have demonstrated elevated all-cause and coronary mortality among men with the metabolic syndrome.

ATP III recognizes the metabolic syndrome as a **secondary treatment target** after LDL cholesterol is controlled. The report recommends treating the underlying causes of metabolic syndrome (overweight/obesity, physical inactivity) by implementing weight loss and aerobic exercise and managing cardiovascular risks, such as hypertension, that may persist despite lifestyle changes. A post-hoc analysis of the Scandinavian Simvastatin Survival Study (4S) showed that patients with high LDL cholesterol, low HDL cholesterol, and high triglycerides benefited more from simvastatin therapy than patients with isolated high LDL cholesterol.

Hypertriglyceridemia

Recent analyses suggest that hypertriglyceridemia is an **independent cardiovascular risk factor**. Hypertriglyceridemia is often observed in the metabolic syndrome, and there are many potential etiologies for hypertriglyceridemia, including obesity, diabetes mellitus, renal insufficiency, genetic dyslipidemias, and therapy with oral

TABLE 30-9. COMPARISON OF ADULT TREATMENT PROGRAM III (ATP III) AND WORLD HEALTH ORGANIZATION (WHO) DIAGNOSTIC CRITERIA FOR THE METABOLIC SYNDROME

	ATP III[a]	WHO[b]
Carbohydrate metabolism	Fasting glucose ≥110 mg/dL	Fasting glucose >110 mg/dL, or fasting insulin in the upper quartile of the nondiabetic population
Abdominal obesity	Men, waist >40 in.; women, waist >35 in.	Waist/hip ratio >0.9, BMI >30 kg/m², or waist ≥37 in.
Dyslipidemia	Triglycerides ≥150 mg/dL; men, HDL cholesterol <40 mg/dL; women, HDL cholesterol <50 mg/dL	Triglycerides ≥150 mg/dL or HDL cholesterol <35 mg/dL
Hypertension	BP ≥130/85 mm Hg	BP ≥140/90 mm Hg, or BP-lowering medication

BMI, body mass index; BP, blood pressure; HDL, high-density lipoprotein.
[a]To qualify for the diagnosis of metabolic syndrome by ATP III criteria, a patient must meet at least 3 of the 5 criteria (hyperglycemia, abdominal obesity, high triglycerides, low HDL cholesterol, high blood pressure).
[b]To qualify for the diagnosis of metabolic syndrome by WHO criteria, a patient must have an abnormality of carbohydrate metabolism and abnormalities in 2 of the other 3 categories (abdominal obesity, dyslipidemia, hypertension).

TABLE 30-10. COMPARISON OF LOW-DENSITY LIPOPROTEIN CHOLESTEROL (LDL-C) AND NON–HIGH-DENSITY LIPOPROTEIN CHOLESTEROL (HDL-C) GOALS BY CORONARY HEART DISEASE (CHD) RISK CATEGORY

Category	LDL-C target (mg/dL)	Non–HDL-C target (mg/dL)
Very high risk	<70	<100
High risk	<100	<130
Moderately high risk	<130	<160
Moderate risk	<130	<160
Low risk	<160	<190

Adapted from Grundy SM, Cleeman C, Merz NB, et al. Implications of recent clinical trials for the National Cholesterol Education Program Adult Treatment Panel III Guidelines. *Circulation* 2004;110:227.

estrogen, glucocorticoids, or beta-blockers. The ATP III classification of serum triglyceride levels is as follows:

- Normal: <150 mg/dL
- Borderline-high: 150–199 mg/dL
- High: 200–499 mg/dL
- Very high: ≥500 mg/dL

Treatment of hypertriglyceridemia depends on the degree of severity. For patients with very high triglycerides, triglyceride reduction through a very low fat diet (≤15% of calories), exercise, weight loss, and drugs (fibrates, niacin) is the primary goal of therapy to prevent acute pancreatitis. When patients have a lesser degree of hypertriglyceridemia, control of LDL cholesterol is the primary aim of initial therapy. TLC is emphasized as the initial intervention to lower triglycerides. Non-HDL cholesterol, a measure of VLDL remnant particle (IDL) cholesterol, is a secondary treatment target. A patient's non-HDL cholesterol is calculated by subtracting HDL cholesterol from total cholesterol. Target non-HDL cholesterol is 30 mg/dL higher than the LDL cholesterol target. LDL and non-HDL cholesterol treatment targets for various degrees of cardiovascular risk are summarized in Table 30-10.

Low High-Density Lipoprotein Cholesterol

One of the modifications from ATP II includes redefining low HDL cholesterol as <40 mg/dL. Low HDL cholesterol is an **independent CHD risk factor** that is identified as a non-LDL cholesterol risk and included as a component of the Framingham scoring algorithm. Etiologies for low HDL cholesterol include physical inactivity, obesity, insulin resistance, diabetes mellitus, hypertriglyceridemia, cigarette smoking, high (>60% calories) carbohydrate diets, and certain medications (beta-blockers, anabolic steroids, progestins). Because therapeutic interventions for low HDL cholesterol are of limited efficacy, ATP III identifies LDL cholesterol as the primary target of therapy for patients with low HDL cholesterol. Low HDL cholesterol often occurs in the setting of hypertriglyceridemia and metabolic syndrome. Management of these conditions may result in a secondary improvement of HDL cholesterol. Aerobic exercise, weight loss, smoking cessation, moderate alcohol consumption, menopausal estrogen replacement, and treatment with niacin or fibrates may elevate low HDL cholesterol.

Lipid-Lowering Therapy and Age

The risk of a fatal or nonfatal cardiovascular event increases with age, and most cardiovascular events occur in patients age 65 years and older. Secondary prevention trials with the HMG CoA reductase inhibitors have demonstrated significant clinical benefit for patients age 65–75 years. The HPS failed to show an age threshold for primary or secondary prevention with simvastatin. Patients age 75–80 years at study entry experienced a nearly 30% reduction in major vascular events. The Prospective Study of Pravastatin in the Elderly (PROSPER) trial found a significant reduction in major coronary events among patients age 70–82 years with vascular disease or CHD risks treated with pravastatin. **ATP III does not place age restrictions** on treatment of hypercholesterolemia in elderly adults.

ATP III recommends TLC for young adults (men age 20–35 years; women age 20–45 years) with an LDL level ≥130 mg/dL. Drug therapy should be considered in the following high-risk groups: (a) men who both smoke and have elevated LDL levels (160–189 mg/dL), (b) all young adults with an LDL ≥190 mg/dL, and (c) those with an inherited dyslipidemia.

TREATMENT OF ELEVATED LOW-DENSITY LIPOPROTEIN CHOLESTEROL

Hydroxymethylglutaryl-Coenzyme A Reductase Inhibitors (Statins)

Statins are the treatment of choice for elevated LDL cholesterol. Available statins are summarized in Table 30-11.

The lipid-lowering effect of statins appears within the first week of use and becomes stable after approximately 4 weeks of use. Common side effects (5–10% of patients) include GI upset (abdominal pain, diarrhea, bloating, constipation), and muscle pain or weakness (which can occur without creatinine kinase elevations). Other potential side effects include malaise, fatigue, headache, and rash.

Elevations of liver transaminases 2–3 times the upper limit of normal are dose dependent and reversible with discontinuation of the drug. Liver enzymes should be measured before initiating therapy, at 8–12 weeks after dose initiation or titration, then every 6 months. The medication should be discontinued if liver transaminases elevate to >3 times the upper limit of normal.

Because some of the statins undergo metabolism by the cytochrome P450 enzyme system, taking them in combination with other drugs metabolized by this enzyme system increases the risk of **rhabdomyolysis**. Among these drugs are: fibrates, itraconazole (Sporanox), ketoconazole (Nizoral), erythromycin, clarithromycin (Biaxin), cyclosporin (Gengraf), nefazodone (Serzone), and protease inhibitors. Statins may also interact with large quantities of grapefruit juice to increase the risk of myopathy, although the precise mechanism of this interaction is unclear. Simvastatin (Zocor) can increase levels of warfarin (Coumadin) and digoxin. Rosuvastatin (Crestor) may also increase warfarin levels.

Bile Acid Sequestrant Resins

Currently available bile acid sequestrant resins include

- Cholestyramine (Questran): 4–24 g PO/day in divided doses before meals
- Colestipol (Colestid): tablets, 2–16 g PO/day; granules, 5–30 g PO/day in divided doses before meals
- Colesevelam (Welchol): 625-mg tablets; 3 tablets PO bid or 6 tablets PO daily with food (maximum, 7 tablets PO/day)

Bile acid sequestrants typically lower LDL levels by 15–30%. These agents should not be used as monotherapy in patients with triglyceride levels >250 mg/dL because they can raise triglyceride levels. They may be combined with nicotinic acid or statins.

Common side effects of resins include constipation, abdominal pain, bloating, nausea, and flatulence. Bile acid sequestrants may decrease oral absorption of many other drugs, including warfarin, digoxin, thyroid hormone, thiazide diuretics, amiodarone, glipizide (Glucotrol), and statins. Colesevelam interacts with fewer drugs

TABLE 30-11. CURRENTLY AVAILABLE STATINS

Name	Atorvastatin (Lipitor)	Fluvastatin (Lescol)	Lovastatin (Mevacor)	Pravastatin (Pravachol)	Rosuvastatin (Crestor)	Simvastatin (Zocor)
Dose range (mg PO/day)	10–80	20–80	10–80	10–80	5–40	10–80
Triglyceride effect (%)	13–32 ↓	5–35 ↓	2–13 ↓	3–15 ↓	10–35 ↓	12–36 ↓
LDL effect (%)	38–54 ↓	17–36 ↓	29–48 ↓	19–34 ↓	41–65 ↓	28–46 ↓
HDL effect (%)	4.8–5.5 ↑	0.9–12 ↑	4.6–8 ↑	3–9.9 ↑	10–14 ↑	5.2–10 ↑

HDL, high-density lipoprotein; LDL, low-density lipoprotein; ↑, increased; ↓, decreased.

than the older resins. Other medications should be given 1 hour before or 4 hours after resins.

Nicotinic Acid (Niacin)

Niacin can lower LDL levels by ≥15%, lower triglyceride levels 20–50%, and raise HDL levels by up to 35%. Crystalline niacin is given 1–3 g PO/day in 2–3 divided doses with meals. Extended-release niacin (Niaspan) is dosed at night. The starting dose is 500 mg PO, and the dose may be titrated monthly in 500-mg increments to a maximum of 2000 mg PO (administer dose with milk or crackers).

Common side effects of niacin include flushing, pruritus, headache, nausea, and bloating. Other potential side effects include elevation of liver transaminases, hyperuricemia, and hyperglycemia. Flushing may be decreased with use of aspirin 30 minutes before the first few doses. Hepatoxicity associated with niacin is partially dose dependent and appears to be more prevalent with over-the-counter time-release preparations.

Avoid use of niacin in patients with gout, liver disease, active peptic ulcer disease, and uncontrolled diabetes mellitus. Niacin can be used with care in patients with well-controlled diabetes (Hgb A1C ≤ 7%). Serum transaminases, glucose, and uric acid levels should be monitored every 6–8 weeks during dose titration, then every 4 months.

Cholesterol Absorption Inhibitors

Ezetimibe (Zetia) is currently the only available agent in this category. Ezetimibe appears to act at the brush border of the small intestine and inhibits cholesterol absorption. The recommended dosing is 10 mg PO once daily. No dosage adjustment is required for renal insufficiency, mild hepatic impairment, or in elderly patients. Ezetimibe may provide an additional 25% mean reduction in LDL when combined with a statin and provides an approximately 18% decrease in LDL when used as monotherapy. It is not recommended for use in patients with moderate to severe hepatic impairment. Coadministration with fibrates is not recommended because the safety and effectiveness of this combination has not been established.

There appear to be few side effects associated with ezetimibe. In clinical trials, there was no excess of rhabdomyolysis or myopathy when compared with statin or placebo alone. There is a low incidence of diarrhea and abdominal pain compared to placebo. Liver function monitoring is not required with monotherapy because there appears to be no significant impact on liver enzymes when this drug is used alone. Liver enzymes should be monitored when used in conjunction with a statin, as there appears to be a slight increased incidence of enzyme elevations with combination therapy.

TREATMENT OF HYPERTRIGLYCERIDEMIA

Nonpharmacologic Treatment

Nonpharmacologic treatments are important in the therapy of hypertriglyceridemia. Nonpharmacologic approaches include

- Changing oral estrogen replacement to transdermal estrogen
- Decreasing alcohol intake
- Encouraging weight loss and exercise
- Controlling hyperglycemia in patients with diabetes mellitus
- Avoiding simple sugars and very high carbohydrate diets

Pharmacologic Treatment

Pharmacologic treatment of isolated hypertriglyceridemia consists of a fibric acid derivative or niacin. Statins may be effective for patients with mild to moderate hypertriglyceridemia and concomitant LDL elevation. [See the sections Nicotinic Acid (Niacin) and Hydroxymethylglutaryl-Coenzyme A Reductase Inhibitors (Statins) for dosing details.]

Currently available fibric acid derivatives include

- Gemfibrozil (Lopid): 600 mg PO bid before meals
- Fenofibrate (Tricor): 54–160 mg PO/day

Fibrates generally lower triglyceride levels 30–50% and increase HDL levels 10–35%. They can lower LDL levels by 5–25% in patients with normal triglyceride levels, but may actually increase LDL levels in patients with elevated triglyceride levels. Common side effects include dyspepsia, abdominal pain, cholelithiasis, rash, and pruritus. Fibrates may potentiate the effects of warfarin. Fibrates (particularly gemfibrozil) given in conjunction with statins may increase the risk of rhabdomyolysis.

TREATMENT OF LOW HIGH-DENSITY LIPOPROTEIN CHOLESTEROL

Nonpharmacologic therapies are the mainstay of treatment, including smoking cessation, exercise, and weight loss. In addition, medications known to lower HDL levels should be avoided such as beta-blockers, progestins, and androgenic compounds. Niacin is the most effective pharmacologic agent for increasing HDL levels. [See the section Nicotinic Acid (Niacin) for dosing details.]

KEY POINTS TO REMEMBER

- Lowering total and LDL cholesterol reduces the risk of coronary death, myocardial infarction, stroke, and the need for coronary revascularization.
- All adults should be screened for hyperlipidemia and treated based on risk assessment. All high-risk patients should be treated to an LDL cholesterol <100 mg/dL, and very-high-risk patients should be treated to an LDL cholesterol <70 mg/dL.
- All patients with elevated lipids should implement TLC.
- Statins are the treatment of choice for lowering LDL cholesterol. Other options for patients who cannot tolerate a statin include bile acid sequestrant resins, nicotinic acid, and ezetimibe.
- The response to therapy should be assessed every 6 weeks until the target LDL level is achieved.
- Nonpharmacologic treatments (e.g., diet and exercise) are very important in the therapy of hypertriglyceridemia.

SUGGESTED READING

Cannon CP, Braunwald E, McCabe CH, et al. for the Pravastatin or Atorvastatin Evaluation and Infection Therapy-Thrombolysis in Myocardial Infarction 22 (PROVE IT-TIMI22) Investigators. Intensive versus moderate lipid lowering with statins after acute coronary syndromes. *N Engl J Med* 2004;350:1495.

Downs JR, Clearfield M, Weis S, et al. for the AFCAPS/TexCAPS Research Group. Primary prevention of acute coronary events with lovastatin in men and women with average cholesterol levels: results of AFCAPS/TexCAPS. *JAMA* 1998;279(20):1615.

Executive summary of the third report of the National Cholesterol Education Program (NCEP) expert panel on detection, evaluation, and treatment of high blood cholesterol in adults (Adult Treatment Panel III). *JAMA* 2001;285:2486.

Grundy SM, Cleeman JI, Merz NB, et al. Implications of recent clinical trials for the National Cholesterol Education Program Adult Treatment Program III Guidelines. *Circulation* 2004;110:227.

The Long-Term Intervention with pravastatin In Ischemic Disease (LIPID) study group. Prevention of cardiovascular events and death with pravastatin in patients with coronary heart disease and a broad range of initial cholesterol levels. *N Engl J Med* 1998;339:1349.

MRC/BHF Heart Protection Study of cholesterol lowering with simvastatin in 20,536 high-risk individuals: a randomized placebo-controlled trial. *Lancet* 2002;360:7–22.

Scandinavian Simvastatin Survival Study Group. Scandinavian Simvastatin survival study. *Lancet* 1994;344:1383.

Sever PS, Dahlof B, Poulter NR, et al. Prevention of coronary and stroke events with atorvastatin in hypertensive patients who have average or lower-than-average cholesterol concentrations in the Anglo-Scandinavian Cardiac Outcomes Trial–Lipid Lowering Arm (ASCOT-LLA). *Lancet* 2003;361:1149.

Shepherd J, Blauw GJ, Murphy MB, et al. Pravastatin in elderly individuals at risk of vascular disease (PROSPER): a randomized controlled trial. PROspective Study of Pravastatin in the Elderly at Risk. *Lancet* 2002;360:1623.

Third Report of the Expert Panel on detection, evaluation, and treatment of high blood cholesterol in adults (Adult Treatment Panel III). http://www.nhlbi.nih.gov/guidelines/cholesterol/index.htm.

REFERENCES

Alberti KG, Zimmet PZ. Definition, diagnosis, and classification of diabetes mellitus and its complications. Part 1: diagnosis and classification of diabetes mellitus provisional report of a WHO consultation. *Diabet Med* 1998;15:539.

Anderson TJ, Meredith IT, Charbonneau F, et al. Endothelium-dependent coronary vasomotion relates to the susceptibility of LDL to oxidation in humans. *J Clin Invest* 1996;93:1647.

Ballantyne CM, Olsson AG, Cook TJ, et al. Influence of low high-density lipoprotein cholesterol and elevated triglycerides on coronary heart disease and response to simvastatin therapy in 4S. *Circulation* 2001;104:3046.

Castelli WP, Garrison RJ, Wilson PW, et al. Incidence of coronary heart disease and lipoprotein cholesterol levels: the Framingham Study. *JAMA* 1986;256:2835.

Chong PH. Lack of therapeutic interchangeability of HMG-CoA reductase inhibitors. *Ann Pharmacother* 2002;36:1907–1917.

Feussner G, Wagner A, Kohl B, et al. Clinical features of type III hyperlipoproteinemia: analysis of 64 patients. *Clin Invest* 1993;71:362.

Ford ES, Giles WH, Dietz WH. Prevalence of metabolic syndrome among US adults: findings from the Third National Health and Nutrition Examination Survey. *JAMA* 2002;287:356.

Genest JJ, Martin-Munley SS, McNamara JR, et al. Familial lipoprotein disorders in patients with premature coronary artery disease. *J Am Coll Cardiol* 1992;19:792.

Grundy SM, Chait A, Brunzell JD. Familial combined hyperlipidemia workshop. *Arteriosclerosis* 1987;7:203.

Innerarity TL, Mahley RW, Weisgraber KH, et al. Familial defective apolipoprotein B-100: a mutation of apolipoprotein B that causes hypercholesterolemia. *J Lipid Res* 1990;31:1337.

Knopp RH. Drug treatment of lipid disorders. *N Engl J Med* 1999;341:498.

Krauss RM, Lingren RT, Williams PT, et al. Intermediate-density lipoproteins and progression of coronary artery disease in hypercholesterolemic men. *Lancet* 1987;2(8550):62.

Kugiyama K, Doi H, Motoyama T, et al. Association of remnant lipoprotein levels with impairment of endothelium-dependent vasomotor function in human coronary arteries. *Circulation* 1998;97:2519.

Lakka HM, Laaksonen DE, Lakka TA, et al. The metabolic syndrome and total and cardiovascular disease mortality in middle aged men. *JAMA* 2002;288:2709.

Loscalzo J, Weinfeld M, Fless GM, et al. Lipoprotein(a), fibrin binding, and plasminogen activation. *Arteriosclerosis* 1990;10:240.

Nissen SE, Tsunoda T, Tuzcu EM, et al. Effect of recombinant ApoA-I Milano on coronary atherosclerosis in patients with acute coronary syndromes: a randomized controlled trial. *JAMA* 2003;290:2292.

Package insert. Crestor (Rosuvastatin). Wilmington, DE: AstraZenica Pharmaceuticals; August 2003.

Package insert. Lescol (Fluvastatin sodium). East Hanover, NJ: Novartis Pharmaceuticals Corporation; May 2003.

Package insert. Lipitor (atorvastatin calcium tablets). Morris Plains, NJ: Parke-Davis Pharmaceutical Research; November 2002.

Package insert. Mevacor (Lovastatin). West Point, PA: Merck and Co, Inc.; June 2002.

Package insert. Pravachol (pravastatin sodium). Princeton, NJ: Bristol-Myers Squibb Company; March 2003.

Package insert. Zetia (Ezetimibe). North Wales, NJ: Merck/Schering-Plough Pharmaceuticals; March 2003.

Package insert. Zocor (Simvastatin). West Point, PA: Merck and Co, Inc.; April 2003.

Podrez EA, Febbraio M, Sheibani N, et al. Macrophage scavenger receptor CD 36 is the major receptor for LDL modified by monocyte-generated reactive nitrogen species. *J Clin Invest* 2000;105:1095.

Sachs FM, Pfeffer MA, Moye LA, et al. The effect of pravastatin on coronary events after myocardial infarction in patients with average cholesterol levels. *N Engl J Med* 1996;335:1001.

Sattar N, Faw A, Scherbakova O, et al. Metabolic syndrome with and without C-reactive protein as a predictor of coronary heart disease and diabetes in the West of Scotland Coronary Prevention Study. *Circulation* 2003;108:414.

Shepherd J, Cobbe SM, Ford I, et al. Prevention of coronary heart disease with pravastatin in men with hypercholesterolemia. *N Engl J Med* 1995;333:1301.

Steinberg D, Gotto AM. Preventing coronary artery disease by lowering cholesterol levels: fifty years from bench to bedside. *JAMA* 1999;282:2043.

Stone NJ, Levy RI, Fredrickson DS, et al. Coronary artery disease in 116 kindred with familial type II hyperlipoproteinemia. *Circulation* 1974;49:476.

Tall AR. Plasma high density lipoproteins. Metabolism and relationship to atherogenesis. *J Clin Invest* 1990;86:379.

Third JL, Montag J, Flynn M, et al. Primary and familial hypoalphalipoproteinemia. *Metabolism* 1984;33:136.

Zioncheck TF, Powell LM, Rice GC, et al. Interaction of recombinant apolipoprotein(a) and lipoprotein(a) with macrophages. *J Clin Invest* 1991;87:767–771.

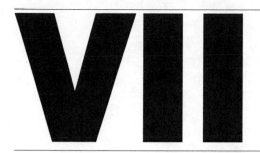

VII

Neoplasms

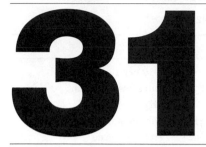

Multiple Endocrine Neoplasia Syndromes

Lamice R. El-Kholy

INTRODUCTION

Multiple endocrine neoplasia (MEN) syndromes are hereditary syndromes of benign and malignant endocrine neoplasms. There are two distinct syndromes, MEN1 and MEN2. The main subtypes of MEN2 are MEN2A, with its variants, including familial medullary thyroid cancer (FMTC), and MEN2B.

The genetic and molecular bases of these syndromes have been identified, allowing better understanding of their pathogenesis. Both syndromes have an autosomal dominant pattern of inheritance and provide examples of different genetic mechanisms of tumorigenesis. MEN1 is caused by loss of function, or inactivation of a tumor suppressor gene. On the other hand, MEN2 is caused by gain of function or activation of a proto-oncogene.

CAUSES

See Table 31-1.

Multiple Endocrine Neoplasia 1

MEN1 is inherited as an autosomal dominant trait. It is rare, with an incidence of 2–20 per 100,000 in the general population. Approximately 10% of mutations arise *de novo*.

The gene responsible for MEN1 has been recently identified. It is located on the long arm of chromosome 11 (11q13). The MEN1 gene functions as a tumor suppressor gene. It encodes a 610–amino acid nuclear protein called menin. The function of menin is not yet fully known, although studies suggest it might have a role in transcriptional regulation. More than 300 different MEN1 germline mutations have been identified, making genetic screening difficult.

Multiple Endocrine Neoplasia 2

MEN2 is a rare autosomal dominant syndrome. It has an estimated prevalence of 1–10 per 100,000 in the general population. It has been identified in 500–1000 kindred worldwide. Two main subtypes are recognized: MEN2A and MEN2B (previously known as MEN2 and MEN3, respectively). MEN2A accounts for 75% of cases of MEN2.

Medullary thyroid carcinoma (MTC) is present in 90–100% of patients, and 25% of patients with MTC have one of the MEN2 variants. Pheochromocytoma is the second most common tumor in MEN2, present in approximately 50% of patients.

The gene for MEN2 has been identified and well studied. It is the RET proto-oncogene, located on chromosome 10 (10q11-2). The product of the RET gene is *RET*, a transmembrane tyrosine kinase–linked protein. A number of mutations have been identified that are linked to the development of the MEN2 syndrome, and unlike in MEN1, there is a high degree of correlation between a specific mutation and clinical phenotype. MEN2A mutations all map to the extracellular portion of *RET*, whereas all MEN2B mutations occur at the intracellular kinase domain of the *RET* receptor.

TABLE 31-1. GENETICS OF MEN1 AND MEN2

	MEN1	MEN2
Incidence	2–20 per 100,000	1–10 per 100,000
Inheritance	Autosomal dominant	Autosomal dominant
Gene	MEN1 gene	RET gene
Location	Chromosome 11 (11q13)	Chromosome 10 (10q11-2)
Function	Tumor suppresser gene	Proto-oncogene
Type of mutation in tumors	Inactivation	Activation
Gene product	Menin, a nuclear protein	RET, a transmembrane tyrosine kinase–linked protein

PRESENTATION
See Table 31-2.

Multiple Endocrine Neoplasia 1
The clinical picture can be variable; however, the three most common features are parathyroid, enteropancreatic, and pituitary tumors.

Parathyroid Tumors
Hyperparathyroidism is the most common endocrine abnormality in patients with MEN1. It occurs in nearly 100% of patients by the age of 50 years. It is usually the first manifestation, with typical age of onset around age 20–25 years. Because the

TABLE 31-2. CLINICAL MANIFESTATIONS OF MEN1, MEN2A, AND MEN2B[a]

MEN1	MEN2A	MEN2B
Hyperparathyroidism (100%)	Medullary thyroid cancer (100%)	Medullary thyroid cancer (100%)
Enteropancreatic tumors (40–75%)	Pheochromocytoma (50%)	Pheochromocytoma (50%)
Gastrinoma (40%)	Hyperparathyroidism (20–30%)	Mucosal neuroma (95%)
Insulinoma (10%)		Intestinal ganglioneuroma (40%)
Others, glucagonoma, VIPoma		Marfanoid habitus (75%)
Anterior pituitary tumors (20–60%)		
Prolactinoma (20%)		
Others, ACTH, TSH, or GH-secreting (rare)		
Adrenal cortical tumors (20–40%)		
Carcinoid tumors (15%)		

GH, growth hormone; TSH, thyroid-stimulating hormone.
[a](%) = prevalence of patients with these manifestations.

hyperparathyroidism is invariably due to hyperplasia of all 4 glands, treatment is parathyroidectomy with removal of 3.5 of the parathyroid glands, or removal of all 4 glands with auto reimplantation of one gland.

Enteropancreatic Tumors

Enteropancreatic tumors are the second most common tumors, with an estimated prevalence of 40–75% in MEN1–affected individuals. They can be functional or nonfunctional. Symptoms of hormone excess usually occur by age 40 years, although with biochemical testing and imaging, asymptomatic tumors in carriers can be identified much earlier.

Gastrinoma is the most common enteropancreatic tumor, present in approximately 40% of MEN1 patients. An initial diagnosis of gastrinoma should suggest MEN1, because 25–30% of all gastrinoma patients have MEN1. The tumor causes hypergastrinemia with increased gastric acid output (Zollinger-Ellison syndrome). It is usually multicentric and has malignant potential. 50% of gastrinomas in MEN1 have already metastasized before diagnosis, although the metastatic tumors in MEN1 are usually less aggressive than sporadic gastrinoma tumors. They are often located in the duodenum and may be associated with pancreatic tumors. Patients may present with peptic ulcer disease, which is usually well controlled with proton pump inhibitors.

Insulinoma is the second most common enteropancreatic tumor, occurring in approximately 10% of MEN1 patients. Most insulinoma tumors arise spontaneously because less than 5% of insulinoma patients have MEN1 syndrome. Patients present with fasting hypoglycemia. The tumors are usually too small to be identified by CT or MRI; however, intraoperative ultrasound usually identifies the tumor within the pancreas. For further details, see Chap. 29, Hypoglycemia.

Pituitary Tumors

Anterior pituitary adenomas are common in MEN1 patients, with prevalence varying between 10% and 60%, and are the presenting tumors in 10–25% of cases. Two-thirds are microadenomas, which are usually functional and commonly secrete prolactin. Less commonly, they can secrete other hormones: ACTH leading to Cushing's disease or growth hormone leading to acromegaly. The diagnosis and management are similar to sporadic pituitary adenomas. (See Chap. 1, Pituitary Adenomas.)

Less Common Tumors

Adrenal cortical lesions, both functional and nonfunctional, occur in 20–40% of patients. Hypercortisolism can be secondary to pituitary adenoma, adrenal adenoma, or ectopic ACTH secretion from carcinoid. Most cases are secondary to pituitary adenomas, but it is important to differentiate between different causes by standard biochemical testing. Hyperaldosteronism from adrenal adenoma has also been described.

Carcinoid tumors are present in 15% of patients. All carcinoid tumors in MEN1 originate in tissues arising from embryologic foregut. Thymic carcinoid is seen predominately in males, can be asymptomatic until a late stage, and tends to be more aggressive than in sporadic tumors. Bronchial carcinoid occurs mainly in females. Gastric enterochromaffin-like cell carcinoids have been found mainly as incidental tumors during gastric endoscopy for gastrinoma in MEN1. They are common, occurring in approximately 10% of patients.

Multiple Endocrine Neoplasia 2

Medullary Thyroid Cancer

MTC is the most common manifestation of MEN2 and is the main cause of morbidity. It occurs in 90–100% of patients and is preceded by parafollicular or C cell hyperplasia. It is usually multicentric. It presents as a thyroid nodule and/or increased serum calcitonin. It tends to be more aggressive in MEN2B, with earlier age of presentation, commonly before age 5 years.

Pheochromocytoma

Pheochromocytoma occurs with an incidence of approximately 50% in both MEN2A and MEN2B. It can be uni- or bilateral. It has a peak presentation in the fourth to fifth decade but can present in childhood. It is rarely malignant. If unrecognized, it can present as hypertensive crisis during surgery early in childhood for MTC. (See Chap. 15, Pheochromocytoma.)

Hyperparathyroidism

Hyperparathyroidism is seen in approximately 20–30% of patients with MEN2A, but is rarely seen in MEN2B. It is usually due to hyperplasia of the 4 glands, although it is less aggressive than in MEN1. (See Chap. 22, Hyperparathyroidism.)

Other Features

Ganglioneuromas occur in 95% of MEN2B patients. They can occur at the lips, eyelids, and tongue, giving these patients a characteristic phenotype that can be apparent at birth. Intestinal ganglioneuroma can manifest as early as infancy with GI motility disorders.

Patients with MEN2B have characteristic **marfanoid features**, but do not have lens subluxation or aortic disease.

MANAGEMENT

Multiple Endocrine Neoplasia 1

To diagnose MEN1 syndrome in an individual, the patient must have 2 of the 3 main MEN1–related tumors: parathyroid, pituitary, and enteropancreatic tumors.

Familial MEN1 is defined as at least one case of MEN1 plus a first-degree relative with 1 of the 3 tumors.

Screening

Once an index case of MEN1 is identified, genetic counseling and testing should be considered in all family members. The age to start screening is still controversial.

Once an individual is identified as high risk for MEN1 (positive gene test or family history) periodic biochemical screening should be carried out. A proposed screening scheme is as follows:

- Serum calcium (ionized) yearly, starting at age 8 years.
- Gastrin, gastric acid output, and secretin-stimulated gastrin: yearly, starting at age 20 years.
- Fasting glucose ± insulin yearly, starting at age 5 years.
- Prolactin (PRL) and IGF-1 yearly starting at age 5 years.
- Radiologic screening can be done, as needed, every 3 years with abdominal CT scan for detecting carcinoid and/or enteropancreatic tumors.

Treatment

- Treatment of individual tumors is the same as in sporadic cases.
- Subtotal parathyroidectomy with transcervical near total thymectomy is the most common surgery for hyperparathyroidism. Alternatively, total parathyroidectomy with autograft to the forearm can be carried out. Minimally invasive parathyroidectomy is not recommended.
- Surgery is the treatment of choice for insulinoma and is usually curative.
- The role of surgery in management of gastrinoma in MEN1 is still controversial. Proton pump inhibitors effectively control hypergastrinemia, but are administered at twice the typical dose (e.g., 40 mg PO qd omeprazole, 60 mg PO qd lansoprazole, 80 mg PO qd pantoprazole).
- Somatostatin analogues can be used for control of other enteropancreatic tumors.

Multiple Endocrine Neoplasia 2

MEN2 syndrome is an example of a genetic disorder in which genetic testing allows for early diagnosis and early preventive surgical intervention. Once a case of possible MEN2 syndrome is identified, the individual should be tested for RET oncogene mutations. If this test is positive, all family members should be counseled and tested.

If an individual tests negative for the RET mutation, he/she is not at risk for development of MEN2 syndrome, and no further testing is needed. Those who test positive should be screened according to the scheme outlined below. RET testing is recommended instead of biochemical testing for MTC.

Thyroidectomy is carried out once the diagnosis is made (by age 6 months in MEN2B and 5 years in MEN2A). After surgery, patients are screened with serial calcitonin measurements to look for residual disease or metastatic tumor.

Those at risk for hyperparathyroidism should be screened annually with ionized calcium and intact parathyroid hormone (PTH). Hyperparathyroidism is managed with subtotal parathyroidectomy or total parathyroidectomy with autotransplant. If evidence of parathyroid hyperplasia is found at the time of thyroidectomy, this should be managed as evidence of hyperparathyroidism, even in the absence of biochemical evidence of disease.

Screening for pheochromocytoma with yearly plasma and/or urinary metanephrine measurements is done in all patients. The age at which to start screening for pheochromocytoma depends on specific codon mutations. Screening should start at age 5–7 years in families with high-risk mutations and later in those with mutations in less high-risk codons. An abnormal biochemical test should be followed by imaging, preferably CT, to localize tumors. Some advocate routine imaging every 3–5 years even in the presence of normal biochemical tests.

Treatment of pheochromocytoma is similar to that in sporadic cases. Alpha-adrenergic blockers (with or without beta-blockers) are used to control preoperative intravascular volume. Those with evidence of unilateral disease should have unilateral adrenalectomy followed by yearly biochemical testing to detect recurrence. Those with evidence of bilateral disease must undergo bilateral adrenalectomy.

FAMILIAL MEDULLARY THYROID CARCINOMA

FMTC is a variant of MEN2A. It is a familial, autosomal dominant syndrome in which MTC is the only manifestation. Mutations in codons 768, 804, and 891 of the RET oncogene are found only in FMTC; however, other mutations can be found in both MEN2A and FMTC. Kindreds with these mutations develop only MTC and are not at risk for other endocrine tumors such as pheochromocytoma or hyperparathyroidism.

Because MTC can present long before pheochromocytoma in MEN2, specific criteria have been suggested to diagnose FMTC to avoid missing diagnosis of other endocrine tumors. These criteria include >10 carriers in the kindred, multiple carriers or affected members over the age of 50 years, and an adequate medical history, particularly in older family members.

FMTC presents later in life, with a peak incidence in the fourth and fifth decade. It tends to be less aggressive than in other forms of MEN. Management is thyroidectomy in individuals who test positive for the mutations.

KEY POINTS TO REMEMBER

• MEN syndromes are rare, autosomal dominant disorders.
• MEN1 is associated with both hormone excess (PTH, PRL, gastrin) and malignant tumors (gastrinoma, carcinoid).
• Surgery is the treatment of choice for hyperparathyroidism and insulinoma, whereas medical treatment is indicated or gastrinoma.
• MTC and pheochromocytoma are the main tumors associated with MEN2A and MEN2B.
• Hyperparathyroidism is present mainly in MEN2A, whereas MEN2B is associated with ganglioneuromas and characteristic habitus.
• Genetic testing is important in the MEN2 syndrome because testing allows for early diagnosis and early preventive surgical intervention.

REFERENCES AND SUGGESTED READINGS

Brandi ML, Marx SJ, Aurbach GD, et al. Familial multiple endocrine neoplasia type 1: a new look at pathophysiology. *Endocr Rev* 1987;4:391–405.

Brandi ML, Gagel RF, Angeli A, et al. Guidelines for diagnosis and therapy of MEN type 1 and type 2. *J Clin Endocrinol Metab* 2001;86(12):5658–5671.

Burgess JR, Greenaway TM, Shepherd JJ. Expression of the MEN-1 gene in a large kindred with multiple endocrine neoplasia type 1. *J Intern Med* 1998;243:465–470.

Chandrasekharappa SC, Guru SC, Manickam P, et al. Positional cloning of the gene for multiple endocrine neoplasia type 1. *Science* 1997;276:404–407.

Doherty GM, et al. Lethality of multiple endocrine neoplasia type 1. *World J Surg* 1998;22(6):581–585.

Eng C, Clayton D, Schffenecker L, et al. The relationship between specific RET proto-oncogene mutations and disease phenotype in multiple endocrine neoplasia type 2. *JAMA* 1996;276:1575–1579.

Gagel RF, Marx SJ. Multiple endocrine neoplasia. In: Larsen PR, et al., eds. *Williams textbook of endocrinology*, 10th ed. Philadelphia: WB Saunders, 2003:1717–1762.

Mulligan LM, Ponder BAJ. Genetic basis of endocrine disease: multiple endocrine neoplasia type 2. *J Clin Endocrinol Metab* 1995;80:1989–1995.

Thakker RV. Multiple endocrine neoplasia type 1. *Endocr Metab Clin North Am* 2000;29:541–62.

Tramp D, Farren B, Wooding C, et al. Clinical studies of multiple endocrine neoplasia type 1 (MEN 1). *QJM* 1996;89:653–669.

Wells SA Jr, Chi DD, Toshia K, et al. Predictive DNA testing and prophylactic thyroidectomy in patients at risk for multiple endocrine neoplasia type 2A. *Ann Surg* 1994;220:237–247.

Wells SA Jr, Skinner MA. Prophylactic thyroidectomy, based on direct genetic testing in patients at risk for multiple endocrine neoplasia type 2 syndromes. *Exp Clin Endocrinol Diabetes* 1998;106:29–34.

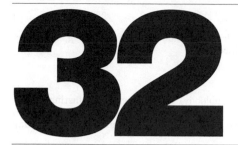

Carcinoid Syndrome

Denise A. Teves

INTRODUCTION

Carcinoid tumors were first described by Lubarsch in 1888. Oberndorffer introduced the term *karzinoide* to describe intestinal tumors that histologically resembled carcinomas but did not behave in their aggressive manner.

Carcinoid tumors arise from neuroendocrine cells. They have positive reactions to silver stains and to markers of neuroendocrine tissue (neuron-specific enolase, synaptophysin, chromogranin). The cells contain granules composed of biogenic amines (serotonin), polypeptides (substance P), and prostaglandins, which cause the symptoms of carcinoid syndrome in approximately 10% of patients with carcinoid tumors. The incidence of carcinoid tumors in the United States has been estimated to be 1–2 cases per 100,000 people.

Carcinoid tumors have been classified according the site of origin: foregut (bronchi, stomach), midgut (small intestine, appendix, proximal large bowel), and hindgut (distal colon, rectum). Histologically, these tumors are classified as well-differentiated or poorly differentiated neuroendocrine carcinomas. 90% of carcinoid tumors originate in Kulchitsky cells of the GI tract, most commonly in the appendix, ileum, and rectum. Carcinoid tumors of the small bowel and bronchus have a more malignant course than tumors of other sites.

In general, carcinoid tumors have a good prognosis. The tumors grow slowly and the 5-year survival is 82%. The best survival rates are for appendiceal (85.9%), bronchopulmonary (76.6%), and rectal (72.2%) tumors. The 5-year survival rate also varies with the extent of the disease: localized tumors (94%), regional lymph node metastases (64%), and widely metastatic tumors (0–27%). The major causes of death are carcinoid heart disease and cachexia due to mesioenteric entrapment. Histologic criteria are poor determinants of malignancy.

CAUSES

No etiologic factors associated with the development of these tumors have been identified. Sporadic foregut carcinoids, as well as multiple endocrine neoplasia 1 (MEN1), display allelic losses at chromosome 11q13, and somatic MEN1 gene mutations have been reported in one-third of sporadic foregut tumors. Midgut carcinoids are not included in the MEN1 syndrome. Deletions on chromosome 18 were found in 88% of midgut carcinoid tumors in a recent report. Among carcinoid tumors, 10% of those in the small intestine, <1% in appendix, and virtually none in the rectum are associated with carcinoid syndrome. Gastric and bronchial carcinoids are associated with atypical carcinoid syndromes. Serotonin is synthesized from its precursor, 5-hydroxytryptophan, and subsequently metabolized by monoamine oxidase to 5-hydroxyindoleacetic acid (5-HIAA), which is excreted in the urine.

The liver inactivates the bioactive products of carcinoid tumors. This may explain why patients who have GI carcinoid tumors have the syndrome only if they have hepatic metastasis. Bronchial and other extraintestinal carcinoids rarely cause the syndrome. However, if the syndrome is present, it does not necessarily mean there is metastatic disease, because the bioactive products are not immediately cleared by the liver.

PRESENTATION

The principal features of carcinoid syndrome include flushing, sweating, wheezing, diarrhea, abdominal pain, and cardiac fibrosis.

Diarrhea

Diarrhea is usually secretory (watery, nonbloody) and persists with fasting. Stools may vary from a few to >30/day and can be explosive. If accompanied by abdominal cramping, diarrhea is due to mesenteric fibrosis. It is usually unrelated to flushing episodes.

Flushing

Flushing is always dry (no diaphoresis) and occurs in 85% of patients with carcinoid syndrome. In midgut carcinoid, flushing is usually of faint pink to red color and involves the face and upper trunk down to the nipples. Flushing is initially provoked by alcohol and food containing tyramines (blue cheese, chocolate, red sausage, red wine). With time, flushing may occur spontaneously. It typically lasts for 1–5 minutes and may occur many times per day. Flushing associated with foregut tumors is more intense, lasts for hours, is frequently followed by telangiectasias, and involves the upper trunk and the limbs. Episodes induced by anesthesia may last hours and can be accompanied by severe hypotension (carcinoid crisis).

Bronchospasm

10–20% of patients with carcinoid syndrome have wheezing and dyspnea, often during flushing episodes.

Carcinoid Heart Disease

Carcinoid heart disease can be seen in up to 60% of patients with metastatic carcinoid. It consists of deposits of fibrous tissue on the endocardium of the heart, valve leaflets, atria, and ventricles. Valvular heart disease is the most common pathologic feature, with tricuspid damage (tricuspid regurgitation) found in 97% of patients and pulmonary valve damage (pulmonary stenosis) in 88% of patients. Clinical manifestations are those of right-sided valvular heart disease and include peripheral edema, ascites, and pulsatile hepatomegaly.

Other Manifestations

Other manifestations can include pellagra dermatosis (hyperkeratosis and pigmentation), Peyronie's disease of the penis, intraabdominal and retroperitoneal fibrosis, and occlusion of the mesenteric arteries and veins. Intraabdominal fibrosis can lead to intestinal obstruction. Retroperitoneal obstruction can result in urethral obstruction. Rarely, carcinoid tumors of foregut or of hindgut origin can cause bone metastases. These tumors can secrete corticotropin-releasing hormone and ACTH (ectopic Cushing's syndrome), or growth hormone (GH)-releasing factor (acromegaly). Gastric carcinoids are associated with MEN1.

MANAGEMENT
Diagnostic Evaluation

The most useful initial diagnostic test for carcinoid syndrome is to measure **24-hour urinary excretion of 5-HIAA** (sensitivity of 75% and specificity of 100%). The patient should not eat serotonin-rich foods, such as bananas, pineapple, kiwi fruit, walnuts, pecans, or avocados, before the test. Patients should also avoid guaifenesin, acetaminophen, salicylates, L-dopa, caffeine, tea, heparin, imipramine, and isoniazid. The normal range of 5-HIAA excretion is 2–8 mg/day. Patients with carcinoid syndrome usually have urinary 5-HIAA levels of 15–60 mg/24 hours (100–3000 umol/24 hours). Chromogranin (A,B,C) concentrations appear to be sensitive markers, but are not used for diagnosis of carcinoid syndrome; however, they can be a predictor of prognosis, as an elevated level of chromogranin A has been shown to be an independent predictor of poor overall survival. Determination of **serum serotonin** is more sensitive than 5-HIAA and may be useful in cases when urinary 5-HIAA results are equivocal. The mean fasting serum serotonin concentration in patients without carcinoid syndrome ranged in one report from 71–310 ng/mL (0.4–1.8 umol/L), and in 10 patients with carcinoid syndrome the fasting concentration ranged from 790–4500 ng/mL (4.5–25.5 umol/L) (Richter G, et al. *Gastroenterology* 1986). However, if a patient is taking SSRI antidepressant medications, the serum serotonin concentration can be reduced. Provocation of flushing using epinephrine or pentagastrin is useful in evaluating patients who describe flushing but have normal or marginally elevated biochemical markers.

Tumor Localization

Once the biochemical diagnosis of carcinoid syndrome is confirmed, the tumor must be localized. Abdominal CT scan is the primary diagnostic procedure for tumor staging. It identifies the primary tumor, mesenteric lymph node enlargement, and liver metastases. MRI is sensitive for the diagnosis of extrahepatic disease. The presence of somatostatin receptors in carcinoid tumors has allowed the use of indium-111 octreotide for tumor imaging (90% sensitivity in patients with carcinoid syndrome and 60% sensitive for identifying the primary tumor site). In addition to tumor imaging, octreotide scanning may be useful in predicting responses to octreotide therapy. Echocardiography can establish the severity of carcinoid heart disease.

TREATMENT

The management of patients with carcinoid syndrome includes removal of the tumor (if metastases have not occurred) and control of symptoms. More than 90% of patients with carcinoid syndrome have metastatic disease (except bronchial and ovarian tumors, which may cause symptoms without metastasis). The treatment of choice for a patient who has a localized carcinoid tumor is surgery. Tumors <2 cm in the appendix can be treated with appendectomy. Larger appendiceal carcinoids require right hemicolectomy. Carcinoids of the small intestine should be removed by segmental resection with mesenteric lymph node excision. Radical excision of the rectum is recommended for rectal carcinoids and radical colectomy for colonic carcinoids. Bronchial carcinoids are usually removed surgically.

The medical treatment of metastatic carcinoid tumors includes the use of the somatostatin analog octreotide (Sandostatin). Flushing and diarrhea resolve in 75–80% of patients treated with 50 mcg of subcutaneous (SC) octreotide three times per day. Side effects of octreotide (anorexia, nausea, vomiting) are avoided if it is titrated carefully to a maximum daily dose of 1500 mcg SC. The addition of interferon-alfa to therapy has been effective in controlling symptoms in patients whose disease is resistant to therapy with octreotide alone.

Cytotoxic chemotherapy (streptozocin, cyclophosphamide, fluorouracil, doxorubicin) has had limited success in the treatment of metastatic carcinoid tumors. External-beam radiation can result in effective palliation of bone or CNS metastases. In uncontrolled trials, hepatic artery embolization can induce marked symptomatic improvement in patients with hepatic metastases, but the response lasts only 1–18 months, and eventually all patients progress.

KEY POINTS TO REMEMBER

- The principal features of carcinoid syndrome include flushing, sweating, wheezing, diarrhea, abdominal pain, and cardiac fibrosis.
- Carcinoid syndrome only occurs in <10% of patients with carcinoid tumors.

- Patients who have GI carcinoid tumors have the syndrome only if they develop hepatic metastases.
- Bronchial and other extraintestinal carcinoids can cause the syndrome in the absence of metastatic disease.
- The most useful initial diagnostic test for carcinoid syndrome is measurement of 24-hour urinary excretion of 5-HIAA.
- The treatment of choice for a patient with a localized carcinoid tumor is surgery.
- The medical treatment of metastatic carcinoid tumors includes the use of octreotide.

REFERENCES AND SUGGESTED READINGS

Fink G, Krelbaum T, et al. Pulmonary carcinoid: presentation, diagnosis, and outcome in 142 cases in Israel and review of 640 cases from the literature. *Chest* 2001;119:1647.

Janson ET, Homberg L, et al. Carcinoid tumors: analysis of prognostic factors and survival in 301 patients from a referral center. *Ann Oncol* 1997;8:685.

Kulke M, Mayer R. Carcinoid tumors. *N Engl J Med* 1999;340:11.

Kvols LK, Moertel CG, et al. Treatment of malignant carcinoid syndrome: evaluation of a long-acting somatostatin analogue. *N Engl J Med* 1986;315:663.

Modlin IM, Sandor A. An analysis of 8305 cases of carcinoid tumors. *Cancer* 1997;79:813–829.

Oberg K. Carcinoid tumors, carcinoid syndrome, and related disorders. In: Larsen PR, et al., eds. *Williams textbook of endocrinology*, 10th ed. Philadelphia: WB Saunders, 2003:1857–1876.

Richter G, et al. Serotonin release into blood after food and pentagastrin. Studies in healthy subjects and in patients with metastatic carcinoid tumors. *Gastroenterology* 1986;91(3):912–918.

Sitaraman SV, Goldfinger SE. Treatment of carcinoid tumors and the carcinoid syndrome. In: Rose BD, Rush J. *UpToDate*, version 12.1. Wellesley, MA: UpToDate, 2004.

Vinik AI. Carcinoid tumors. In: DeGroot L, Jameson JL, eds. *Endocrinology*, 4th edition. Philadelphia: WB Saunders, 2001:2533–2546.

Index